THE SINGLE SOURCE CANCER COURSE

Volume 2:
Treatment and Survival

By

S. Wilking Horan

ISBN-10 1439275564
EAN-13 9781439275566

Praise for

The Single Source Cancer Course

DR. MICHAEL ENGELBERG,
Medical Oncology, Comprehensive Cancer Center, Cedars-Sinai Medical Center, Los Angeles, California:

"Includes the best analysis of breast cancer I've read. I have no doubt this book will prove to be of great value to many people."

PHYLLIS DILLER,
Legendary comedienne, actor and author:

"Susan's Layering Effect is brilliant!"

MARY BUFFETT,
Bestselling author of *Buffettology* and *The Tao of Warren Buffett*, Simon and Schuster:

"I loved this book because every page offers a gem of advice that only someone who has gone through the experience can give you. Quite often, Susan's wit and insights get you through the hard part. This is by far one of the best books I've read on diagnosis, recovery and positive spirit because it so deftly packages Susan's ideas in a form that anyone can identify with. A great read that you will want to keep by your side, to refer to over and over."

JAMES CROMWELL,
Academy Award nominated actor and activist:

"*The Single Source Cancer Course* is a thoroughly researched, comprehensive encyclopedia of cancer facts - an essential and invaluable resource for anyone."

GREG MOODY,
Author and thirty year veteran of radio, newspaper, television and online reporting, *Critic At Large,* KCNC-TV, Denver, Colorado:

"I come from a family of cancer survivors. And, the greatest difficulty in dealing with cancer is simply finding information. Where do you look? Who do you listen to? What information is nonsense, what is anecdotal, what is hard fact? The truth is, we search thousands of places to bring together the information we need to comfort ourselves, our friends, our families. Until now. Susan Wilking Horan has created the ultimate reference guide for all of us. Thousands of facts, contacts and information sources are suddenly at your fingertips in a highly readable, easily referenced format. The book also includes some of the most sensible common sense I've ever found in ANY medical reference text. You'll simply be amazed at the things we do daily – mindlessly – that can adversely affect our health. You're not alone. You're no longer in the dark. Information is at hand and you can find it right here."

Thanks

Thanks to he following people for their patience, input and answers to my numerous questions, many of which were posed completely out of context:

Dr. Michael Engelberg, Oncology, Los Angeles, California; Dr. Edward Share, Gastroenterology, Los Angeles, California; Dr. Steve Horan, Orthopedics, Denver, Colorado; Dr. Lisa Becker, Obstetrics & Gynecology, Littleton, Colorado; Kate Horan, Ultrasonography, Denver, Colorado; Peg Horan, Speech and Language Pathologist, Insurance Referrals; Toborcia Bedgood, Radiological Therapist, Los Angeles, California.

With additional thanks to the following people for additional reasons:

Dr. Joseph Yadagar, Dr. Mitchell Karlin, Dr. Kristi Funk, Dr. C. Michelle Burnison, Terry Magnatta, Erin Rogers, Jim Agee, Michael Garrett, Kristi Blicharski, Mark Fleischer and my computer guru Evan Leonard who kept all my computers and printers running throughout the long writing and re-writing process.

DISCLAIMER

The information contained within this book and all related materials is intended only as an educational aid. This information is not intended as medical advice for individual treatments or conditions, nor is it intended as a substitute for advice by a physician or any other health care practitioner. Readers should consult their personal medical professionals to properly evaluate the comprehensiveness and utility of the information within this book. Readers who suspect they may have a specific medical problem should consult their physician to secure a proper diagnosis and determine a safe and effective course of treatment. And, of course, in the event the information or advice within this book differs from information or advice provided by a health care professional, readers should always follow the recommendation of the health care professional.

Who Should Read This Book?

I will begin by stating that I am not a medical doctor. I have never been to medical school nor did I study pre-med courses in my undergraduate years. Rather, I studied Psychology in college and graduated in 1988 with a Bachelor of Arts Degree from the University of California, Northridge. I then went to law school and graduated in 1993 with a Juris Doctor Degree from Loyola Law School, Los Angeles.

I believe this is important because this book is not a textbook. It's not designed by a doctor to be read by other doctors. It's not written in dense medical terms that only those with a specialized education can understand. It's not a publication or treatise written to gain promotion or tenure. And it's not associated with, nor does it promote, any particular medical organization, community or business over another.

Quite simply, this is a "how-to" book written by one ordinary person for the benefit of other ordinary people. I have survived three different cancers over the last fifteen years. I have spent more time in hospitals, doctors' offices and medical facilities during that time than I care to remember. My expertise on the subject comes primarily from personal experience. And I have taken this experience, combined it with my research and writing skills as an attorney and my knowledge of psychology to produce this one-stop-shopping guide to a better understanding of cancer and its many related issues.

Just as important is the fact that I do not advocate anything in this book. I do not advocate one cancer treatment over another or one scientific study over another or one course of action over another. I do not present information that reflects one school of thought over another. While I do present that information upon which the most re-spected medical organizations and publications the world over appear to agree, I also present information that is in controversy and scientific findings that are contradictory. For information is not static, but fluid and ever-changing. There are many experts on cancer and not all of them are in agreement, and findings that state one thing today will often state something completely different tomorrow.

To that end, I have done my best to present a comprehensive layperson's guide to preventing, treating and surviving cancer as we understand it today. I have utilized the most reliable and up-to-date sources available and have distilled their vast oceans of information into the pages before you. I simply present information and ask the reader to reach her or his own conclusions. For if I advocate anything in this book it is that each individual take full responsibility for her or his personal life and health. I advocate that each individual be as fully informed as possible. I advocate that each individual become pro-active rather than re-active. I advocate that each individual make her or his own decisions based upon thorough research, consultation and analysis. And, I hope this book will make that task a little easier.

Cancer is common. Eventually, it will affect everyone in one way or another. Everyone will either wage her or his own personal battle against the disease or be drafted into the personal battle of another. Accordingly, the person who should read this book is one who:

1) Desires concise information on cancer-related issues in an accessible, user-friendly format;
2) Is at present engaged in a battle with the disease;
3) Knows someone who is engaged in battle with the disease;
4) Requires clear information regarding cancer treatments;
5) Has survived cancer and requires guidance in navigating the health care and legal systems, and;
6) Seeks a better understanding of the nature of the disease and common-sense steps to help in its prevention.

How to Read This Book

When it comes to cancer we are surrounded by a world of information. Literally, truck loads exist. Indeed, I have an entire guestroom filled to the ceiling with research materials that attests to that fact. Yet, too much information is just as confusing as too little. Perhaps, it's even more confusing. The trick is to understand what information is essential to the cancer process. This information must be separated from the excess and the facts must be distinguished from the fiction. It must then be reduced to its essence and presented in a user-friendly source that is comprehensive without being unnecessarily cumbersome.

This is what I hope my book has accomplished--at least, to some small degree. It's the result of years of personal research, years of personal experience and years of listening to and counseling others. In the interest of accessibility, it has been divided into two Volumes. The first is entitled "Prevention" and the second is "Treatment and Survival." Clearly, readers who have never had cancer may wish only to read Volume 1, while readers who now have or have had cancer in the past may wish to read both. And, although each volume contains approximately 400 pages, please trust me when I say that each is written in simple language that's easy to understand.

So, let's discuss the progression of this book in the same manner in which it was written. We'll start with the first volume and proceed to the second, with each chapter laying the foundation for the next. We'll move slowly and logically through the information one small step at a time.

Volume 1

"Prevention" begins with a short history of cancer and a thorough discussion of what we believe cancer to be. This is important because we need to understand the basics of what cancer is and how it begins if we ever hope to prevent it. I believe one of the biggest obstacles my readers will face will be overcoming unfounded fears and outdated misconceptions of the disease. It's necessary to replace fear with knowledge, for knowledge truly is power. And, it's crucial for you – the reader - to remove the paralyzing blinders often associated with cancer, and to arm yourself with the latest information and universally accepted facts and figures.

Once we've broken the ice, Volume 1 moves on to a discussion of statistics. That's right, statistics. Now, this has nothing to do with mathematics so please don't panic. Rather, this section discusses the way in which scientific studies are conducted and findings are presented. This is important to understand because new information on cancer is always emerging. New studies are always being published and quite often, the results of one will contradict the results of another. This section will help train us to ask the right questions about such studies and to reach our own conclusions by applying common sense and logic.

Next, we will dive into an exploration of those things that are believed to cause cancer. Now, it's very difficult to establish a direct link between many commonly accepted causes of cancer and the disease itself. Accordingly, this book will present the terms "cause" or "causes" in quotes. I do this simply to remind the reader that it's hard to "prove" something causes cancer. Rather, it is more accurate to say that certain things have been associated with or linked to the development of cancer. These are the things we will explore in this book.

Indeed, I have organized this particular material into thirteen different areas of exploration. These include:

1) Heredity

2) Solar Radiation
3) Air Pollution
4) Water Pollution
5) Pesticides and Chemicals
6) Viruses

7) Drugs
8) Ionizing Radiation
9) Hormones

10) Occupation
11) Diet
12) Alcohol
13) Tobacco

As you can see the first area, **Heredity**, is in a category of its own. The second area includes the five major **Environmental** "causes" of cancer. The third includes those "causes" associated with **Medical Conditions and Treatments**. The last includes those "causes" associated with **Lifestyle**.

Indeed, these "causes" are those that have been studied extensively and have been generally accepted as those most associated with the development of cancer.

Of course, new agents are always coming under suspicion within the cancer research community, but those listed here will give the reader a solid understanding of the usual suspects. And, once this is established, we will thoroughly discuss the major cancers that are implicated by these thirteen areas of concern.

Now, having this foundation of knowledge is essential. Understanding the connection between the most commonly accepted "causes" of cancer and the cancers related to them will allow us to evaluate our own lives and bodies and our own possible risk for some cancers. In fact, this is so important that it is presented twice in this book; first in a short, superficial way and then in an in depth, detailed way beginning with many of the ground-breaking cancer studies of the 1980s and the 1990s.

This leads us to a section of the book I call "The Layering Effect" which, in my opinion, may be the most important section. The Layering Effect is an exercise which allows us to assess the **possible** cancer risks for an individual. It's presented in the same way as our previous section on "causes" and related major cancers. First, we profile three hypothetical individuals and their lifestyles. We apply our "Layering Effect" in an effort to identify known cancer risks each individual may face. We add the "layers" of risk together and then list the possible cancers for which the individual may be at risk. Based upon this, we make suggestions as to how each individual may decrease or mitigate his or her potential risk.

Now, the first two profiles will be simple. The second three, however, will be much more detailed. And once we've done this, we'll evaluate our own risk by applying "The Layering Effect" to ourselves with a personal worksheet included in the chapter. Of course, this exercise isn't perfect and it's not infallible. For as we will say many times, we cannot predict with certainty what cancers may or may not affect us. But, this exercise is an effective tool that will help us understand our **potential** risk for different cancers and the ways in which we may decrease or mitigate that risk.

Of course, Volume 1 would not be complete without a thorough discussion of the most common screening and detection procedures for the most common cancers. Prevention is pro-active. It is not re-active. It's vital to monitor our own health and well-being by utilizing all the tools available to us. Yearly exams, regular visits to our physicians and age and risk-related tests must become a part of our regular health-care routine. For fighting cancer is very much like certain sporting events. The best defense is a strong offense. Let's not live in fear but, rather, act confidently with the benefit of knowledge.

Finally, both volumes of this book are dotted with several personal notes from my own experience and several synopses of scientific studies. The former notes help to illustrate specific points in our discussion and the latter studies help to test our knowledge and teach us to think for ourselves and come to our own conclusions.

Volume 2

Congratulations! If you've finished Volume 1 you now have a better understanding of cancer and its "causes" than probably ninety percent of the general population. You're learning to evaluate information and to reach conclusions based upon your own knowledge and common sense. And, you're aware of the importance of screening procedures and regular medical check-ups according to your personal risk profile. Yet, having a firm knowledge of cancer and incorporating preventive measures into everyday life does not guarantee any individual will remain cancer-free.

Volume 2 addresses this very issue. Suppose you've taken advantage of every applicable screening procedure **and** you've undergone regular and necessary medical exams **and** you still develop some form of cancer. What do you do now?

To begin, it's important to understand that developing cancer even when you've been careful and responsible **does not mean your preventive measures have failed**. Rather, it means that if a cancer does develop, your preventive measures in all likelihood will have detected it early when the cancer is highly treatable. It also means that because of your good health practices, you are probably in fairly good physical condition at the time of diagnosis. And this, of course, means that you'll be better able to withstand any treatment that might be required. All of these things are extremely important if and when your battle with cancer becomes personal.

Now, most cancers will require some form of surgery. Accordingly, the first section of Volume 2 addresses this issue. We discuss several of the most common cancers and the surgical procedures typically recommended. After surgery, many cancers will require chemotherapy, radiation or both.

As these two latter treatments are the most common, we discuss each in great detail. We'll explain what they are, how they work and how they're administered. We'll also examine the possible side effects and discuss the potential dangers of each treatment. We'll discuss the short-term and long-term conditions you might face from undergoing these treatments including the ways in which each impacts reproduction. This is an honest and frank discussion that I refer to as "all the things you need to know that no one wants to tell you." For I believe one must be fully informed before one can make responsible choices and decisions. Then we'll finish this section by discussing some additional therapies also commonly used in treating cancer.

Next, we'll move on to a section entitled, "Basic Medical Know-How." For if you or a loved one has cancer, knowing the ins and outs of your medical community and how it functions is a necessity. We'll begin by discussing the role of the technician. The technicians, by the way, will be responsible for most of your day-to-day care. It is they who will monitor your regular check-ups, conduct your necessary procedures and interface with your doctors. You need to understand what their job is, what you should expect from them and how far their responsibility extends.

Then, we'll discuss the role of the doctor. After all, your life is in the hands of this professional. So I caution you, never take anything for granted. Never just hand your well-being over to another individual without careful consideration. Accordingly, the importance of this section is to instill in you the need to think for yourself. Its purpose is to make you aware that no one should be allowed to make decisions about your life without your input. You must work in concert with your physician. You must question her or his actions. And, you must take responsibility for your own well-being. In so doing, one of the most important relationships of your life, in one of the most crucial times of your life, will be successful and rewarding.

And of course, this leads us to our next discussion of your role as the patient. So far we've examined the responsibilities your technicians and doctors have toward you. Now we'll examine the responsibilities you have toward them. We'll also discuss in great detail your legal and privacy rights as you move through the medical network.

Now that we have the basic nuts and bolts of your treatment out of the way, we'll spend a little time on pain management. While this is not typically an issue with cancer itself, it's often an issue that results from the treatments of cancer. We start by clearing up the confusion that exists on the subject of narcotics. We'll discuss the various drugs that are available and why some are legally sanctioned and others are not. Apart from these drugs, we'll also examine additional procedures and techniques for treating pain or discomfort. Then we'll finish this section up with a discussion of several alternative and complementary medical techniques.

At this point, we'll move our discussion from cancer patient to cancer survivor. This is a big transition, and this new role encompasses issues quite different from those we've already investigated. First, we'll discuss the physical concerns. The focus here, of course, is to maintain health and monitor for any future occurrence or a recurrence, for as a survivor, you must be vigilantly aware. You must engage in strict post-cancer check-ups, blood tests and screening procedures. You must adhere to a positive, healthy lifestyle. And, you must be dedicated to simple, yet essential, good health practices in your daily routine for the rest of your life.

Second, we'll discuss the emotional concerns associated with cancer survival, of which there are many. We'll examine the anger, anxiety, grief and depression that can result from a battle with cancer. We'll examine how your personal relationships with family, friends and lovers may be affected. We'll also examine how your relationships in the workplace may change, what your legal rights within your workplace are and how you can protect those rights.

Third, we'll discuss the financial concerns of a cancer diagnosis. This is a most important issue, for a battle with cancer can devastate the life savings of an entire family. In this section you will learn how to make the system work for you. You'll become an expert on medical insurance issues and how they may apply to your case. You'll become familiar with federal and state sponsored insurance programs as well as private plans. You'll learn how to extend your insurance, change your insurance and protect your insurance. For those who don't have insurance, you'll learn how to help yourself by utilizing other available programs, funds and foundations.

We'll also discuss disability benefit programs and survivor benefit programs. We'll discuss your medical rights and the procedures in which you can appeal a negative decision from your insurance carrier. Then, we'll discuss medical facilities, how they differ from one another and how you can protect yourself from treatment and billing mistakes.

Of course, the United States passed a new Health Care Bill in March of 2010. I don't profess for a second to fully understand it, nor have I spoken to one other person who believes they fully understand it. Indeed, it may be years before the full impact of this Bill becomes clear. Nevertheless, I have included a small section in this volume that attempts to clarify some of the aspects of this bill and how they may relate to the issues we have discussed. Finally, Volume 2 ends with a list of organizations that can help you through every step of your cancer experience as well as a synopsis of cancer research and its future.

Now, I've included a list of sources for the information found within these pages in the reference section of each Volume. It's just not possible, however, for me to list *every* source that may apply. If I were to do so, the reference section of this book might be longer than the text. Accordingly, I typically list one or two sources. When discussing scientific studies, I sometimes cite the initial work that laid the foundation for the area of study. Sometimes I cite a few of the ground-breaking studies, many of which were conducted in the 1980s and the 1990s. And, sometimes when there are far too many studies and researchers to list, I simply cite the pages of a comprehensive source.

Moreover, readers will notice the term "Id." appears often in the reference section. Id. is an abbreviation of the Latin term "ibid." It simply means that a citation is identical to the previous citation or "the immediate past one." Typically, in legal documents Id. is only used when the previous citation contains one source. This book, however, is not a legal document. As a result, and in the interest of brevity, I have used Id. even when the previous citation contains two or more sources. This means that the text being referenced comes from *all* the same sources as the previously referenced text.

Similarly, other citations within this book may not always conform to the rules of the legal profession. The rules and opinions for citing information continue to change as does the technology for gaining information. And, sometimes certain information is just not available. As a result, some citations may lack a page or section number, or an author's name or full date. Other citations may appear as they were cited in a previous publication, correct or not. In any event, they remain sufficient enough to point those readers who wish to conduct their own research on a topic in the right direction.

Much of the basic cancer information within this book can be found in the literature of many organizations including the American Cancer Society, the National Cancer Institute and the World Health Organization. For readers who want more information on specific subjects, one internet search will probably yield several pages of additional references. And for readers who wish to know more about scientific studies, there are a few websites in particular that contain data on nearly every cancer study that's been conducted. These are wonderful reference tools and two of my favorites are:

PubMed
   (http://www.ncbi.nlm.nih.gov/pubmed/) and;
Journal of the American Medical Association Archives
   (http://pubs.ama-assn.org/).

Finally, direct quotes found within the text of this book have been credited, of course, to the specific source in which they were found.

I want to end this section by once again offering my heartfelt congratulations to each and every one of you who has the courage and the determination to read this book. It's not easy to face our fears. And, it's not easy to tackle this particular subject. But in reading this book, you are arming yourself with the most powerful weapon on earth-- knowledge. And as you continue to expand your knowledge, you continue to expand your ability to protect yourself and your loved ones.

Remember, we are engaged in a war. And the best way to win any war is to learn everything you can about the enemy. Let's not stand helpless on the sidelines. Let's not stick our heads in the sand and hope the enemy passes us by. Let's not ignore its presence and convince ourselves we are immune. Let's not allow it to surprise us and catch us off guard. Rather, let's be prepared! Let's meet this enemy head-on with confidence and power! Let's be pro-active! Let's go after it before it comes after us! Together we can save lives. And, together we can halt the march of this enemy and turn the tide in our favor! For this, I applaud you all!

Introduction

To know the road ahead, ask those coming back.
Chinese Proverb

I've been through colon cancer, skin cancer and breast cancer. And I'm still here. I was a healthy, young, athletic, slim, non-smoking vegetarian when I was diagnosed with colon cancer ten years ago. During the next decade, while recuperating not only from that disease but from the treatments I received, including chemotherapy and radiation, I also developed skin cancer. And to top it all off, I was diagnosed with breast cancer in 2007. I was ill prepared for my first cancer, better prepared for my second and firmly prepared for my third, for I did my homework. I studied. I researched. I know what it takes to survive. And the full benefit of my knowledge lies within the pages of this book.

As anyone who has experienced the same can tell you, the road from cancer prevention to recovery and survival is difficult, filled with unexpected turns, detours and a multitude of pitfalls and obstacles. And not knowing my way the first time, I took every wrong turn, got lost with every detour, fell into every pitfall and stumbled over every obstacle. For the great problem with cancer is that when one or a loved one is diagnosed with the disease, time becomes a critical issue. One must gather information quickly. One must make decisions quickly. One must act quickly. And to further compound this unavoidable reality, cancer is a subject that doesn't lend well to simple phrases, immediate comprehension or easy choices. Rather, cancer is a complicated subject that must be dissected carefully to be understood. It's a disease that raises enormously important questions for which clear answers are not always evident. And, it's a disease the existing information for which is far too vast to be adequately collected, sorted and digested in a limited period of time.

In addition, a diagnosis of cancer often leaves one in a state of emotional turmoil in which one's ability to make objective and logical decisions becomes clouded and compromised. And, of course, the diagnosis is only the beginning, for the road that leads one from diagnosis to survival and recovery can be long and arduous. Each step requires one to be fully aware and informed, regardless of the fear, doubt or confusion one may encounter along the way.

Accordingly, this brings us to the purpose for this book. It's a handbook, really. It's one source that contains just enough of the essential information necessary to guide one from cancer prevention to cancer survival. In Volume 1 of this book, we'll discuss the history of cancer; describe what it is, how it begins and why. We'll discuss our deep-rooted fear of the disease and many of the misconceptions that surround it. We'll discuss the field of statistics, how statistical information applies to cancer, and the ways in which we can analyze that information to separate fact from fiction. We'll discuss the known risk factors associated with cancer, first from the perspective of the risks themselves, then from the perspective of the major cancers they implicate. We'll supply tools that will enable one to objectively determine her or his potential cancer risks and provide examples to illustrate the usefulness of these tools. We'll outline the ways in which one can protect oneself from cancer through lifestyle choices, screening procedures and early detection.

In Volume 2, we'll move on to discuss a diagnosis of cancer and a variety of the cancer surgeries and treatments that may follow. Not only will we describe these surgeries and treatments, we'll be extremely frank in discussing the problems they may create and the ways in which one may prepare for, avoid or mitigate such problems. We'll explore the roles of both patient and medical personnel, the importance of these relationships, as well as the patient's legal protections and privacy rights. Moreover, we'll discuss the many issues one will face as she or he makes the transition from cancer patient to cancer survivor. We'll discuss the necessary follow-up programs that one must adhere to, and the physical and emotional issues that may surface. And, of course, we'll discuss the financial aspects of cancer including insurance, disability, employment rights and other legalities. We'll discuss the differences among treatment facilities, hospital billing practices, clinical trials and the resources through which one may find additional help. We'll punctuate each section with personal notes and a variety of news headlines to drive our points home and hone our analytical skills. And we'll emphasize the importance of personal responsibility and the necessity of thinking for oneself throughout.

In essence, this book is a compilation of cancer basics. It provides a solid starting point, sure footing and a useful map for the road ahead for those who wish to protect themselves from cancer, as well as those fighting cancer. And while this book is an essential source, it's not an exhaustive source, for it simply isn't possible to include all of the world's information on cancer and all its aspects within one source. Furthermore, some of this information is constantly changing. Accordingly, I apologize in advance to those whose questions may not be answered in this book. I apologize to those whose specific cancers may not be discussed in this book. And I apologize to those who seek information that may be beyond the scope of this book.

I also apologize for the fact that much of the information within this book pertains primarily to the developed and industrialized countries of the world. This is in no way a statement about the relative importance of one country or population compared to another. Rather, this is a practical reflection of reality in that cancer information and cancer statistics typically are more current and available in the developed and industrialized countries of the world. It's within these regions of the world that most of the populations generally know how to read and have access to the luxury of books through their homes, schools or libraries. As a result, these are the populations that may most benefit from the information within this particular book.

Moreover, as a citizen of the United States, some of the statistics and information relating to certain matters such as insurance and finances will be unique to the United States. Finally, as a resident of California, some of the examples within this book will be limited to that particular state, only because the information needed to make the point may have been, in some cases, more accessible.

Having said this, I nevertheless hope that most readers will find the answers and information they seek within these pages. I hope that some of the fear associated with this disease will be dispelled. I hope that the many ways in which one can protect oneself from this disease will be incorporated into one's life. And I hope that those who strive to prevent cancer, have been diagnosed with cancer, are currently fighting cancer or have survived cancer will themselves find hope, knowledge and inspiration within these pages. For, this is the book that I wish I had had when I was diagnosed with my first cancer.

I've been down this road before. Indeed, I've been down this road three times. I know the way. I can help shed light on the path and illuminate the darkness. I can help one navigate the terrain, avoid the wrong turns, negotiate the detours, anticipate the pitfalls and sail over the obstacles. I've already jumped through all the hoops, and if just one reader can benefit from my mistakes, or learn from my experience, the purpose of this book will be served.

S. Wilking Horan

TABLE OF CONTENTS
Volume 2: Treatment and Survival

Part 4: From Patient to Survivor: The Big Transition

Part 5: Hope for the Future

Volume 2: Treatment and Survival

Part 1:
A Diagnosis of Cancer—Now What?

I'm not afraid of storms,
for I'm learning how to sail my ship.
Louisa May Alcott

The results of the test are back and the screening procedure, or blood test, or biopsy that was conducted has confirmed the presence of cancerous tissue. The first thing of which an individual will be advised is, of course, where in the body the cancer has been detected. We know that different cancers are named for the body part in which they begin and, accordingly, any cancerous tissue found in the breast will be called breast cancer, any cancerous tissue found in the lung will be called lung cancer and so on.

Yet, simply because a cancer begins in a specific body part is no guarantee that it will stay there. As we know, some cancers, especially in an early stage of development, will be small and will only affect the tissues in one part of the body. We also know that these cancers are referred to as "localized" cancers or cancer "in situ."

On the other hand, cancers that aren't detected early have more time to grow and as the cells multiply they often spread, or metastasize, into nearby tissues. Individual cells of the cancer also can break off and travel through the body either through the blood of the circulatory system or through the lymphatic system and reappear in a body part far from the initial site. Clearly, the difference between these two scenarios of localized or metastasized cancer and what each will mean to the individual is staggering in terms of treatment and survival.

Chapter 1:
Cancer Treatments

Similar to everything else about cancer, the decision about how to treat the disease must be determined on a case-by-case basis. No two individuals are exactly the same, and accordingly, no two treatment programs will be exactly the same. Of the many individual factors that must be considered when deciding upon cancer treatment are the patient's age, sex, general health and menopausal status if the patient is female. Treatment also will depend upon the type of cancer diagnosed and whether or not the cancer has remained localized in one tissue or has spread to surrounding tissues and additional body parts.

Surgery: The First Step

With many cancers, some type of surgical procedure typically will follow a diagnosis of the disease. These procedures are all designed to remove the affected tissues or organs and will range from minimally invasive inconveniences to major operations. To illustrate the variety of possible procedures, we'll once again move through a few of the most common cancers and briefly describe the surgical procedures typically associated with each.

Breast Cancer

We'll begin with breast cancer, a disease for which surgery is the most common treatment and for which several surgical treatment options exist. The least invasive options are known as **breast-sparing,** or **breast-conserving,** surgeries and include the **lumpectomy** and the **segmental,** or **partial mastectomy**. These procedures, performed when the cancer appears to be localized, are designed to remove the tumor while preserving the breast.[1]

A small incision is made in the breast, and as the tumor is removed, so too is a minimal amount of normal tissue that encircles the cancer. The surgeon also will make a small separate incision under the armpit located on the same side as the affected breast, known as an **axillary lymph node dissection**, to remove and test the lymph nodes for any cancer that may have spread.

With some types of breast cancer **cryosurgery,** or **cryoablation,** also may be an option. This technique is becoming more common in treating precancerous conditions and early stage cancers, including those of the liver, prostate and skin. In treating breast cancer, this out-patient procedure essentially freezes the abnormal tissue with cold argon gas pumped through a probe. An ice ball forms around the tumor, then is allowed to thaw.[2]

This cycle of freezing and thawing is repeated and within a few weeks the former tumor is transformed into dead tissue, which is absorbed by the body's immune system. Cryosurgery doesn't require a large incision, is virtually pain free and allows the breast to retain its normal shape and contour. The long term effectiveness of this procedure, however, isn't clear at this time.

Lumpectomy: A Process More Than a Procedure

More and more younger women today are being diagnosed with early stage breast cancer. Whether this phenomenon is a reflection of compounded genetic evolution, the environment, compromised food or water supplies, more precise imaging techniques and early detection, a combination of all these factors or something else entirely is unclear. In the majority of cases in which the tumor appears to be localized the lumpectomy, or partial mastectomy, has become the surgery of choice. This surgery, however, is only one step in a series of procedures that precede as well as follow the actual surgery itself. So step by step, let's go through this entire process from the beginning.

Typically, the first step following one's decision to undergo a lumpectomy is a procedure known as a **bi-lateral breast MRI.** This particular MRI has the ability to detect small breast lesions sometimes missed in mammography and not felt during a physical exam. It requires a contrast agent injection to insure that the images of the breasts are as clear and readable as possible. An IV, therefore, will be inserted, often into one's arm, before the patient is taken into the imaging room.

Now, this procedure is similar to any other MRI except the patient lies on her stomach on a table that has a cut-out area into which her breasts drop. As the table moves into the chamber each breast is imaged individually, a process that takes approximately half an hour. Like any other MRI, the patient typically will be provided ear plugs to obscure the noise and a blanket to keep warm. The patient also may request a "head rest" so that her face is lifted off the table. It may take a few days before the MRI has been completely reviewed by a radiologist, at which time the images won't only confirm the existence of the cancer in question, but also will "pick up" any additional areas in either breast that may appear to be abnormal.[3]

This information is essential to the surgeon who relies upon the MRI for her or his surgical plan. For example, the results may indicate that a slightly smaller or larger area of tissue may need to be removed around the original cancer. Or, the MRI may pick up another suspicious spot in the same breast, or an additional spot in the other breast.

If additional pick ups are confirmed, one of two things may occur. If the pick up is near the original cancer, the surgeon simply may choose to remove this additional tissue during the lumpectomy and wait for post-surgery pathology to determine if it's malignant or not. In contrast, if the additional pick ups are numerous, some distance from the original cancer or in the other breast, a biopsy may be performed to determine if the lumpectomy is still a viable surgery. If these additional pick ups are malignant, it may be necessary to resort to another form of surgery.

It's important to remember, however, that the bi-lateral breast MRI is an extremely sensitive procedure prone to false positives. In particular, pick ups located close to the original tumor site may be nothing more than a swelling or inflammation of the tissue, a completely normal physical response to the nearby cancer. Indeed, it's been estimated that seventy-five percent of the additional pick ups found by this MRI are false positives while only twenty-five percent actually turn out to be cancers.

Once this step is completed, and the findings indicate that the lumpectomy still appears to be the proper form of surgery, the patient typically will undergo a **sentinel lymph node biopsy** and **needle localization**. These procedures are performed on the day of surgery in the radiology department before the patient is taken into the operating room.[4]

To begin, we know that within the breast there is a network of lymphatic vessels that drain cells and fluid from the tissue into the bean-shaped lymph nodes located in the axilla or armpit. If cancer cells escape from a primary tumor site in the breast, they'll enter this lymphatic system and travel to the under arm lymph nodes. The first lymph node they reach is known as the "sentinel" node, or the node that guards or watches over the other nodes. Now, the only way to know which node is the sentinel node is to mimic or trace the pattern of drainage from the breast tissue into the lymphatic system. This is done by numbing the breast with a local anesthetic and injecting (typically around the nipple) a tracer substance that travels through the lymphatic system of the breast.

This tracer may be a blue dye known as **methylene blue**, a radioactive substance known as **technetium-99**, or both. In the first case, the dye will be traced visually, and in the second case the radioactive isotopes will be traced with a gamma ray or Geiger counter. Separately, or together, these methods will reveal the exact location of the sentinel nodes.[5]

At this point, the surgeon can make a small incision, excise the sentinel (as well as perhaps a few surrounding nodes) and through a frozen section (which only takes a few minutes) examine for cancer. If the results are positive, the removal of more nodes in the area may be required. If the results are negative, however, the cancer hasn't spread beyond the breast, and it's unnecessary to perform an extensive dissection of the regional lymph node area.

In addition to the above, for small tumors, especially those too small to be felt by the surgeon, a needle localization also will be performed. It's imperative to precisely locate the tumor within the breast, for the breast is composed primarily of fatty tissue, and a small tumor can sometimes "get lost" in the surrounding healthy tissue.

First, breast tumors are located externally by assigning a "clock face" to the breast. From the front, the breast is imagined to be a clock with the nipple at the center, twelve o'clock at the top of the breast and six o'clock at the bottom. Accordingly, tumors are described as being at one o'clock, seven o'clock, ten-thirty, and so on. Internally, however, a more precise location must be determined, and the needle localization is just another way to accomplish this.

Typically this procedure will be performed at the same time the sentinel node injection is performed. The patient is awake, either sitting upright or lying down, with the breast area numbed. A mammogram or ultrasound will locate the abnormality and the radiologist will insert a thin wire into the area. In addition, a small amount of the same methylene blue dye will be injected into the tissue providing the surgeon with yet another localizing marker.

In this way, the tumor is targeted in three separate ways, once by the metal tag implanted during the biopsy, once by the needle localization and once by the methylene blue, all of which help insure the surgeon will remove precisely and completely the area in question. And ladies, please note, this dye will turn your pee and poop blue for a few days, and your breast tissue blue for a few weeks.

Finally, the patient is ready for surgery. A lumpectomy is performed under an intravenous sedation and usually takes between one and two hours. The surgeon makes a small incision in the breast, removes the tumor, the localization needle and the biopsy metal tag. She or he also may move or shift the breast tissue surrounding the excised area to "reconstruct" the breast and insure a rounded and attractive post-surgery shape. The incision will be closed with sutures placed beneath the skin and are absorbed into the tissue over time. Finally, a small band aid, or **steri strip,** will be placed over the incision and the patient will be wheeled into the recovery room where she'll remain for approximately one hour.

Incredulously, in spite of the rather long and arduous nature of the lumpectomy process, it remains an out-patient procedure that only requires a designated driver for one's return trip home. And, even though the lumpectomy necessitates some form of follow-up radiation, women need to realize that when a breast tumor is found early, is localized and has not spread, surgery alone basically is the cure.

In some cases, however, a woman may develop more than one tumor within the tissue of a single breast. Should this occur, the most appropriate procedure may be a **total** or **simple mastectomy**.[6] First, these names are rather inadequate as it's confusing to refer to the least severe form of mastectomy as "total" and there's nothing "simple" about a major surgery that removes a part of the human body. We, therefore, will refer to this procedure as a **simplified mastectomy**.

All forms of mastectomy involve the removal of the breast, yet while this mastectomy removes the breast, it doesn't remove the two chest wall muscles known as the pectoralis. This is important because these muscles will facilitate and provide the foundation for prosthetic breast reconstruction should it be desired. The simplified mastectomy may or may not involve the removal of the nearby armpit lymph nodes based upon the individual case. This mastectomy also is sometimes an elective procedure chosen as a prophylactic measure in extreme cases by women whose risk profiles indicate a particularly high risk for breast cancer.

Although not used for treating cancer, a **subcutaneous mastectomy** is another procedure that's used strictly for prophylactic measures. In this surgery only the underlying breast tissue is removed, while the skin, nipple, areola, chest wall muscles and lymph nodes are retained. A breast prosthesis can then be inserted under the skin and into the area formerly occupied by the natural breast tissue.[7]

In cases where the cancer has spread to the lymph nodes, a **modified radical mastectomy** may be recommended. In this procedure the entire breast will be removed, most of the lymph nodes under the arm and, in many cases, the lining over the chest wall muscles or pectoralis. It also may include the removal of the smaller of the two chest muscles to facilitate the removal of the lymph nodes.[8]

The last type of mastectomy is referred to as a **radical mastectomy,** or a **Halsted radical mastectomy**. In this procedure the breast, both of the chest muscles, all of the lymph nodes under the arm as well as additional fatty tissue and skin will be removed. This is an extreme surgery that is not only disfiguring, but results in significant swelling and diminished use of the affected arm. While it was for many years considered the standard treatment for all women with breast cancer, it is only used today in rare instances in which the cancer has spread to large portions of the chest wall muscles.[9]

If a woman does undergo a mastectomy and wishes to maintain her female figure, two choices will be available to her. First, if she doesn't wish to subject herself to additional surgery she may decide to wear a prosthetic breast. Such a prosthesis is shaped like a breast, is usually fashioned from rubber or a similar material and fits into a specially designed brassiere. The second choice is to undergo breast reconstruction surgery which may be performed at the same time as the mastectomy or some time following.

There are various procedures used to reconstruct the female breast although the most common involves the use of implants. These implants may be made of saline or silicone and, while the salt water filled saline implants are universally considered safe, some controversy still exists about the safety of silicone implants. Indeed, silicone breast implants have been banned in several countries. In 2006, the United States changed its strict regulations regarding these implants by granting approval for their use to two manufacturers, Allegen and Mentor. The new regulations include several requirements that must be met by these manufacturers, and allow silicon implant usage by women who are at least twenty-two years old for breast augmentation, and women of any age for breast reconstruction.[10]

Whichever implant is used, however, it will be placed underneath the remaining chest wall muscles. At this time, the surgeon also can reconstruct the areola and nipple, an important fact as using one's own nipple tissue may increase a woman's risk for a recurrence of the disease. Moreover, in the rare instance that a radical mastectomy has been performed and the chest wall muscles have been removed, the surgeon still may be able to reconstruct the breast by shaping a breast from the skin, fat and muscle tissue taken from the woman's abdominal wall or chest. This procedure also may be used for women who have their chest wall muscles intact, but don't wish to have implants. Regardless of the method of reconstruction, however, medical techniques have vastly improved over the years and tens of thousands of women have had excellent results from every method in use.

Special Concerns

Clearly, any surgery will cause pain and tenderness around the surgery site for varying lengths of time. Every surgery also involves certain risks such as possible infection, excessive bleeding, slow healing or even uncomfortable or dangerous reactions to the anesthesia. In addition, complications are always possible in any major surgery, and the procedure itself may take longer than expected.

If either of these latter events should occur, a blood transfusion may become necessary. Although the world's blood banks continue to become increasingly safe and dependable, some patients may prefer to use blood from someone they know. If so, it may be advisable to have a friend or family member who is blood type compatible donate a few pints of blood before the surgery. Doing so may offer the patient a greater level of comfort and insure that blood from a known donor is available for immediate use should a transfusion become necessary.

In addition, women who undergo a mastectomy can expect a number of possible complications unique to the procedure. First, the removal of a breast can cause a woman's weight and balance to shift. This imbalance, especially in women with large breasts, may create pain and discomfort in her back and neck as the spine attempts to compensate for the lost tissue. In addition, the shoulder and arm muscles around the surgery site may be extremely stiff, and movement may be limited. Some women may experience a permanent loss of strength in the affected arm, and if nerves are severed or injured during surgery, she also may experience temporary or permanent numbness or tingling in the chest, arm and shoulder area.

Another problem a woman may face if the lymph nodes under the arm are removed is a build up of fluids within the affected arm. As we know, the lymph system is a circulatory system that returns water and proteins from the tissues back to the blood. The fluid transported through this system is called **lymph,** and the lymph nodes are essential to this process. If the nodes in a particular part of the body are reduced in number or completely removed, the process of moving the lymph is compromised and the fluid may accumulate in the affected area.

This complication, referred to as **lymphedema,** may be reduced, however, or even prevented with specific exercise. It also may be alleviated through medication, massage or by wearing an elastic sleeve on the arm designed to improve circulation. In any event, a mastectomy is a major surgical procedure that will require extensive mental and physical rehabilitation before a woman can expect a full and complete recovery.[11]

Headline:

Antibiotic Use Linked to Breast Cancer[12]

This link was first proposed in 1981, but it didn't gain widespread recognition until it was revisited in a study conducted in 2004. Over ten thousand women participated in this subsequent study which concluded that those who used the greatest amounts of antibiotics doubled their chances for developing breast cancer, that the risk increased with the number of prescriptions and that the risk applied to all types of antibiotics.

This association might be explained by the effect antibiotics can have on bacteria within the intestinal tract, an effect that may impact the way certain foods that help prevent cancer are broken down in the body. Antibiotics also may impact the body's immune system and its response to inflammation both of which may be related to the development of cancer. Or the association may be due to the underlying conditions that led to the antibiotic use in the first place such as immunodepression or hormonal imbalances.

Further, it has been theorized that because different types of antibiotics work in different ways it's unlikely that all antibiotics would create the same overall increased risk for the same type of cancer. On the other hand, attempts to explain the increase of breast cancer among these women as the result of heredity factors or hormone use failed.

So while the research results are not without controversy, they cannot be dispelled either. Physicians must continue to prescribe antibiotics judiciously and cautiously, and women must, of course, continue to take the necessary life-saving medications for bacterial infections when required. But a definitive answer to the question of whether a link between antibiotics and breast cancer exists, and what the details of that link might be, will be forthcoming only after much additional research is conducted.

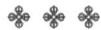

Colorectal Cancer

The appropriate surgical procedure for colorectal cancer also depends upon whether the cancer has been detected early or not. As we know, this cancer typically begins in the form of a polyp within the intestinal lining. If such polyps are detected during a colonoscopy or siegmoidoscopy, they'll be removed during the procedure and sent to a laboratory for further testing. Even if the polyps are determined to be cancerous, if there's no indication they've spread into the deeper tissue of the intestine, additional surgery may not be necessary.

On the other hand, if the cancerous tissue has spread into the wall of the intestine major surgery most likely will be required. Typically, this surgery will remove the tumor and a portion of the healthy colon surrounding the affected area. Then, after removing the affected section, the surgeon will attempt to reconnect the two healthy ends of the colon in a procedure known as a **resection**. In most cases, this procedure will be successful, and the patient's digestive tract, although somewhat reduced in length, will continue to function normally.[13]

In years past, a resection typically involved an incision in the abdomen that extended from the base of the sternum to the pubic bone. Today, this incision may be much smaller thanks to new technology and the advent and widespread use of **laparoscopic surgery**. "Lapara" is the Greek word for "loin" and "skopein" is the Greek for "to look," a term applicable to many of the procedures we have discussed.[14]

This particular one utilizes a **laparoscope**, which consists of an endoscope or tube, and an illuminated optical system. It allows the surgeon to make a small incision at the point of injury or illness, and examine the surrounding tissue. This procedure can be used in a number of different situations, including the inspection or removal of reproductive organs, female sterilization, gall bladder surgery and the detection of cancer.

In the latter case, the laparoscope allows the surgeon to take a close look at suspect tissues or at a tumor that previous tests have already confirmed. The surgeon then can determine the exact size and location of the tumor and in so doing may be able to spare the patient from an unnecessarily large incision wound. This is particularly important with colorectal cancer as the procedure may make the difference between an incision running the full extent of the abdominal cavity from breastbone to pubic bone and an incision half that size, beginning at the navel. Similarly, **robotic** procedures utilize tiny computerized instruments that operate inside the patient as they mimic the movements of the surgeon's hands outside the patient.[15]

While initially developed to facilitate abdominal surgeries, both types of procedures are now being used in patients with a variety of different cancers. Once again, the benefits of these less invasive techniques include reduced pain, less blood loss and scarring, shorter hospital stays and quicker recoveries.

For a variety of reasons, however, a resection for colon cancer isn't always possible. Should this be the case, the surgeon will have to perform another procedure known as a **colostomy**. Remember, if the intestinal tract cannot be reconnected, the patient won't be able to pass waste material through the length of the colon, into the rectum and out the anus. As a result, a new pathway for the elimination of body wastes must be surgically provided, and it's the colostomy that will accomplish this.

First, a surgical opening called a **stoma** is made through the wall of the abdomen. The upper end portion of the colon is then pulled into this opening and surgically secured while the lower end will be closed off. With a small pouch tightly fastened on the outside of the abdomen, this new opening will allow waste to move through the colon and leave the body. Clearly, a colostomy will require time before an individual fully adjusts to the mental and physical changes created by the procedure. Initial discomfort around the stoma, getting used to a new method of elimination and the need to periodically empty the pouch and cleanse the stoma may prove somewhat difficult, or at the very least, inconvenient. Yet, a permanent colostomy is another medical miracle that saves lives, and thousands of individuals who have undergone the procedure simply incorporate it into their active and productive lifestyles.[16]

Moreover, new medical technologies have greatly improved the efficiency and ease of the procedure that, by the way, is necessary in only about fifteen percent of all colorectal cancer patients. Actually, it's more likely to be performed in male patients because the structure of the male pelvis is smaller than that of the female. As a result, there's less room within the male pelvis for a surgeon to operate and a resection can be more difficult to perform. Additionally, a temporary colostomy may be performed in patients of both sexes to allow the lower portion of the colon to heal after primary surgery and before a resection is attempted.

Personal Note

My surgery for colon cancer was expected to last four hours. It actually lasted over eight. In addition, I was anemic. Fortunately, one of my forward thinking sisters had taken it upon herself to give a few pints of her matching blood just in case it might be needed. When my surgeon decided it was, my own personal supply was right by my side, ready and waiting. I admit, the knowledge that my transfusion came from a member of my own family provided me with a complete sense of comfort, security and, of course, lasting gratitude.

Special Concerns

The primary surgery and resection for colorectal cancer are extremely technical and exacting procedures. While previous procedures have confirmed the cancer site within the intestinal tract the surgeon still needs to inspect for additional problems. This requires the surgeon literally to scoop the large intestine, or colon, out of the abdominal cavity and, with both hands, carefully go through every inch of the tract. The intestine is then replaced within the abdomen, the affected section or sections are removed and the resection is performed. Regardless of a successful outcome, however, this time consuming process is not without significant additional concerns.

First, and with apologies to practitioners of geometry, the large intestine is shaped like a three-sided square. It begins on the right side of the abdomen where it connects with the small intestine and moves up toward the liver. It then crosses the abdomen from right to left and moves downward to the sigmoid that connects it to the rectum. When a resection is performed, however, the shortened colon cannot be placed into the abdominal cavity exactly as it was prior to surgery.

It also may be necessary for the surgeon to move other organs during the procedure to prevent the new placement of the colon from twisting or collapsing in some way. The bladder, for instance, may be moved slightly back in the abdomen to support the sigmoid area if a portion of the lower colon has been removed. Organs also may be moved slightly away from the surgical site in an effort to protect them from exposure to additional treatments. For example, a woman's uterus and ovaries may be moved away from the resection site if a course of radiation therapy to the area is anticipated.

In any event, moving the organs in this way often creates special problems for the patient. If the bladder is pushed against the colon it may be difficult to determine when the bladder is full and needs to be emptied. Unusual pressure on any part of the colon may cause problems with digestion, diarrhea or constipation. If the cervix is pushed back against the rectum it may be somewhat difficult for a woman's physician to conduct a PAP test.

In addition, the colon is a large and powerful muscle that moves in a manner similar to that of a caterpillar. Known as peristalsis and similar to the motion of the esophagus, the colon contracts and expands in a coordinated rhythm that forces food to move through the digestive tract. When handled, however, the colon temporarily loses its ability to move and essentially becomes paralyzed. As a result, it may be days after surgery before the digestive tract begins to work properly.

Indeed, the first sign that normalcy is returning is the patient's ability to pass gas. Often referred to as "the big event" this is a momentous occasion greeted with both jubilation and relief as it indicates that the resection was successful and the new and improved colon is beginning to function properly. The length of time it takes for this normalcy to return, however, depends upon many factors, including the general health of the patient, the amount of the colon removed and the location of the resection. The type and amount of pain medication the patient has received post surgery also greatly influences this return as many pain relievers are narcotics, and narcotics slow the digestive process, impede peristalsis and cause constipation.

In any event, colorectal cancer surgery alters the body in ways that will require time and patience on the part of the patient. One may not be able to eat as much or may not be able to eat certain foods. Bowel habits may change, and the new placement of organs may create general pressure and discomfort in the abdominal area for months or even years after surgery. Indeed, such adjustments will be an individual process in which each patient must learn how her or his new body works and how to take care of it.

Personal Note

One of my two uncles who developed colon cancer underwent the typical surgery to remove the malignancy and then underwent a colostomy. This colostomy was temporary and was only in place for a few months. My mother, however, reminded me recently that during this time we all had taken a vacation to the beach. My uncle dearly loved the ocean, and there was no way that a colostomy was going to interfere with his desire to swim each day. So, he simply covered the stoma with a bandage while he spent hours walking in the sand and playing in the water.

This occurred decades ago when the technology of such surgery was much less sophisticated and living with it was much more complicated. Yet, even with his colostomy, my uncle managed to live a normal life replete with hobbies and sports. He refused to let his condition compromise his personal freedom or enjoyment. And, if my dear uncle managed this well so long ago, imagine how well one can manage today.

Lung Cancer

Once again, the appropriate surgery for lung cancer depends upon many factors, including the size of the tumor, the location of the tumor and the general health of the patient. In addition, surgical options will depend upon the type of cancer detected. Although there are many different types of lung cancer, we know they can be divided into four basic groups. If the cancer is one of the small cell varieties, surgery may not be an option as these cancers typically spread too quickly to be completely removed surgically. On the other hand, if the cancer is one of the large celled varieties a number of surgical procedures may be performed.

If, for example, the tumor is small and accessible, an operation called a **segmental,** or **wedge resection,** may be performed to remove the affected tissue. If the tumor is no longer localized and has spread to a larger portion of the lung a **lobectomy** may be required to remove an entire lobe, or large rounded section, of the lung. And, in situations where the cancer is extensive the entire lung may be removed through a procedure known as a **pneumonectomy.**[17]

Additional surgeries may include **cryosurgery**, often used to freeze and destroy cancer tissue in the later stages of large cell lung cancers, and **laser surgery**, which may be used to destroy tumors that obstruct airways and cannot be surgically removed. Laser stands for **light amplification by stimulated emission of radiation,** and each type of laser derives its name from the substance it uses to operate. These substances, which may be gas, liquid or solid, are encased within a tube and are stimulated to emit light. A laser beam is created when this light is reflected between mirrors, and as the wavelength of the beam varies so too does the beam's strength. Clearly, of course, the strength of the beam will depend upon the type and size of the tissue to be removed.[18]

In addition, the surgeon may perform one of two procedures that will help determine if the lung cancer has spread into the nearby lymph nodes. In a **mediastinoscopy** the surgeon makes a small incision in the patient's neck through which a lighted scope is inserted. This scope allows the surgeon to examine the center of the patient's chest as well as the lymph nodes. A second procedure known as a **mediastinotomy** also allows the surgeon to examine the patient's chest and lymph nodes, although the incision in this case is made in the chest. Both procedures require a general anesthetic and the removal of tissue samples for laboratory examination.[19]

Special Concerns

In addition to the typical risks associated with other surgeries, unique problems may arise in the case of lung cancer. First, most lung cancers occur in individuals who have smoked heavily for many years. As a result, even if cancer is found only in one lung the cancer-free lung may still have been damaged by emphysema. If this is the case, a partial or complete removal of the cancerous lung may not be possible as the remaining lung may be incapable of providing the individual with the necessary oxygen.

To determine the existence of possible breathing problems, therefore, the individual must undergo additional tests prior to the cancer surgery. If these tests indicate the patient's general health is good and surgery still appears to be the best option, she or he can often expect to resume normal activities within four to six weeks.

Ovarian Cancer

As one of the silent cancers, and one often advanced at the time of diagnosis, major surgery is the typical treatment for this disease. Usually, the ovaries, fallopian tubes, cervix and uterus are removed in a procedure known as a **hysterectomy** with **bilateral salpingo-oophorectomy**. While the first procedure is familiar to most women there are actually two types of hysterectomy.

The first is a **total hysterectomy**, which involves the removal of the uterus and cervix, and the second is a **radical hysterectomy** in which the ovaries, the abdominal lymph nodes and lymph channels are removed in addition to the uterus and cervix. The second procedure refers to the removal of the fallopian tube and ovary on either one side, or in the case of a bilateral procedure, on both sides.[20]

Additionally, ovarian cancer often spreads to the thin fold of tissue that covers the stomach and large intestine known as the omentum. In many cases, therefore, the surgeon will remove this tissue as well. Finally, for women whose profiles indicate a high risk for developing ovarian cancer, the ovaries are sometimes removed as a preventative measure through a procedure known as a **prophylactic oophorectomy**.[21]

Special Concerns

In addition to the pain and tenderness that a woman may feel at and around the surgical site, surgery for ovarian cancer may include significant side effects. Because so many organs are held within the abdominal cavity, it's extremely difficult to operate on one without affecting another. For several days or weeks after a woman undergoes a hysterectomy, for example, she may experience difficulty emptying her bladder and colon. In most cases, ovarian cancer also requires the removal of both ovaries, and when this occurs a woman loses her ability to become pregnant.

Moreover, removing the ovaries removes the female body's source of natural estrogen and progesterone production. Accordingly, menopause and all its related symptoms may appear within weeks of the surgery and as these changes occur quickly, they don't give a woman much time to adjust. Each patient will have to decide what measures she wishes to take to improve and preserve her quality of life.

Professional counseling, for instance, may be helpful in learning to accept her inability to have children. Hormone replacement therapy typically has been used to alleviate menopausal symptoms in years past, yet this type of estrogen exposure has been linked to the development of both breast and endometrial cancer. Guidance regarding new or natural methods of treating such symptoms, therefore, may be necessary. Clearly, surgery for ovarian cancer will create unique physical and emotional changes in a woman's life that will require careful evaluation and physician assisted decisions.

Headline:

Hysterectomy: A Viable Preventative[22]

Yes, for some women predisposed to two types of reproductive cancers, the removal of their ovaries and uterus can be a powerful preventative measure. In particular, a genetic disorder known as Lynch Syndrome is detected in one out of every one thousand women. These women have a sixty percent chance of developing endometrial cancer compared to a three percent chance for women without the disorder. These women also have a twelve percent chance of developing ovarian cancer compared to the one to two percent chance shared by women without the disorder.

Lynch Syndrome is usually not detected until a woman, or one of her family members, develops cancer, typically colon cancer, at an early age. This makes sense, as we already know that colon cancer diagnosed at an early age is very likely the result of hereditary factors. We also know that women who develop colon cancer that appears to be genetically related have a greater risk for developing endometrial cancer as well.

Further, women who are at a high risk for breast cancer also may be at a greater risk for developing ovarian cancer. For all women, therefore, who share a greater than average risk for either endometrial or ovarian cancer based upon past or present cancers, a hysterectomy may prove a valuable preventative tool in the fight against specific future cancers.

Prostate Cancer

In the event that this cancer is diagnosed early and hasn't spread to the surrounding tissues or organs, surgery is the most common initial form of treatment. Indeed, if the cancer is localized it can often be cured through a variety of surgical procedures. Depending upon the size and location of the tumor, a portion of the prostate may be removed in a procedure known as a **prostatectomy**.[23]

This sometimes is accomplished through a **transurethral resection of the prostate,** or **TURP,** procedure in which the surgeon inserts a special instrument into the urethra. This instrument has a small wire loop on one end that transmits an electric current capable of cutting the cancerous tissue from the prostate. This procedure is especially useful in removing a tumor that may be blocking the flow of urine within the urethra.

If it appears necessary to remove the entire prostate the surgeon will perform a **radical prostatectomy**, a procedure commonly performed in one of two ways. In a **radical retropubic prostatectomy** the surgeon will remove the prostate and nearby lymph nodes through an incision in the abdomen. In a **radical perineal prostatectomy**, however, the surgeon will remove the prostate by making an incision between the scrotum and the anus, and will remove the nearby lymph nodes through a second incision in the abdomen.[24]

Yet, it's not uncommon in prostate cancer cases for the surgeon to remove the lymph nodes for examination before performing a prostatectomy. This allows the surgeon to determine if the cancer has spread from the prostate into the nodes and surrounding tissue, and, if this is the case, surgery may not be an appropriate treatment. If surgery is appropriate, however, the patient will face a number of post-surgical complications.

Clearly, he'll experience pain and discomfort at the surgical site and may feel extreme fatigue for several days or weeks. In addition, normal urination may not be possible for a period of time following the surgery so it'll be necessary for the patient to have a tube, known as a catheter, inserted into the urethra to drain urine from the body.

While these are short-term and temporary complications, long-term and even permanent complications also may result from prostate cancer surgery. Among these, a patient may experience urinary incontinence and lose his ability to control his bladder. Rectal injuries that occur during surgery may create problems with elimination and, in extreme cases, a colostomy may be necessary to correct these problems.[25]

Of course, every patient as either a temporary or permanent condition will experience impotence. In an effort to reduce permanent impotence, however, the surgeon may use a new technique known as **nerve-sparing surgery**. This technique combines the traditional prostatectomy with a method of prostate removal that cuts around the major nerves that control erections.

When this technique is utilized and the surgery is completely successful, the patient may experience only temporary impotence. Yet, this technique may not be an option for men who have been diagnosed with large tumors or tumors that are close to the major nerves. **Cryosurgery** that utilizes liquid nitrogen to freeze and kill cancer cells may be an option for some men with smaller tumors, although this procedure also can cause erectile dysfunction.[26]

In addition, men who have undergone a prostatectomy lose their ability to produce semen. As a result, patients who regain their ability to have erections and orgasms will experience what is known as a **dry orgasm**. In other words, the physical sensation of orgasm will be the same, but there will be no ejaculation of fluid. Accordingly, this type of prostate cancer surgery also results in the patient's inability to father children. Clearly, there is much to consider when faced with a diagnosis of prostate cancer for there are no easy choices when it comes to treatment. In light of this, it's sometimes recommended that certain patients forego surgery in favor of **watchful waiting**. As its name implies, this requires the physician and the patient to carefully monitor the growth of the cancer rather than engage surgery or another form of treatment. This approach may be recommended for men whose cancer appears to be slow growing, for those with certain medical conditions and for older men. Certainly in the case of older individuals, the substantial risks and the changes in one's quality of life resulting from surgery, and other cancer treatments, may not outweigh the possible benefits.[27]

On the other hand, watchful waiting may limit one's control over the cancer should it continue to grow and spread. Should this occur, surgery or any other treatment, for an older individual in particular, will become more and more difficult to manage as he continues to age. Once again, the decision to have surgery after a diagnosis of prostate cancer must be considered carefully with a full awareness of both the benefits and the risks.

What's New?

As research on cancer vaccines continues, one for advanced prostate cancer was introduced in 2009. Utilizing a drug known as **Provenge**, this vaccine stimulates the immune system to fight advanced cancers that don't respond to anti-androgen treatments. In a study of 512 men with advanced cancer of the prostate, the overall survival rate of those receiving Provenge was significantly increased. This drug is not without side effects including headaches, vomiting, fatigue and fever. Yet, the promise of an effective new treatment for this late stage cancer is generating excitement and optimism.[28]

Skin Cancer

Basel cell is the most common, the least invasive and the most easily treated of the skin cancers. As always, the treatment for this form of cancer will depend upon the size, depth and location of the tumor. If the tumor is small, for example, the physician may remove it by first **scraping** the area with a sharp instrument, then burning the area in a procedure known as **cauterization**. Similarly, a series of microscopically controlled shaved excisions may be used to remove the tumor in a **Mohs' surgery**.

In other situations, the tumor may be removed through **cryosurgery**, which uses sub-freezing temperatures, often in the form of liquid nitrogen, to destroy the tissue. With this type of skin cancer **laser surgery** can be used to treat a precise target area by gently burning the surface of the skin without harming surrounding normal tissue. When a variety of wavelengths is used, a pulsed light is created, and it's this type of laser that provides the safest and most efficient treatment for skin disorders.[29]

Finally, in cases where the tumor is somewhat larger or deeper, a small **surgical incision** may be required to remove the cancer and a small amount of the surrounding tissue. In any event, the surgical treatments for basel cell cancer are among the easiest to perform, carry the least risk and rarely need to be followed by additional treatments.

The size, depth and location also will determine the surgical options for **squamous cell** cancer as well as whether or not the cancer has metastasized. Once again, Mohs' surgery may be used to remove the diseased tissue. **Surgical excision**, however, may be required not only to remove the tumor, but also to remove the skin surrounding it. Indeed, when the removal of skin is extensive the patient may require a skin graft to replace that which has been excised.

If a skin graft is required, a separate procedure will be performed in which skin is removed from another area of the body and used to replace the excised skin. Often, grafts will be removed from a flat surface of the skin such as the abdomen, thigh or back with an instrument called a **dermatome**. The size and thickness of the graft will vary depending upon the location in which it's to be used and, of course, the amount of skin that must be replaced. Yet, most grafts typically will be removed and sutured into place using a local anesthetic and all successful grafts will be firmly established within a three-day period.[30]

Clearly, the more serious nature of squamous cell skin cancer dictates surgical procedures that may be somewhat more complicated than those for basel cell cancers. It also may be necessary to follow these surgeries with other cancer treatments, such as topical chemotherapy in which the anticancer drugs are contained in a lotion, and radiation therapy.

Melanoma, of course, is the most serious of the skin cancers and will, therefore, require more extensive treatment. This form of skin cancer typically will be removed through **surgical excision** similar to that used for squamous cell cancer. With this cancer, however, the surgery will remove the tumor and a large amount of normal tissue as well. This may result in disfigurement and once again, a skin graft to the affected area may be necessary. In addition, melanoma is more likely spread than other skin cancers and, as a result, the nearby lymph nodes typically will be removed for additional laboratory examination. If this is the case, the surgery most likely will be followed by additional cancer treatments.[31]

What's New?

Progress in cancer research and treatment often seems to move at glacial speeds. Every once in a while, however, a new development is announced that shatters this perception and elevates research to a new level. To illustrate, scientists have announced a new drug for the treatment of advanced melanoma. Known as **ipilimumab** or "ipi" for short, this drug has been used in clinical trials on patients with stage 4 melanoma. In these trials, those receiving the drug increased their life spans from six months to ten. Moreover, twenty to thirty percent of the patients with metastasized cancer found their tumors significantly decreased in size or disappeared completely. While "ipi" doesn't cause the typical nausea or hair loss of many chemotherapies, it does hyper-stimulate the immune system. This means the patient could develop a variety of autoimmune diseases including colitis and rheumatoid arthritis. The good news, of course, is that this drug already has the ability to extend lives and fight existing tumors. It is a dramatic discovery that holds great promise for not only treating melanoma, but for treating other cancers as well.[32]

General Concerns

Although numerous other surgical procedures exist for treating cancer, the above examples offer some insight into their variety. It's important to note that the need to perform either a minor procedure or a major surgery will depend upon whether or not the cancer was detected early in its development. Clearly, cancers diagnosed early will require the least treatment. In these cases, it's entirely possible that the surgery alone will cure the disease.

In contrast, cancers that are more developed or cancers that have spread from the initial site to other body tissues will require more extensive treatment. In these cases, surgery will attempt to remove all of the affected tissue although this may not always be possible. In the event that the cancer is too large or too widespread to be completely removed, a technique known as **tumor debulking** will be used. The goal of this technique is to remove as much of the cancer as possible to increase the effectiveness of other treatments such as chemotherapy and radiation. Yet, in the event the cancer has remained undiagnosed, it may not be possible to perform surgery and the patient will be forced to rely entirely upon the success of other treatments.[33]

Staging and Grading

Surgery has long been considered the cornerstone of cancer treatment and some form of it will almost always follow a diagnosis of the disease. Yet, in most cases surgery is just the beginning. With the exception of cancers that by their very nature are widespread, such as the leukemias, which affect the blood system, the goal of surgery isn't just to remove a diagnosed cancer tumor, but to determine the extent of its growth as well.

For example, through surgery the physician can see if the cancer is only on the surface or lining of an organ, or if it has moved into the deeper tissues of the organ as well. Surgery also allows the physician to inspect the surrounding organs and tissues for cancerous growths. By removing the lymph nodes near the surgical site, the physician can determine if the cancer has spread into the lymphatic system. If so, the cancer also may have spread to other areas of the body, a possibility that can be confirmed by examining additional lymph nodes throughout the body.

This diagnostic process of determining if and how far a cancer has spread is an essential element of every cancer diagnosis. Known as **staging**, this process varies somewhat according to the type of cancer. The most commonly used system of staging, however, is known as the **TNM** system. T determines the size of the tumor and whether it has spread to local tissues. N determines if the cancer cells have spread to the nearby lymph nodes. And, M determines if the cancer has spread to distant areas of the body.[34]

Breast cancer, for example, includes five different stages of development. The first is called Stage 0 where the cancer cells are localized or "in situ" in a small portion of the breast. This is followed by Stage I in which the cancer is still in the early stages of development and hasn't spread beyond the breast, although the tumor is larger and may be an inch across.[35]

Stage II is a little tricky in that it includes three different scenarios. The first involves a tumor less than an inch across, yet the cancer has spread to the nearby lymph nodes. The second involves any tumor between one and two inches in size whether or not the cancer has spread to the lymph nodes, and the third involves a tumor more than two inches across, but hasn't spread to the lymph nodes.

Stage III also is called locally advanced cancer and refers to a tumor more than two inches and has spread to the lymph nodes and/or other tissues near the breast. Finally, Stage IV, or metastatic cancer, refers to cancer that has spread beyond the breast, into the lymph nodes and through the lymphatic system to other parts of the body.[36]

Similarly, colorectal cancer has five different stages of development, ranging again from 0 to IV. If the cancer is determined to be at Stage 0, the disease was caught early and was found only in the innermost lining of the colon or rectum. A Stage I diagnosis indicates the cancer has moved from the inner wall of the colon or rectum and into the deeper tissues of the intestinal tract. Stage II indicates the cancer has spread through the outer wall of the colon or rectum and into some of the nearby tissue. Stage III also indicates that the cancer has spread through the outer wall of the colon or rectum to surrounding tissue and into the nearby lymph nodes. Finally, a Stage IV diagnosis indicates the cancer has not only moved through the intestinal wall to nearby tissue and lymph nodes, but has been carried by the lymph system to other parts of the body as well.[37]

The phases of staging will remain fairly constant regardless of the type of cancer with which one has been diagnosed. In other words, the first stage will always be the best situation in which the cancer is localized or in situ, typically the result of early detection. In the next stage, the cancer still will be found only within the affected organ. The following stage will indicate that nearby tissues are cancerous as well as the organ in question, and this is followed by a situation in which the lymph nodes are also affected. The last stage will identify a fully metastasized cancer with the organ, the nearby tissue, the lymph nodes and additional body parts all affected by the disease. Clearly, this last situation requires the most extreme treatment and offers an individual the least opportunity for a complete recovery.

In addition to staging, the **grade** of the cancer also must be determined. This term refers to the appearance of the cancer cells when they're examined under a microscope. It's the appearance of these cells that will help identify the possible growth rate of the tumor and its tendency to spread into other tissues. For example, if the cancerous tissue looks much like the surrounding normal tissue, the grade of the cancer is considered to be lower or less aggressive. These cancers are more likely to be slow growing tumors that aren't likely to spread quickly.

On the other hand, cancer that appears to be quite dissimilar from normal tissue is graded higher. Such cancers are considered more aggressive and have the ability to transform the structure and appearance of normal body cells much faster than less aggressive cancers. Clearly, the aggressive cancers typically will require treatment that is more intense or lengthy than other cancers.[38] Determining the stage and grade of a cancer is a laborious and time-consuming process. In addition to the tissue samples removed during the initial surgery, other tissues may need to be removed and examined as well. Additional CT scans, MRIs or other laboratory examinations also may be required to complete the patient's diagnostic profile. For example, an MRI may be required for one diagnosed with prostate cancer to help determine the most effective and yet the least invasive treatment. This post-surgery analysis is completely normal, and the patient shouldn't be alarmed if it takes several days, or even weeks, to complete.

A thorough and accurate diagnosis of the cancer is essential and forms the foundation upon which the patient's entire treatment program will be based. As we stated, surgery and tissue analysis is often only the beginning in a long process of cancer treatment. Depending upon the stage and grade of the cancer, the size and location of the cancer and numerous other factors unique to the individual, treatments in addition to surgery may be required. So, let's explore the most common of these additional treatments, beginning with the two most common, chemotherapy and radiation, and discuss some of the benefits and risks associated with each.

Chemotherapy

As defined earlier, chemotherapy is simply the treatment of any infection or disease through the use of chemical agents. There is evidence that humans have attempted to treat cancer with drugs since the time of the ancient Egyptians. Modern chemotherapy, however, dates from World War II when an American ship carrying poisonous mustard gas was bombed near the coast of Italy. It was later discovered that the mustard gas had destroyed the lymph cells in the blood of those who perished in the blast. As a result, a new drug derived from mustard gas was developed and used to treat cancer of the lymph nodes.[39]

Today, many different drugs are used to treat many different cancers. Remember, cancer is fast growing tissue in which the cells divide without restraint. Accordingly, modern chemotherapy drugs have the ability to detect these fast growing cells within the body. Rather than killing the cells directly, however, chemotherapy drugs impair the ability of the cells to multiply by interfering with the DNA and RNA activities associated with cell division. Further, chemotherapy doesn't always involve the use of a single drug. Indeed, the more common treatment will combine a number of different drugs that all work together to destroy the malignancy.

Most cancer treatments can be divided into two groups, those used to treat a small area of the body and those that treat the entire body. Surgery and radiation belong in the first group and are referred to as "localized" treatments. Chemotherapy, on the other hand, belongs in the second group and is known as a "systemic" treatment. Accordingly, it's often recommended in cases where the cancer was initially localized, then metastasized to other parts of the body. It also is used, however, in situations where lymphoma or leukemia has been diagnosed and the cancer itself typically is widespread by nature. It's even helpful in relieving the symptoms of advanced cancers that may be inoperable.

Basically, chemotherapy is used in one of two ways. In the first, it's used to target and attack cancer cells that still may remain in the body following surgery or radiation therapy. When used in this way, the treatment is referred to as **adjuvant chemotherapy**, which comes from the Latin word "adjuvans" meaning "to aid." Technically, this type of chemotherapy is a preventative measure almost always used in cases where the cancer has spread to the lymph nodes, the surrounding tissue or additional body parts. It's often used as well, however, in post-surgery cases in which there's no indication the cancer has spread to the lymph nodes or additional tissues. For, even if it appears that the cancer has been completely removed through surgery, it's always possible that a few cancerous cells, or even one, have escaped undetected.[40]

In the second, chemotherapy is administered before any other treatment is attempted. In these cases, the chemotherapy is referred to as **neoadjuvant**, or "upfront" therapy, and is used when it's not possible or practical to administer other treatments immediately following a cancer diagnosis. Often used with cancers of the head and neck, this method weakens a tumor and renders it more sensitive to subsequent treatments. Chemotherapy used in this way could destroy the malignancy, or at the least, reduce the size and growth rate of the tumor so that smaller and safer doses of radiation, or other treatments, can finish the job.[41]

When, Where and How

As we know, the type of cancer and the extent to which it has or hasn't spread are significant factors in determining which anticancer drugs will be used in each patient's chemotherapy. These factors also help determine how long one's treatment will last and if the chemotherapy will be administered once a day, once a week or once a month. In any case, however, chemotherapy is given in cycles where the treatments are balanced with periods of rest. For example, anticancer drugs known to be mild and produce a minimum of side effects may be given on a daily basis for a week, and stopped for several days before beginning again. In contrast, more potent treatments may be limited to once a week allowing the body six days to rest and build new healthy cells before undergoing another treatment. In situations where the treatment is especially strong, the body may need a full month to recover from one session. In any event, the treatments will continue until their job has been accomplished. And, throughout the process, the patient's response to the anticancer drugs will be monitored closely and the schedule of treatment will be adjusted if necessary.

In addition to the schedule of treatment, the location of treatment also must be determined. This will depend upon the potency of the anticancer drugs in use, the frequency with which they're administered and several other factors including the patient's overall health and her or his proximity to the treatment facility. The physician's need to observe and oversee the patient also must be considered as well as the desires of the patient and the patient's family. Lastly, the patient's insurance coverage, if applicable, is an important part of the equation as different policies set forth different guidelines and limitations concerning cancer treatment procedures.

In most cases, however, chemotherapy is given on an out-patient basis, which allows the patient to return home immediately following each treatment. Indeed, some treatments may be given in the patient's home, yet most will be conducted in a hospital, cancer center, clinic or hospice. This decision will depend not only on the factors already mentioned, but on the method of delivery as well. For, chemotherapy can be administered in several different ways including oral or topical application, injection and a variety of intravenous methods.[42]

First, some drugs contained in typical chemotherapy treatments actually can be given by mouth in the form of capsules or liquids. If this is the case, the patient simply adheres to a schedule and takes the medications as prescribed. Second, some anticancer drugs come in a liquid or lotion form that can be applied directly to the skin. This method is utilized in photodynamic therapy, also known as photochemotherapy, where the effect of the applied drugs is enhanced by exposing the skin to ultraviolet light.

Third, chemotherapy can be administered to a patient by injection. Using a needle and syringe, anticancer drugs can be injected intramuscularly into a muscle, subcutaneously under the skin or intralesionally in which the drugs are injected directly into a malignant skin lesion. For example, chemotherapy drugs utilized in the fight against ovarian cancer can be injected directly into the abdomen through intraperitoneal delivery.

Lastly, however, most chemotherapy is given as an intravenous or IV treatment where the liquefied anticancer drugs are injected into a vein. Typically, this form of chemotherapy requires the patient to be in a hospital, clinic or medical center during the therapy. Receiving chemotherapy in this way usually takes two to four hours, and as such, it's important for the patient to be comfortable. She or he will either sit or lie down while a needle is inserted into a vein, connected to an IV tube and bag, and the drugs are slowly pumped into the patient's bloodstream. The patient is fully alert during the session and many spend the time visiting with family and friends, sleeping, watching television or catching up on her or his reading. When the session is over, the needle as well as the IV is removed and the patient is free to go home. Indeed, sedatives aren't necessary for this procedure, and therefore the patient may drive her or himself to and from the session unless she or he is experiencing uncomfortable side effects.[43]

When receiving chemotherapy in this way, it's always advisable for the patient to check the drugs to be administered before the treatment begins. In most cases, the names of the anticancer drugs used in a particular chemotherapy will be labeled on the container or the IV packet along with the patient's name. While it's the job of the attending nurse or technician to make sure the correct drugs are being used, human beings make mistakes and tragedies, while rare, do occur.

Indeed, in any medical situation the patient should always make sure the medical practitioner checks one's bar code bracelet before administering any medication. Similarly, one must always know the name of every medication before taking it as well as the dosage. By assuming responsibility for oneself, one can rest assured that the proper treatment is being administered. Additionally, it's always a good idea to schedule treatments on the same day or week of the month and, if possible, at the same time. This greatly increases the chance that the patient will have the same medical team, one familiar with the patient and the case, each time one's treatment is delivered. If the medical personnel are not the same when one arrives for a scheduled therapy, one shouldn't hesitate to explain the details of one's particular case and treatment.

Finally, the cancer specialist, or **oncologist**, in charge of one's case typically won't be present when the patient is receiving the prescribed chemotherapy.[44] Accordingly, patients should always communicate with their oncologist the day before treatment is scheduled to discuss any problems the patient may be experiencing. If, for example, one is experiencing diarrhea, severe nausea or pain, the scheduled treatment may be canceled until the condition dissipates. A telephone call the day before can save the patient an unnecessary trip to the treatment facility where the nurse or technician, precisely for these reasons, may themselves cancel the treatment.

As with any medical procedure, however, complications can arise from this intravenous form of chemotherapy. It's possible for the anticancer drugs to leak from the needle into the tissues surrounding the vein rather than going directly into the bloodstream. To avoid this possibility, the patient must report any unusual sensation of coolness or burning at the injection site when the needle is inserted. It also is necessary to report any reaction that occurs at the site after the needle is removed such as swelling, pain or discoloration.

Further, this procedure requires the nurse or technician to find a thick vein that has the strength to receive the anticancer drug effectively. Such veins usually can be found on the arms or hands; however, repeated use of a vein for this purpose is likely to damage, change or collapse the vein. After many needle injections, therefore, the strength of the vein may be compromised, and it may lose its ability to receive a needle and transport the anticancer drugs. It also is possible for the skin at the injection site to become sore or irritated and, if either of these conditions occurs, a new vein and site must be found.

In many cases, a patient simply runs out of preferred veins for the procedure and smaller veins must be used. It's more difficult to deliver the drug when a small vein is used, yet it can be done. Indeed, this is often necessary when the patient is an infant or child, or an older individual whose veins may be fragile and more vulnerable to damage. Should this be a necessity, a specialized needle called a **butterfly** can be used for the IV. A butterfly is a small needle capable of piercing a small vein without puncturing the walls of the vein, causing it to "blow out."[45] While they're just as effective as larger needles, their small size and the fact they're inserted into smaller veins mean that the infusion of drugs must be done more slowly. As a result, each session may take a little longer, but the patient's comfort once again will be maximized.

In the alternative, for intravenous procedures such as iodine-enhanced CT scans or MRIs in which a butterfly may not be appropriate, a "baby" needle may be used. Just as its name suggests, this is a needle typically used for infants. This needle, however, also is good for fragile veins and for smaller veins often found in the hands or wrists. This is important as the veins of the hands and wrists often are used as a last resort in many chemotherapy patients who have experienced collapsed veins in other parts of their bodies. The veins of the hands and wrists aren't a first choice as they're quite small, and puncturing these veins may prove to be more uncomfortable than puncturing other veins as the hands and wrists are home to numerous nerve bundles and typically are quite sensitive.

If one must use these veins, therefore, it is good to keep in mind that regular blood testing will continue for several years, if not for the rest of one's life. Should this be the case, one must protect those veins and avoid procedures that may cause them damage. For example, saline injections that typically are used on the hand to reduce the size of a vein and create a smoother appearance in the skin should be avoided by those who rely upon these veins for medical purposes.

Many of the problems associated with the health of one's veins can be avoided, however, by administering intravenous chemotherapy through specialized **catheters**, **ports** and **pumps**. First, a catheter is a thin, flexible tube surgically placed directly into one of the body's large veins. It's left in this position for as long as treatment continues and eliminates the need to use a needle for each session. An IV is simply connected to the catheter and the anticancer drugs are administered.

A catheter also can be used to draw blood from a patient and to give additional drugs, all without the need for further needles and injections. While a catheter can be placed in any artery or large vein, most are placed within one of the large veins of the chest and are known as **central venous catheters**. Others that are placed in the large veins of the arm are called **peripherally inserted central catheters**, or **PICCs**. Yet, some catheters are placed in other parts of the body, such as an **intracavitary catheter**, located in the abdomen or pelvis, and an **intrathecal catheter**, which delivers anticancer drugs directly into the spinal fluid.[46]

In some cases, the catheter is placed into a vein, then attached to a device called a **port**. This port is a small round disc made from metal or plastic placed under the skin.

A catheter with or without a port, however, still requires the patient to be immobilized for the period of time it takes to administer the treatment. In contrast, when a catheter again, with or without a port, is used in combination with a **pump** the patient remains mobile and free to conduct their daily business in a normal fashion.

A pump is a device that contains a small storage area for the drug and regulates the amount that a patient receives. They're attached to the patient in one of two ways, the first of which remains outside the body and is called an **external pump**. This type may be attached to the catheter or port and automatically dispenses the drug, as treatment is needed. Many external pumps also are designed to be portable, and many can be worn on a special belt or on one's clothing. The pump is connected to the catheter or port, and as the patient goes about her or his normal daily activities, the drug is delivered in measured doses.

The second type, known as an **internal pump,** is surgically placed inside the body typically just under the skin. While the placement of these pumps differs according to type, they both work in exactly the same way supplying anticancer drugs to the patient in a consistent and regulated manner.[47] The fact that one can remain physically mobile in most cases by using a pump makes this type of intravenous chemotherapy attractive to many patients. Yet, this method also requires that the patient be attached in some way to a permanent device be it a catheter, a pump or a catheter and a port. This means that one will never be free physically from the machinery of chemotherapy, and some patients may not want to be reminded of the cancer and the treatment every moment. This is a psychological consideration of which every patient should be aware.

In contrast, chemotherapy administered through a typical IV with a needle is something the patient can leave completely behind each time a session is completed. In any event, each method of treatment has pros and cons that must be weighed carefully by each individual and her or his oncologist before committing to one or another.

Headline:

Stomach Cancer: The Second Deadliest Cancer in the World[48]

Yes, according to some sources, stomach cancer is the second leading cause of cancer deaths the world over. At least, it is for men. Yet, every source will agree that this particular cancer is a major threat in many parts of the world, with the highest death rates occurring in Japan and China. This cancer, however, typically isn't a major threat in most of the industrialized countries of the world. It appears that a low incidence rate of this cancer is associated primarily with good refrigeration. Refrigeration reduces the growth of bacteria in foods and allows access to fresh fruits and vegetables throughout the year. It also has reduced the need for other methods of food preservation, such as salting and smoking, both of which are associated with higher rates of stomach cancer.

Indeed, irritants such as salt can promote the harmful effect of local carcinogens. The bacterium Helicobacter pylori or H. pylori which is transmitted through fecal/oral or oral/oral contact, a source of which often is water contaminated with human waste, also can increase one's risk for developing some forms of stomach cancer. Overall, increasing a diet rich in fresh fruits and vegetables as well as decreasing salted, smoked, pickled foods and tobacco use will reduce one's risk for this cancer significantly.[49]

❧ ❧ ❧

Wrestling the Octopus

Before we begin our discussion of chemotherapy, radiation and the numerous ways in which each can change one's body either intentionally or unintentionally, we'll offer an analogy that can be useful in understanding these changes and their complicated and often frustrating nature. Wrestling is a popular sport the world over, and in the Western world it's a sport that requires one participant to contain or "pin" the shoulders or arms of the other. In this sport, it's an accomplishment to gain control over one arm of an opponent and an even greater accomplishment to gain control over both. In theory, therefore, the more arms one must contend with, the more difficult the goal of control is going to be.

Now, the thought of applying this sport and its goal to an octopus with eight arms seems a ludicrous proposition. Yet, wrestling an octopus is exactly what many cancer patients face when trying to manage the effects and side effects created by the various cancer treatments. Imagine for a moment holding such a creature and trying to control each arm simultaneously. For every arm over which we gain control, we lose control over two. In grasping the two, we lose control over four others. As we regain control over these four, one more slips out in front, then two more in the back, and so on.

Similarly, the problems that may result from cancer treatments often are like the arms of a large, slippery octopus all of which the patient attempts to control at the same time. There will be many instances in which a patient will find a way to control one physical problem only to discover that the remedy aggravates another. And in an attempt to reduce the aggravated condition, an entirely new problem may be created.

Just as it's difficult to control all the arms of an octopus at the same time, it often is difficult to control and manage all the symptoms and side effects of cancer treatment at the same time. What may help one problem may harm another. What may reduce one problem may increase another. What may eliminate one problem, may give rise to another. Even though it may be possible to simultaneously control the side effects and physical problems that result from cancer treatment, it remains a tricky proposition. Keeping this in mind, therefore, let's begin our discussion of the various cancer treatments and their . . .

Effects and Side Effects

*In the depths of winter I finally learned
there was in me an invincible summer.*
Albert Camus

While chemotherapy is necessary in most cases and recommended in many, it's not without significant complications. Indeed, it's not uncommon for many patients undergoing chemotherapy to feel that the treatment is much worse than the disease. It's vital, therefore, to remember that while chemotherapy may prove unpleasant, uncomfortable and a miserable temporary impediment to one's quality of life, when administered properly, it won't kill you. Cancer, on the other hand, can. This being the choice, let's discuss the many problems that one might experience while undergoing chemotherapy and more importantly, the ways in which one might reduce the impact of these problems.

First, let's develop a clear understanding of why so many medical problems arise with the use of chemotherapy. To begin, the side effects of chemotherapy don't result from the anticancer drugs attacking and impeding cancer cells. Rather, side effects occur when these drugs attack healthy cells within the body. To review, we already know that cancer is basically a cell or cells that grow fast and continue to multiply without stopping. We also know that chemotherapy is successful in treating cancer because the drugs used in the therapy have the ability to "sniff out" fast growing cells, and once these cells are targeted, the drugs attack and interfere with the cell's ability to divide.

Yet, there are other cells within the human body that also are "fast growing," and these include the cells of the hair follicles, the finger and toe nails, the digestive tract, the blood cells formed in the bone marrow and the cells of the reproductive system. As a result, the anticancer drugs found in chemotherapy often will attack these cells as well as the cancer cells. For, chemotherapy anticancer drugs cannot distinguish between normal, healthy fast growing cells and abnormal fast growing cancer cells.[50]

This is exactly why a patient's hair sometimes falls out during chemotherapy. The anticancer drugs attack the fast growing cells of the follicle. The cells lose their ability to thrive and multiply, and as they die, the hair within the follicles becomes loose and susceptible to the slightest pressure from a comb, a brush or one's hands. Further, hair loss from chemotherapy may occur on a patient's head or it may affect hair on any other part of the body. It's not uncommon for those undergoing chemotherapy to lose hair on the arms and legs, the pubic area, the face or the underarms. Similarly, as the fast growing cells of the finger and toenails are attacked, the nails may change color, become brittle and lined, or completely fall off.

In addition, the digestive tract, which includes the mouth, esophagus, stomach and intestines, is packed with fast growing cells that aid digestion and elimination on a daily basis. When the cells within the mouth or throat are attacked, the mucous membrane responsible for maintaining a normal balance of moisture is compromised. As a result, these tissues may become more susceptible to sores or prone to dryness, which may hinder a patient's ability to eat and chew food comfortably. Indeed, one's ability to taste certain foods also may be compromised or one may experience a bitter or metallic taste when eating.

This may be further complicated by the destruction of cells lining the esophagus, which can create severe dryness and interfere with the process of swallowing. Cells lining the stomach are prone to a similar attack and when this occurs the stomach cannot operate or process food properly. In addition, the delicate balance of producing the necessary and adequate amount of acids needed for digestion may be impaired. When the cells lining the small and large intestine are attacked each loses its ability to absorb nourishment and engage in normal peristalsis. As a result, the entire digestive tract from intake to elimination may be compromised and a patient may experience discomfort, stomach upset and nausea, pain and cramping, sluggishness and constipation, or dehydration and diarrhea all within a single course of chemotherapy.[51]

This concept of fast growing cells also helps us understand why cancer patients often experience severe fatigue. The red blood cells formed in the bone marrow are responsible for carrying oxygen to all parts of the body. It's this essential oxygen that allows the tissues and muscles of the body to operate properly. In addition, the red blood cells, like cancer cells, divide and multiply quickly, and as a result they too are prime targets for the anticancer drugs used in chemotherapy. When the red blood cells are attacked by these drugs, their quality and quantity is diminished, and their ability to do their job is compromised. As a result, the body tissues don't receive enough oxygen to remain strong, and the patient may experience shortness of breath, headaches, dizziness or confusion and a general state of weakness.[52]

Yet, the red blood cells aren't the only blood cells affected by chemotherapy. The white blood cells that form in the bone marrow are fast growing cells and targets for anticancer drugs as well. It's these cells that defend the body against all foreign material such as bacteria and viruses. From our discussion of leukemia, we know that these cells include the granulocytes, the monocytes and the lymphocytes. We also know that the lymphocytes include the B cells that produce antibodies and the T cells that attack foreign and diseased cells.[53]

When the white cells themselves, however, come under attack by anticancer drugs their quality and quantity, like the red blood cells, is compromised. This fact renders the patient more vulnerable and more likely to develop a number of various infections in addition to severe fatigue. Further, the bone marrow also is responsible for the production of platelets, which are necessary for proper blood coagulation and clotting, a process that will be interrupted as well by the anticancer drugs.[54]

Lastly, of course, the fast growing cells of the reproductive system are particularly vulnerable to the toxic effects of anticancer drugs. Indeed, the complications that affect reproduction and fertility are significant and, as such, will be discussed in detail in a separate section.

While these fast growing healthy cells of the human body are the most vulnerable to anticancer drugs, each patient's experience with chemotherapy will differ. Some may experience every complication we've mentioned and some may experience none. Some may experience discomfort of a severe nature and others may be only slighted affected. The type of side effect and its severity will depend largely upon the types of anticancer drugs used in a patient's personal chemotherapy treatment.

Referred to as a **chemo-cocktail**, the proper recipe for each individual's program will depend once again upon the many factors already discussed including the characteristics of the cancer as well as the personal characteristics of the patient.[55]

If a cancer is caught early, for example, the chemotherapy drugs typically used will be of a mild nature. Clearly, however, if the cancer has spread from its initial site to other body parts, stronger anticancer drugs will be necessary to fight the malignancy.

As these stronger drugs attack the cancer with greater force, they attack the fast growing healthy body cells with equal force. In such cases, therefore, the patient is much more likely to experience the serious side effects associated with the hair and nails, the digestive tract, the blood and the reproductive organs. Understanding the complications of chemotherapy, while informative, isn't really useful unless we also have the necessary tools to deal with these complications. So, let's address each of these major side effects one at a time and discuss the ways in which their impact upon the patient may be minimized, if not wholly avoided.

The Hair: Alopecia

Alopecia is the term that refers to any hair loss regardless of whether the loss is total or partial in nature. Physically, the hair is composed of keratin, the same material found in the finger and toenails and the outer layer of human skin. Similar to human skin, the hair also contains melanin, the substance that determines not only skin color but hair color as well. The hair shaft or strand is that part that rises out of the skin and its numbers will reach approximately 100,000 strong on a healthy, typical adult human head. Each strand consists of three layers of keratin that include the outermost layer or cuticle, the middle layer or cortex and the innermost layer or medulla.[56]

It's the cortex that contains the melanin granules and just as melanin determines the color of one's skin, it also determines the color of one's hair. Those with few granules in the cortex, for instance, will be blond while those with many will be brunette. In addition, it's the cortex that determines if one's hair will be curly or straight. The hair root of each strand lies just below the surface of the skin and is enclosed in a "sac" known as the hair follicle, the nourishment and health of which is provided by tiny blood vessels and nearby oil producing glands.[57]

Similar to skin cells, human hair grows and sheds regularly. The average rate of growth for hair is about half an inch a month and after growing steadily for two to six years, each strand will rest and then fall out. At this point, the follicle will produce a new strand of hair and the process will be repeated. A healthy human being, therefore, will have about eighty-five percent of her or his hair growing and fifteen percent resting at any given time, and can expect an average loss of fifty to one hundred strands per day.[58]

When illness strikes, however, this typical process of hair growth can be greatly altered. In the case of cancer, in fact, hair loss is often the side effect that people worry about the most. It also is a concern that isn't limited to the chemotherapy patient. For the question, "Is your hair going to fall out?" is often the first asked by well meaning family members and friends. And while hair loss can occur on any part of the body, this concern and query are focused directly upon the hair one has on her or his head. Nor is this a rational concern that arises from a fear of permanent physical disfigurement, such as the loss of a finger, or a leg, or a breast. For the hair one loses as a result of chemotherapy will, with very rare exceptions, always grow back.

Rather, this concern of hair loss arises from deep-rooted psychological issues and cultural expectations. Some cultures, for example, consider a lock of hair to be the ultimate gift of love and others consider a woman's hair a thing of beauty to be revealed only to her husband. Throughout time societies the world over have revered the importance and beauty of human hair. Poetry and literature are filled with references to one's "crowning glory" or to an individual's "one great beauty" and pay homage to sacrificing heroines whose shorn locks are sold for the benefit and well being of loved ones. Human hair has been regarded as a symbol of strength in the story of Sampson. It has been likened to a lion's mane, symbolizing vitality and nobility. And, the lack of hair, replaced with serpents in the mythological figure of Medusa, has been associated with disfigurement, corruption and fear.

Today, a full head of hair is highly prized and regarded as a shining symbol of beauty, health and well being. Indeed, the industrial countries of the world are home to vast commercial enterprises whose sole purpose is to produce and distribute products to maintain and improve the look of one's hair. Fortunes are spent on drugs developed to increase hair growth and prevent hair loss. Additional fortunes are spent developing wigs, toupees and sprays designed to disguise thinning hair and balding heads. Billions of consumer dollars are spent lightening, darkening, straightening, curling, styling and transplanting the hair on our heads.

Our hair has become an important element of our personal self image. It represents to a large extent, the way we see ourselves and the way we want others to see us. Indeed, the state of our hair has even become a part of our modern vernacular where one's well being is often described by the terms "a good hair day" or "a bad hair day." One's hair can represent youth and sex appeal, vigor and vitality, self-expression, beauty and love, and when we lose our hair, the subconscious irrational fear is that we lose all those things as well.

Moreover, some patients choose not to share the state of their health with others. Some patients with cancer choose to battle their foe privately. When one's hair falls out as a result of this battle, this private and personal matter is literally uncovered for all to see. Many patients are left feeling uncomfortable, vulnerable and naked. And, unless steps are taken to once again "cover" the condition, one's personal battle with the disease becomes public in a very obvious way. It's not surprising, therefore, for a patient faced with chemotherapy to experience apprehension and anxiety about this one, single side effect perhaps more than any other.

Clearly, it's essential to put the specter of hair loss into perspective. For every cancer patient must focus on fighting the disease and required chemotherapy is an important part of the battle. It can save lives, and if a patient's hair falls out in the process, it's a small price to pay. The loss of hair is temporary and unimportant compared to the larger issues at hand. When we see a different image in the mirror, one that reflects a less than perfect picture of health due to cancer, we need to remember that this image also reflects a survivor. It reflects the face of a warrior, and the qualities instilled in that image are those of perseverance, resilience, fortitude and courage. Indeed, it's a badge of courage, an image that should spark inspiration and pride in each and every individual who possesses it and each individual who bears it witness.

Helpful Hints

Having said this, adjusting to a new physical image as a result of any situation remains a challenging and difficult task. When the situation involves hair loss resulting from cancer and its treatments, our primary concern must be for the comfort and well being of the patient. It's important, therefore, to discuss some of the ways in which the physical and psychological discomfort of this side effect can be minimized. As mentioned, whether or not a patient loses her or his hair will depend upon the anticancer drug or drugs used in the chemotherapy, a decision to be made by one's oncologist. Accordingly, the first thing each patient must do is become familiar with her or his own personal chemo-cocktail and the drugs it contains. Together, the oncologist and the patient can review each drug and identify those typically associated with hair loss, be it mild or severe.

If it appears that hair loss is inevitable, the patient may wish to take some preventative measures. For example, if the individual has long hair, she or he may wish to cut it short so that the eventual loss is less shocking and easier to manage. Some patients may choose to shave their heads before beginning treatment. This choice not only removes the anxiety about when hair loss will begin, but it can provide the patient with a psychological boost by placing her or him in control of the situation.

One also may choose to cover her or his head once hair loss begins, and if so it's advisable to purchase or borrow wigs, hairpieces, turbans, hats or scarves prior to treatment. By preparing for this side effect before it takes place, the patient's overall emotional stress during treatment may be reduced. With this accomplished, the patient is left free to concentrate on the other important issues she or he will encounter during the course of treatment.

Once treatment does begin, however, there are other ways in which a patient can maximize her or his level of comfort concerning hair loss. As is the case with most side effects resulting from chemotherapy, this can be accomplished largely by exercising a little common sense. It's important, for example, to treat the hair gently during this period of time. While hair remains on one's head, mild shampoos such as those formulated for infants should be used. Metal and course bristled hairbrushes should be replaced with brushes that have soft bristles, and women should avoid using brush rollers to style their hair. If possible, hair should be allowed to dry naturally after shampooing, and if a hair dryer is used, the heat should be kept low.[59]

Clearly, it's important to avoid chemical contact with the scalp during therapy and the use of hair dyes, bleaches, curling and relaxing products should be temporarily removed from one's beauty regimen. Finally, it's essential to protect one's scalp, whether hair remains or not, from the adverse effects of the sun by using sunscreens and protective clothing whenever UV-B exposure is anticipated. Indeed, one should continue to protect the scalp after chemotherapy is completed and hair is beginning to regrow, a process, by the way, which may result in hair of a different color or texture if the cortex has been affected by the anticancer drugs. By limiting one's use of hair products, using only the mildest formulas when needed and protecting the scalp from unnecessary irritation, the patient can get through this period of time with a minimum of discomfort and a maximum of self-confidence.[60]

Personal Note

I underwent weekly chemotherapy treatments for a year, yet the hair on my head didn't fall out. It did become a little thinner for a year or so, but my particular "chemo-cocktail" wasn't considered to be of an aggressive nature and the drugs I received typically did not result in severe hair loss. My pubic hair, however, did fall out. While this particular hair loss isn't uncommon with chemotherapy, my particular loss was probably due to the combination of chemotherapy and abdominal radiation therapy that I underwent simultaneously.

The Nails

Side effects that affect the nails during chemotherapy aren't as common as alopecia. Yet, this may be an issue for patients whose chemo-cocktail contains anticancer drugs of a more potent nature. First, the physical structure of the nail is similar to that of the hair. The body of the nail is known as the nail plate. It's formed in the nail fold, a pocket of skin that actually resembles a hair follicle. The nail also consists of three layers of keratin, which include the topmost or dorsal layer, the middle or intermediate layer and the bottom or ventral layer. The finger tissue that supports the nail is called the nail bed and the area that generates keratin and nail growth at the back of the nail is called the root, or nail matrix. Finally, the extension of skin that surrounds the back of the nail plate is called the cuticle.[61]

While they share many physical similarities, human nails and hair don't undergo the same cycle of growth. Unlike the hair, the nails grow continuously throughout a human's life with fingernails replacing themselves every five to seven months at a rate of one half to one millimeter each week. The middle fingernail grows the fastest followed by the fourth, second and fifth fingers, and finally the thumb. Further, fingernails grow more quickly on the right hand of right-handed individuals, and more quickly on the left hand of left handed individuals. All nails appear to grow more quickly during the summer months, yet toenails grow much more slowly than those of the finger, at approximately one third to one half the growth rate.[62] Accordingly, the faster growing nails of the fingers are more likely to be affected by anticancer drugs than the nails of the toes.

When any nail is injured and falls off, a new nail at the same average growth rate typically will replace it. If, however, the matrix or root of the nail is damaged, the new nail also is likely to be damaged and distorted in some way such as color or shape. If the matrix is destroyed, a new nail won't grow in at all. Accordingly, when anticancer drugs affect only the fast growing cells of the nail plate, one's nail may become discolored and brittle, or the nail may completely fall off.[63]

In either case, however, the nail will resume natural and healthy growth when the cancer treatment is over. On the other hand, if the anticancer drugs also attack the fast growing cells of the matrix, depending upon whether or not the damage is total, the nail will grow back distorted or not all. While it may not be possible to determine if, or to what extent, the nails will be affected by chemotherapy, it's possible to take protective measures to maximize nail health and minimize damage.

Helpful Hints

Once again, common sense will help dictate the proper care for a patient's nails during her or his therapy. And, once again, the most obvious measure is to avoid chemical contact with the nails as much as possible during treatment. For example, it's advisable to refrain from using nail polishes and lacquers. While nail polishes, especially those that contain nylon fibers, can protect the nail surface and add strength to fragile nails, their use necessitates the use of nail polish removers. And, these removers contain chemicals that can dry and damage the nails.[64]

It's a better idea, therefore, to gently buff the nails to reduce ridges or cracks on the nail surface and provide a subtle cosmetic sheen. Buffing, which should be done in the direction of nail growth rather than back and forth, also can help stimulate blood flow to the nails, which is essential for tissue health and strength. In addition, it's particularly important to keep the nails short during this time to prevent unnecessary snagging and breaking. To shape the fingernails, use a fine file or emery board, always filing the nail tip from the corner to the center. Once again, a back and forth motion should be avoided as this can cause ridges in the nail that can lead to splitting. And, regardless of what one may have been told, the nails aren't related to the development of bone tissue, and as a result, brittle or thin nails cannot be strengthened by calcium or gelatin supplements.[65]

Also, individuals undergoing treatment may want to avoid prolonged exposure to wetting and drying of the nails as this also can cause brittleness and make the nails more likely to split and break. Further, keratin is a protein that is at its hardest and healthiest when its **potential hydrogen,** or **PH,** is slightly acidic. As many detergents, cleaners and soaps are alkaline based products they actually loosen the keratin fibers in the nail, making them more susceptible to damage. Accordingly, one should always wear cotton lined rubber gloves when doing the dishes or other chores that expose the nails to these products and require the hands to be in water for long periods of time. Wearing gloves also will help reduce the potential for bacteria to become lodged under the nail tip and within the nail tissue. In addition, it will be helpful to wear gloves or mittens outdoors during cold weather to protect the nails from harsh weather conditions and avoid using one's fingertips for simple chores.[66] For example, patients shouldn't use their fingers to pick up objects from hard surfaces but instead, should slide the object off with one hand and into the other. In addition, rather than using one's fingers and nails, one should use a pen or pencil to punch the numbers on a telephone or other keypad, use a letter opener for envelopes and use scissors to cut tape and open packages.

It's Not Just a Hangnail

Clearly, nail care is important during one's therapy and while one's toenails are not typically as visible as one's fingernails, they too need special care. Both finger and toenails should be treated after one's bath or shower when the tissues are more pliable, yet because toenails are usually thicker than fingernails, this routine becomes especially important. The same rules for fingernails apply to toenails and buffing should replace the use of polishes and polish removers during treatment. Once again, the nails should be buffed in the direction of growth and after trimming the nail tips straight across, rough edges should be removed by gentle filing from the corners to the center. For both fingers and toes, however, it's important to refrain from cutting or trimming the cuticle because it's the cuticle that provides a protective barrier around the nail from bacteria. The human body in general is more vulnerable to bacteria and infection during this time, and it's important to take the necessary steps in nail care to avoid potential harm. Not only does the cuticle help protect the nails from invading bacteria, but tissue that has been nicked or damaged by scissors or clippers may result in a difficult and lengthy healing process.[67]

It's possible for minor scrapes and scratches to become infected during treatment and any cutting of the tissue, including that of a hangnail, must be performed carefully. For hangnails, as well as other nail problems, often result from dry skin and are prone to tearing, a condition that can result in pain and possible infection. While a mild cuticle softener may help keep this tissue moist and pliable, the cuticle still shouldn't be pushed back with a metal instrument as metal will scrape away the protective cells of the nail surface. Of course, mild hand creams and lotions can help moisturize the cuticle and other tissues of the finger and toenails and reduce the risk of small injuries.[68]

If, however, in spite of this focused care the patient still experiences nail loss, the following steps may prove helpful. First, the finger or toe may be extremely tender after losing a nail. It's important, therefore, to prevent additional harm to either by using the finger as little as possible, or by wearing loose and comfortable shoes. After consulting with one's physician, it may be helpful to apply an antibacterial ointment on and around the nail bed and to wear a Band-Aid or bandage for protection until the tenderness subsides.

Once this occurs, however, there's little one can do while waiting for the new nail to grow in. In the first stages of growth the nail may be misshapen and discolored until it's replaced by nail tissue that is more normal in appearance. This growth is a slow process that may take many months before the individual sees improvement. Of course, if the matrix of the nail has been damaged the new nail may never appear quite normal and, if the matrix has been destroyed, the nail won't grow back at all. Even in this case, however, the fingertip or toe will improve greatly in appearance over time and will only require patience on the part of the individual.[69]

The Digestive Tract

Mucositis or Stomatitis

Problems of the mouth and throat are fairly common in patients undergoing chemotherapy, however, the degree of severity each experiences will differ greatly. Again, this difference will depend primarily upon the potency of the anticancer drugs in each patient's chemo-cocktail. Regardless of the potency, there are many things every patient can do to avoid or minimize these side effects and insure a greater level of personal comfort. Sores that may appear in the mucous membranes of the mouth and throat distinguish the condition known as **mucositis** or **stomatitis**.[70]

Similar to ordinary canker sores, these specific sores can be very painful, they can be numerous and slow to heal once they appear. In addition, these sores are subject to infection because the mouth is home to a multitude of germs, and the patient's ability to fight infection during chemotherapy is compromised due to a decreased white cell count.[71]

The combination of simple prophylactic measures and common sense, however, once again can greatly reduce the impact of this condition.

First, cancer patients typically have at least a few weeks between their cancer surgery and the onset of additional treatments. Remember, this is the period of time in which the staging and grading process of the cancer is conducted. It's during this time that the specific program of chemotherapy, radiation or other treatment will be determined by the physician. This also is the period of time that can be used by the patient to prepare for the recommended treatment.

When chemotherapy is anticipated, the patient should see her or his dentist as soon as possible and as far in advance of the treatment's onset as possible. At this time, any existing problems such as cavities, gum disorders or ill-fitting dentures can be addressed. One's teeth can be cleaned and the dentist can advise the patient on the proper oral care regarding brushing and flossing as well as product use during the chemotherapy. The teeth are more likely to develop cavities during treatment and as a result, one's dentist also may recommend special brushes, toothpastes or mouthwashes that may minimize this particular problem.

During treatment, it's important to clean the mouth regularly by brushing the teeth and rinsing the mouth after eating. For brushing, it's advisable to use a soft bristled brush in a motion recommended by one's dentist. Special toothpastes that are formulated for sensitive teeth and gums, and those containing cavity-fighting agents such as fluoride also may be advisable. For rinsing, it's important to use a mild solution that won't further irritate the vulnerable tissues of the mouth. This may be best accomplished by a home-made formula of warm salt water, or a gentle solution of water and sodium bicarbonate. In any event, the patient should refrain from using harsh over the counter mouthwashes containing alcohol that can irritate sensitive tissues.[72]

One also should avoid any food product that may irritate the mucous membranes of the mouth and throat. As such, foods that are spicy or salty, and foods high in acid content such as citrus fruits and juices should be avoided. While the reasonable consumption of alcoholic beverages may be permissible during some chemotherapy programs, it should be avoided if side effects of the digestive tract such as mucositis exist. Foods that are hard to chew or abrasive to oral tissues such as toast and hard breads, crunchy cereals and many snacks like chips or popcorn also should be avoided. It's even advisable to avoid foods known for their roughage or fiber content, including raw fruits and vegetables, as these also can irritate and scratch the inside of the mouth.[73]

Additionally, it's better to consume foods at room temperature rather than when they're hot. Proper nourishment remains an important issue for every patient during treatment as well. Accordingly, one should blend or puree non-citrus fruits and cooked vegetables and take advantage of their healthy attributes in liquid form. Other soft foods including eggs and yogurt, puddings, cooked cereals, slow cooked stews or soups and even baby foods can help a patient maintain proper nourishment during this time. By incorporating these dietary suggestions, mouth sores actually may be avoided during treatment or at the very least, their discomfort may be reduced.

Headline:

Tea Drinking Reduces Risk of Ovarian Cancer[74]

This is, of course, the type of headline that women would love to believe. And, it's true that the results of one specific study conducted by Swedish researchers suggest this may be the case. The study, which involved over 61,000 Swedish women, questioned the participants about their dietary habits, then tracked each participant through the year 2004 for an average of fifteen years. During this time, three hundred and one of the participants developed ovarian cancer.

The study determined that those participants who habitually drank two or more cups of tea daily were forty-six percent less likely to develop this cancer than those who drank no tea. Moreover, the study suggested that participants who drank less than two cups of tea a day also decreased their risk of developing the disease, although to a lesser degree. Now, this study didn't clarify the type of tea each participant consumed, but it did acknowledge that most of the tea consumed was black tea.

Indeed, this is interesting as black tea, as well as green tea, is known to contain polyphenols, which are substances believed to block the cell damage that can lead to cancer. Other studies on this particular subject, however, have yielded conflicting and inconsistent results that indicate the results of the Swedish study might be due to a variety of factors other than a woman's tea drinking habits. In any case, this is a subject that warrants further investigation as ovarian cancer is the seventh deadliest cancer among the world's female population.

Dry Mouth

Yet another side effect that chemotherapy patients may face is that of an uncomfortably dry mouth or esophagus. In this situation, some of the above suggestions for mucositis also will prove helpful. For instance, soft and pureed foods will be easier to consume and swallow than hard and dry foods. Moisture added to any food in the form of broths and sauces also will help alleviate problems associated with a dry mouth or esophagus and will facilitate chewing and swallowing. Some patients may find that sucking on hard candy or chewing gum may help this condition as well as drinking plenty of water and other liquids.[75]

Keeping our "octopus" in mind, one also needs to remember that the teeth are more susceptible to cavities during treatment and, therefore, these products should be sugar free if possible.

Unfortunately, some of these products contain ingredients that may cause additional problems for the rest of the digestive tract, including the intestines. For example, if the intestines are already being adversely affected by the chemotherapy and the patient is experiencing severe or prolonged diarrhea, sugar free products may only contribute to the problem and may need to be avoided. It also may be helpful to use a moisturizer or petroleum jelly on the lips for persistent dryness and keep bottled drinking water available at all times to aid the body in hydration.

Nausea

As the fast growing cells lining the esophagus and stomach are attacked by the anti-cancer drugs of chemotherapy it's not uncommon to experience stomach upset and nausea as well. At one time, in fact, these side effects were among the most common of those associated with chemotherapy. Fortunately, a plethora of new drugs have greatly reduced the occurrence and the severity of this unpleasant and sometimes painful duo. Known as **antiemetic** or **antinausea** drugs, these medications typically are administered to the patient as a part of her or his chemo-cocktail.[76]

One's physician or oncologist usually will begin with one drug such as compazine, then change or add to the drug as dictated by the patient's need. It may take a few treatments to find the correct drug or combination of antiemetics for each patient, but persistence can result in treatment that's virtually nausea free. If stomach upset and nausea persist, however, many physicians suggest that the patient avoid consuming liquids and solids at the same time. Instead, small amounts of liquids may be consumed an hour or two before or after a meal.

It also may be helpful to eat and drink slowly and to eat small amounts of food throughout the day rather than large, regular meals. Further, foods consumed at room temperature not only decrease the potential for mucositis, they also lack strong smells that may be nauseating for a chemotherapy patient. Finally, chewing solid food well before swallowing will help protect the stomach and reduce the amount of acids it must produce to aid digestion. While eating foods such as plain toast or saltine crackers typically can reduce nausea, these remedies often are not the answer for chemotherapy patients.[77]

Once again, however, we must keep our "octopus" in mind. If the patient already is experiencing mucositis or dry mouth, toast or saltines may increase the discomfort of these side effects even if they do relieve nausea. Similarly, while certain carbonated drinks often reduce nausea, they can produce gas that may increase intestinal distress. Once again, we're in tricky territory where the health of the entire digestive system must be considered. Accordingly, simple experimentation may be the only way an individual can find the proper diet for her or himself, one that will alleviate one symptom without aggravating another.

Diarrhea and Constipation

When the fast growing cells that line the intestines are affected by the anticancer drugs in chemotherapy, the body loses its ability to absorb and digest food properly. As a result, a patient will often experience some degree of intestinal distress, including diarrhea or constipation and cramping or bloating. Of course, as with every other side effect, the degree of distress will depend upon the type and strength of the anticancer drugs in the patient's chemo-cocktail.

The first of these side effects, diarrhea, is a common ailment that has affected nearly every individual at one time or another whether they have undergone treatment for cancer or not. Typically, however, it's an ailment temporary in nature and a "passing" inconvenience at most. For cancer patients, however, this common ailment may become a constant and persistent condition that may continue sporadically for weeks or months at a time. It's one that may completely upset one's regular routine and greatly interfere with daily life. Indeed, it may be debilitating to the point where the resulting loss of body fluids and nutrients require hospitalization and intravenous replacement.[78]

Forget the Fiber

As one's life begins to revolve around the bathroom, however, there are several things one can do to reduce her or his discomfort. Once again, many of the dietary suggestions recommended for reducing the impact of other digestive side effects will help with diarrhea as well. For example, consuming small amounts of food several times throughout the day will aid the intestines in digestion and absorption without overloading the system. Further, these foods should be low in fiber and easily digestible to avoid unnecessary irritation to the intestinal lining.

These foods might include bananas and other soft fruits rich in potassium, well-cooked fish and chicken or turkey without the skin, creamed cereals and stewed vegetables. Dairy products, such as eggs and yogurt, may be consumed unless, of course, they appear to make the patient's condition worse, a phenomenon that's not uncommon. Above all, however, one should avoid high fiber foods that are difficult to digest and can cause intestinal discomfort.[79]

Remember, the last thing a patient with severe diarrhea wants to do is add bulk to the digestive tract that will only increase one's need for elimination. This isn't a time when the bowels need encouragement to do their job. Accordingly, high fiber raw fruits and vegetables, whole grains and once again, snacks including chips, nuts or popcorn should be removed from one's diet during this time. Similarly, other foods that can cause diarrhea and cramping such as spicy or greasy foods should be avoided as well as sugar, caffeine and alcohol.

If in spite of these efforts, however, diarrhea persists, one's physician may suggest a temporary clear liquid diet in an attempt to regain digestive equilibrium. In addition, patients also need to drink adequate nutrient filled fluids to compensate for those lost as a result of the diarrhea. These might include water, broths or a variety of sports drinks formulated to replace the body's store of minerals and vitamins. It's advisable to avoid carbonated drinks, however, as these can cause gas and cramping that may only make matters worse and create more discomfort for the patient. Once again, it's important to chew foods well to reduce the workload for the intestines, as well as the stomach, and foods and liquids should be consumed slowly and at room temperature.[80]

Bathroom Habits

Finding the right diet during chemotherapy is an individual process that must be explored by each patient in concert with her or his physician. One must wrestle the octopus and juggle the pros and cons of each food and the effect it will have on the different body parts and stages of digestion. Until this delicate balance is achieved, however, each individual will be challenged to find and maintain a level of comfort in which daily life can be lived. For in addition to dietary issues, severe diarrhea can create other physical problems that require special attention.

For instance, the tissue around the anus can become irritated as a result of frequent elimination and cleansing. The first thing one can do to ease this problem is to use the softest toilet paper available. The paper also should be unscented, white and free from dyes. Now some paper tissues, including many "baby wipes" contain moisturizing products such as aloe. It might be better, however, to use those that are free from such products so be sure to check with your physician first. Irritation can be kept at a minimum simply by dipping the plain tissue in water, lukewarm, if possible, before patting the anal skin gently. Most toilets are within an arm's length of a sink, which makes this a fairly easy thing to do. If one isn't able to reach the faucet from the toilet, however, it's helpful to place a small plastic bowl of water on the toilet tank or on the floor for easy access.

By moisturizing the tissue in this way every time before touching the anal area, painful and irritated skin can be kept to a minimum and thorough cleansing can be insured. It also may be helpful to apply a gentle lotion or cream to the area such as those prescribed for diaper rash in infants. Again, this should be done only after consulting one's physician as some medicated products may actually burn sensitive skin and others may increase the risk of infection. Chemotherapy patients already are at an increased risk for developing infections, and products such as petroleum jellies, for example, that don't allow the skin to breathe may actually increase this risk.[81]

In addition to irritated skin, however, diarrhea also can lead to other problems of the anal area, including hemorrhoids. Hemorrhoids are enlarged internal or external blood veins in the rectum that can be quite painful. While they often are caused by constipation and straining during elimination, they also can be caused by the increased pressure on the veins that results from intense diarrhea. If and when this type of problem occurs, expert medical advice can always guide one to the proper care and treatment.[82] Further, during episodes of severe diarrhea the bowels are tender and unpredictable, and their movement can create explosive results. Accordingly, out of respect for others, and to avoid personal embarrassment, it's always a good idea to flush twice during this time.

Days and Nights

Digestive distress and severe diarrhea also may necessitate other changes in a patient's life. When the intestinal tract becomes extremely irritated, the tissues can become swollen and bloated. If this happens, the intestines can create pressure on surrounding organs and tissues as well. As a result, the patient may feel discomfort and may lose her or his ability to control other organs such as the bladder. One may not even be able to feel when the bladder is full. Indeed, it's not uncommon for the bladder to empty unexpectedly as the patient stands, walks or sits.

This lack of control is known as **incontinence**, a condition that applies to either the bowels or the bladder.[83] Whether this condition is severe or not, it can greatly impair one's ability to live a normal life. Running simple errands, going to work and engaging in any public situation carries the risk of having an accident. It's a good idea, therefore, for patients experiencing this distress to avail themselves of any number of incontinence products on the market today. Often called adult diapers, these products exist for a reason and they are used by a surprising number of individuals in a variety of circumstances.

In spite of their unfortunate image, most of these products are comfortable to wear, undetectable in use and compact enough to fit in one's bag or briefcase. They offer physical protection from unwelcome surprises and provide an increased level of psychological confidence and security. One disadvantage that may be experienced when using these products, however, might be skin irritations or rashes, and chafing. This may be particularly true for those taking diuretics in an effort to relieve the edema and swelling sometimes associated with chemotherapy. Diuretics, of course, force the body to expel excess liquids. This can create a situation in which one constantly needs to urinate, and when this is combined with incontinence, even these products will be constantly wet. It's important, therefore, to change them as often as possible.

In the alternative, some men in this situation may prefer to use an **external** or **condom catheter** rather than a diaper product. Similar to a condom, this device is a plastic "glove" that fits over the penis. A tube connects the end of the condom with a small plastic bottle that can be attached to one's belt or hidden in one's pocket. In this way, the urine collects in the bottle, which is periodically emptied, and one's clothing remains dry and unsoiled.[84]

In addition to these daytime concerns, however, one affected by severe diarrhea and/or nausea also may have great difficulty getting through the night. When these side effects are severe, one may need to make numerous trips to the bathroom every night. The simple act of running back and forth from the bedroom to the bathroom can be very debilitating. It expends energy the patient typically doesn't have and robs her or him of the essential rest necessary for healing.

Accordingly, it may be helpful to place a "doggie bed" in the bathroom during the most difficult nights. Specifically made for pets, these usually are well padded, cotton or natural fiber beds that come in a variety of shapes and sizes. They can be squeezed into the smallest of spaces and can provide a comfortable place for one to rest. Sleeping in the bathroom in this way will provide immediate access to the toilet and sink, conserve one's energy and eliminate the need to run between rooms all night. Paired with a blanket or pillow, a doggie bed in the bathroom can be the perfect solution for treatment patients already weak from diarrhea, nausea, and fatigue.

The Flip Side

There are, of course, medications that can help relieve severe diarrhea. One must be careful using these products, however, because while they may stop the diarrhea, they may create our second problem, constipation. Once again, the intestinal tract at this time is sensitive and what is known as the "usual dosage" for these medications may not apply. The body may react to the drug only after a substantial dose, or it may over-react to a small dose that may completely stop peristalsis. Moreover, some chemotherapy drugs cause constipation in and of themselves.[85]

As anyone knows who has experienced constipation, this condition can be as uncomfortable and difficult as the diarrhea. It also is important to remember that during bouts of diarrhea, one's intake of fiber usually has decreased or ceased completely, and one is probably not spending a great deal of time exercising, two conditions that contribute to constipation. Of course, adding more fiber to one's diet and drinking warm or hot fluids may help relieve the symptoms of constipation. Yet, doing so may only increase other discomforts one is already experiencing such as mucositis, stomach upset or nausea, as well as the initial diarrhea one is trying to treat.

Further, it's not advisable to use other products such as laxatives, stool softeners, enemas or suppositories without consulting one's physician as these may irritate the sensitive anal tissue. Like many situations one faces in cancer treatments, this is another delicate balancing act that may require a careful process of trial and error before a satisfactory result is found.

The Bone Marrow and Blood Cells

Anemia–Red Blood Cells

One of the most debilitating side effects of chemotherapy, however, may be the extreme fatigue, or **anemia,** that often accompanies it. When this occurs, the ability to live normally and simply get through each day in typical fashion becomes a luxury of the past. As the fast growing red blood cells within the bone marrow are attacked by the anticancer drugs of chemotherapy, their numbers decrease. This decrease means that there are fewer cells to carry oxygen to other parts of the body.[86]

When the body tissues are starved for oxygen they cannot perform their functions properly. The muscles of the body become weak, making simple movements and everyday tasks difficult. The compromised lungs create a shortness of breath and an inability to breathe deeply. In addition, it appears that this loss of oxygen may affect the brain tissue and result in dizziness, memory loss, confusion, depression and an inability to process information efficiently. It is believed, however, that this condition, affectionately known as **chemo-brain**, also may be the result of toxins produced by some of the drugs in certain chemotherapy treatments.[87]

Until recently, it was believed that the brain was immune to the toxicity of chemotherapy because it was protected from invading large molecules in the bloodstream by a layer of cells known as the "blood brain barrier," a highly specialized network of tiny blood vessel cells. Apparently, however, certain chemotherapy drugs can penetrate that barrier, an occurrence that may help create or aggravate this condition. Fortunately, in most cases chemobrain will dissipate once chemotherapy is completed. In other cases, however, it's possible for the condition to continue long after treatment is completed, which means it may take several years before an individual fully regains her or his pre-cancer cognitive abilities.[88]

Clearly, it's important to monitor a patient's red blood cell count on a regular basis throughout treatment. This is accomplished by a simple test in which blood is withdrawn from one's arm. A needle is inserted into a vein while the technician fills a number of different vials. Each vial will be examined in the laboratory to determine several things, one being the patient's red blood count. In some cases, if the patient experiences great difficulty with anemia and the red cell count has fallen to an unacceptable level, one's physician may prescribe a medication known as **erythropoietin**. This is actually a hormone typically synthesized in the kidneys and used to increase the oxygen carrying capacity of the blood.[89]

In rare cases, a severe problem with anemia may necessitate a blood transfusion for the patient. In most cases, however, the patient simply is advised to make small changes in her or his everyday life. Once again, this requires little more than common sense to implement and may include limiting one's activities during the day and resting whenever possible, recruiting help with daily chores, eating properly and drinking plenty of fluids.

Infection–White Blood Cells

As mentioned, the white cells produced by the bone marrow also are affected by many anticancer drugs used in chemotherapy. As their quantity and quality are compromised, the body's ability to fight infection is diminished. While an infection may occur in any part of the body, most begin from bacteria found on the skin or in the mouth, intestines and genital tract.[90]

As it turns out, these areas also are composed of fast growing cells and are vulnerable to the anticancer drugs of chemotherapy. Accordingly, by following the recommended guidelines for maintaining the health of these tissues, including the hair, nails, mouth, intestines and anal area, one can greatly reduce the potential for these tissues to develop chemotherapy-related infections.

Dos and Don'ts

Unfortunately, infections aren't limited to these areas. It's important, therefore, to adhere to a specific program that may help reduce the occurrence of any infection during chemotherapy. Above all, one needs to stay clean. Hands must be washed several times during the day and always right before eating, and a warm bath or shower is a daily necessity that should be followed with a gentle skin oil or moisturizer. Small scratches and scrapes should be cleaned immediately and regularly with soap, water and a mild antiseptic, and blemishes should be allowed to heal naturally without interference. If blemishes are excessive, always consult a physician before using any medicated soap or medication for severe skin problems.

Both men and women may want to reduce the possibility of cuts and nicks by using electric shavers during this time rather than razors. It also is advisable to avoid, if possible, any situation in which bacteria can be spread such as changing diapers or litter boxes, cleaning standing water out of bird baths or fish tanks, and eating raw seafood, meat or eggs. Similarly, one with a low white blood cell count should avoid contact with individuals who recently have received a "live virus" vaccine, including those for chicken pox and oral polio as chemotherapy patients may contract the virus.[91]

Of course, one should avoid contact with individuals who have any illness considered to be contagious. The white cell count also is monitored by regular blood tests, and if one's count becomes unacceptably low, one's physician may suggest medication to improve the situation. These medications, known as **colony stimulating factors,** are growth factors that help the white cells reproduce and counteract the effect of the chemotherapy anticancer drugs. By raising the white cell count in this way, the risk for further infection is greatly reduced.[92]

Clotting Problems–Platelets

The bone marrow also is responsible for producing platelets that are the smallest cells in the blood. And, anticancer drugs can significantly impair their production. Platelets are disc-shaped cells, and while they contain no hemoglobin like red cells, they're essential for the coagulation of blood. When their numbers are reduced during chemotherapy, the blood's ability to clot properly is compromised.

Accordingly, one may bruise more easily, bleed more easily and heal from minor injuries more slowly. The platelet count also will be monitored on a regular basis through blood tests and if it falls too low, a platelet transfusion may be recommended to increase the count. In most cases, however, colony-stimulating factors are the typical remedy prescribed to increase the platelet count and hopefully avoid some of the above problems.[93]

A Few More Things

Nerves and Muscles

We already know that when the brain is deprived of oxygen-carrying red blood cells, one's ability to think clearly and process information may be impaired. Unfortunately, for reasons that aren't clear, additional parts of the central nervous system also may be affected by chemotherapy. For example, a patient may develop **peripheral neuropathy**, a condition in which the nerves that connect to the central nervous system become damaged or inflamed. This may result in muscle weakness as well as numbness, tingling or pain in the limbs, hands or feet depending upon the nerves that are affected. One also may develop tenderness or soreness in the muscles similar to the aches and pains of a typical flu.[94]

Unfortunately, these side effects can be slow to dissipate and may continue long after one's treatment has ended. Until they do subside, however, one should move carefully, exercise caution in handling objects that might be dangerous, such as hot pans or sharp knives, use handrails and canes when possible and consult with one's physician if the discomfort becomes severe. In addition, some extremely potent anticancer drugs may affect the large muscles of the heart and lungs and significantly inhibit their ability to function properly.[95] As always, any change in one's body or ability to function must be communicated to one's physician immediately so that the condition can be monitored and corrected.

Bladder and Kidneys

Chemotherapy also may affect the bladder and kidneys in a variety of ways depending upon the anticancer drugs used. Some of these drugs may change the color of one's urine to red or green or produce a strong metallic or medicinal odor in the urine. Such side effects, however, are harmless and mild as well as temporary in nature. Unfortunately, other anticancer drugs are known to cause more severe side effects to these organs.[96]

These may include an inability to feel when the bladder is full or an inability to empty the bladder completely while urinating. Some drugs may create muscle weakness resulting in incontinence or damage to the kidneys that renders them incapable of fully performing their function of filtering the blood and eliminating waste. While these effects also may be temporary, particularly potent anticancer drugs may cause damage that's long-term or even permanent. In addition, it isn't uncommon for patients undergoing chemotherapy to retain fluid and gain weight. The combination of a compromised bladder or kidneys, the anticancer drugs, hormonal and other body changes due to the therapy may contribute to this condition.[97]

Accordingly, one may need to eliminate salt from her or his diet and in some cases, may need to use a prescribed diuretic. Once again, the potential for developing any of these side effects from chemotherapy may largely be determined by analyzing the contents of one's chemo-cocktail with one's physician. In any event, fluid retention not withstanding, it's vitally important to drink plenty of water and other appropriate fluids during treatment. For even small amounts of fluid taken continuously throughout the day will help cleanse the body of toxins, flush the anticancer drugs from the bladder and kidneys and encourage their proper functioning.

Sun Sensitivity

The skin is another organ composed of fast growing cells and as such it, too, is extremely vulnerable to the effects of chemotherapy. During treatment, the skin may react to the anticancer drugs by becoming extremely dry and flaky. It may become irritated easily and develop rashes or changes in pigmentation. It also may become sensitive to sunlight and as such will require special care during treatment.[98]

This care once again will be dictated by common sense and should include all the recommendations for skin protection already mentioned in the section on solar radiation. These include the avoidance of strong sunlight, the use of protective clothing such as hats, long sleeves and sunglasses, and always the application of a good sunscreen. Of course, every chemotherapy patient, regardless of skin color, should follow these recommendations to insure healthy skin and reduce potential problems that may occur as a result of the treatment.

Weight Fluctuation

Either directly or indirectly, chemotherapy may contribute to weight loss or weight gain. Weight loss may be related to several of the other side effects we've discussed, including poor appetite, nausea, vomiting or diarrhea and dehydration. If weight loss should become significant one's physician will suggest ways in which one can increase her or his caloric and/or protein intake. Antinausea and antidiarrheal medications may be prescribed, and one may consult a nutritionist who can help tailor a diet more palatable to the individual's taste.

On the other hand, chemotherapy can result in unusual weight gain. This may occur indirectly as the result of one's decreased physical activity and exercise during treatment. It also may be the direct result of the specific drugs contained within one's chemo-cocktail as some actually increase one's appetite and others increase fluid retention or edema within the body. Some chemotherapies also contain steroids, which can increase the body's fatty tissues and create bloating and fullness in the face.[99]

Taking these possibilities one at a time, therefore, individuals undergoing chemotherapy should, if possible, maintain their optimal level of physical activity and exercise when tolerable. Once again, a nutritionist can help one with an increased appetite by modifying one's diet to decrease high caloric foods and increase healthy, low calorie alternatives. Fluid retention can be decreased as well through diet modification and the reduction of one's salt intake.

Further, one should avoid standing for long periods of time and elevate one's feet as often as possible. When sitting, one shouldn't cross her or his legs and one should avoid wearing tight clothing except for medically prescribed stockings or hosiery which often are recommended for severe leg swelling. And, if the weight gain is due to long-term chemotherapy related steroid use, one's physician may prescribe a diuretic to control the weight gain, although, this condition typically will dissipate naturally when the treatment is discontinued.

Apart from these possibilities related to chemotherapy, however, weight gain also may occur in specific body areas when lymph nodes in the area have been removed during surgery. These nodes aid in proper drainage of the tissues, and when they're removed from areas such as the abdomen, the surrounding area may become bloated due to fluid build up. Unfortunately, apart from maintaining a proper diet and exercising, there is little one can do to alleviate this type of localized weight gain.[100]

Radiation Therapy

In addition to chemotherapy, radiation therapy is one of the most widely used and commonly known cancer treatments. Indeed, at least half of all cancer patients will undergo radiation therapy either as a lone treatment or in combination with other therapies. Known by several names including radiotherapy, x-ray therapy, irradiation and cobalt treatment, radiation therapy uses directed high-energy radiation to destroy or damage cancer cells.

Unlike chemotherapy, which is a systemic treatment, radiation therapy is a localized treatment that only affects cancer cells in a specified area. It also is a versatile treatment that may be used in a number of different situations. For example, it may be used alone when surgery isn't feasible, or to treat small tumors that might be found in the lymph nodes or vocal cords. It also may be the only treatment used to treat the early stages of certain cancers such as those of the prostate or rectum.[101]

Radiation therapy may be used before surgery to shrink tumors, or after surgery to stop the growth of any cancer cells that might remain in the area. In **intraoperative radiation** the therapy is used in conjunction with surgery where the radiation is given directly to the affected area after the tumor is removed and before the incision is closed. Even in cases where the cancer has metastasized, the ability of radiation to shrink tumors, known as **palliative care** or **palliation**, can result in less pressure or pain for the patient, and also may stop certain tumors from bleeding.[102]

Radiation therapy can be administered to a patient in one of two ways known simply as **external radiation** and **internal radiation**. The first and most common of these is external radiation, which utilizes a machine to direct high-energy radiation rays directly to the affected body area. These machines include a variety of designs that all operate and work in different ways. For example, some are used to treat cancers located near the surface of the skin while others are used to treat cancers located deeper in the body tissues.[103]

Most of these machines, however, are similar in that they utilize the radioactive isotope known as cobalt to produce high-energy electromagnetic waves such as x-rays or gamma rays. In contrast, other machines work by producing beams of electron, proton or neutron particles. The most common of these machines, however, is known as a **linear accelerator**, which is effective for a variety of different cancers, located in a variety of body tissues. Yet, the final choice of machine will depend upon the type of cancer one has and how far into the body the radiation must penetrate.[104]

External Radiation

Before external radiation can be administered, the patient must undergo a process called **simulation** in which the area to be irradiated is mapped on the body. To do this, the patient must lie on an examination table while a special x-ray machine pinpoints the target area. This area is called the **field of radiation,** or the **treatment port**. In some cases, the patient will have only one field to which the radiation will be aimed. In others, depending upon the location of the cancer, more than one field may be defined. This might occur, for example, if one has a malignancy deep within the abdominal cavity where the area may be best targeted from two or three different angles.[105]

Simulation also may include the use of imaging procedures such as CT scans to properly identify the precise area to receive the treatment. At this time, the radiation therapist or technician will mark the field on the patient's skin with small tattoos drawn with dots of permanent ink. These tattoos literally "mark the spot" and will insure that the radiation beam is directed to the same area with each treatment. Once the field has been fully defined and tattooed, an **immobilization device** may then be designed for the patient. This is simply a tool that insures the patient will remain still during treatment and typically is in the form of a body mold or frame fitted to the individual.[106]

During simulation, it's helpful for the patient to remember that she or he will only be clothed in a hospital gown and that rooms used for any type of x-ray procedure can be quite cold. Also, the machine can be very large, its movement very noisy and the treatment room lighting very low. The patient is left alone for most of the process and, as a result, the overall atmosphere during this time can be quite uncomfortable and intimidating.

Moreover, by the time many patients are ready for radiation therapy they're already recovering from surgery and/or chemotherapy. Indeed, many patients undergo chemotherapy and radiation treatments over the same period of time. Many, therefore, are already battling side effects from other treatments such as nausea and diarrhea. In these cases, it can be extremely difficult for one to remain immobile on a cold table for the required length of time while one technician fiddles around with one's body and others watch through a window.

In addition, it's often necessary for the technician to touch and place temporary "markers" on sensitive body areas, or slightly within body cavities such as the rectum, before applying permanent tattoo ink. To avoid embarrassment and adding insult to injury, therefore, patients who are experiencing problems like nausea or diarrhea must communicate that fact to the technician in charge. The patient should know where the nearest bathroom is located and should feel comfortable about interrupting the simulation process if necessary. At the least, the patient should request a few extra towels and an empty trash can just in case an accident occurs.

While a good technician may foresee these potential problems and take the appropriate action to make the patient feel secure and comfortable, the patient shouldn't count on it. One should never assume that someone else is going to perceive a problem and take steps to solve it. Primary responsibility for one's comfort in health-related issues must first be acknowledged by the patient, and then communicated to her or his health caregiver.

This entire process of simulation may take one to two hours, and once completed, the patient's dosage of radiation will be determined. This determination will be a combined effort involving one's **radiation oncologist**, a **radiation physicist** and a **dosimetrist**. The first of these is a physician who specializes in treating cancer with radiation, the second is a specialist who insures the machines are working properly and delivering the correct amount of radiation and the third is a specialist who calculates the proper dose of radiation for each patient's treatment.[107]

Typically, external radiation treatments last six to eight weeks and usually take place once a day, Monday through Friday. In this way, radiation therapy is similar to chemotherapy in that both are scheduled to allow the body tissues brief periods of rest between sessions. In the alternative, radiation may be given two or three times a day in smaller doses. Known as **hyperfractionated radiation**, this method is becoming more common as new research indicates it may be more effective than single daily doses and may reduce the risk for long-term side effects resulting from the radiation.[108]

In any event, the routine for receiving external radiation remains the same regardless of the dosage or the number of sessions per day. First, to maintain the integrity of the treatment, it's important to avoid the use of lotions, deodorants, perfumes and any other product on the area of the body to be treated. Depending upon the area of the body, the patient may be required to wear a hospital gown or robe during the session. For this reason, it's helpful to wear clothing easy to remove and shoes that slip off. Indeed, even if one isn't required to disrobe, it's important to be comfortable during each session, which typically lasts for about thirty minutes.

Once in the treatment room, the patient will be instructed to lie on a treatment table or sit in a special chair. Then, using the patient's previously made tattoos and body molds, the radiation therapist will position the patient correctly on the table or chair. At this time, additional special radiation shields may be placed on or around certain parts of the patient's body to protect healthy organs and tissues from unwanted radiation exposure. When these steps are completed, the patient will be left alone in the treatment room.

The patient will be monitored, however, on a television screen or through a window in an adjoining control room. While operating the radiation machine from this control room, the attending physicians also will be able to communication with the patient through an intercom. The only other sound in the treatment room will be the rumbling noise produced by the radiation machine as it's positioned and moved around the patient.

While this can be a slightly strange and unsettling experience, one needs to remember that the physicians are controlling the situation. The machine, which is under constant surveillance to insure proper performance, may be stopped at any time, and concern voiced by the patient will be heard and responded to immediately. Even though the entire session may take half an hour, the patient only receives radiation for a few minutes, and when the procedure is completed, the patient is free to go home.

Internal Radiation

The second method of treatment known as internal radiation places the radiation source within the cancerous tissue rather than using beams from a machine to irradiate the tissue. In this method, the radioactive material itself may be **cesium**. This is a substance that produces gamma rays and has recently replaced radium in this type of application. It also may use metallic elements such as **iridium** and **palladium**, nonmetallic chemical elements such as **phosphorus** or the radioisotopes of the nonmetallic element **iodine**.[109]

In any case, the material is sealed within a catheter, a tube or a thin wire and then surgically planted within the affected tissue. Medical experts refer to this general method of internal radiation as **brachytherapy** although there are different ways to place internal radiation sources and each method is known by a different name. For example, when an implant is placed directly into the tumor the procedure is called **interstitial radiation**. This process uses a catheter, capsule or seed to hold the radioactive material in place as it's gradually dispensed into the tissue. If the material is held within a small container and placed inside a body cavity such as the uterus or testicle the treatment is called **intracavity radiation**.[110]

Similarly, **intraluminal radiation** places the container of radioactive material within a body passage such as the esophagus and simple **surface brachytherapy** is a procedure in which the material is placed against an existing tumor. And, if a patient undergoes **remote brachytherapy**, a computer is used to guide the radioactive material into a catheter, which is placed near the malignancy. The radiation specialists then view the procedure and the patient on a closed circuit screen and communicate with her or him via an intercom.[111]

In addition, internal radiation may be given by injecting the radioactive material directly into the bloodstream or a body cavity in a process known as **unsealed internal radiation therapy**. Regardless of the method of internal radiation application, however, most patients will need to be hospitalized for the procedure and will receive a local or general anesthesia depending upon the placement required.[112]

In all forms of internal radiation, however, the implant will either be temporary or permanent. This determination will depend upon how much radiation is needed to fight the cancer and how long the process will take. Of course, these issues depend upon the many factors we've already discussed such as the type of cancer, the location of the tumor, the stage and grade of the tumor, and the patient's age and overall health. If the implant is temporary, it will be either a **low dose-rate,** or **LDR,** implant or a **high dose-rate,** or **HDR,** implant. Typically, a low dose-rate implant will be left in place for several days or weeks while a high dose-rate implant will be removed within a matter of minutes. In any case, removal of a temporary implant is a fairly simple procedure usually done in the patient's hospital room without the use of an anesthetic.[113]

On the other hand, if the implant is permanent, the patient typically will be confined to a hospital room for the first few days following implantation. This may be required because the radioactive material is extremely potent in the first few days of treatment, and it's important to observe the patient as well as protect others from its adverse effects. The level of radioactivity, however, decreases each day and eventually the patient will be released from confinement and allowed to return home. Over time, the implant will gradually dispense the radiation throughout the affected tissue. Eventually, the implant will lose its radioactive properties yet the vehicle for implanting the material, be it a capsule or seed, will remain within the patient's body.

Personal Note

Over the last ten years I've encountered numerous individuals who either had a direct experience with radiation therapy or had a friend or family member who did. I've heard story after story about the problems these individuals, or their loved ones, experienced. Terrible body sores. Ongoing pain. One doctor insisted that his eighty-year-old wife had survived colon cancer and chemotherapy only to die from the radiation therapy.

In every instance, these individuals were under the impression that in their particular case, something unusual had occurred. They thought their stories were rare and exceptional. They surmised the equipment wasn't working properly, the technician was inexperienced, the dosage was incorrect, and so on and so on. What I came to realize, of course, was that these stories weren't unusual. They weren't exceptions to the rule at all, but indeed appeared to be the rule. They were typical accounts commonly reported by the majority of radiation patients.

Proceed with Great Caution

As discussed, radiation therapy, alone or in combination with other therapies, is one of the most common of all cancer treatments. Now that we understand how radiation therapy is delivered, however, it's vitally important to review what it is. First, radiation therapy utilizes ionizing radiation created from a radioactive source. "Ionization" is the process in which a neutral atom or molecule gains or loses electrons and acquires a positive or negative electrical charge.[114] This means that the process of ionization actually alters matter on an atomic or molecular level, a process that also can result in cell death and cell mutation.

"Radiation" is the emission of ionizing energy in the form of waves, rays or beams from a radioactive source. Relatedly, "radioactive" refers to any material that emits such energy as atomic nuclei within the material disintegrate. Ionizing radiation, therefore, is a radioactive source of energy that has the ability to destroy or mutate the cells of living tissue or any other matter through which it's directed.[115] Accordingly, radiation therapy is a potent, deadly and irreversible treatment that must be considered carefully by every cancer patient before submitting to its use.

We already have discussed the nature of chemotherapy and its potential for creating uncomfortable and even painful side effects. Yet, most of these unwanted conditions will dissipate either when the chemotherapy is completed or shortly thereafter. The anticancer drugs will eventually be flushed from the body and the experience, although far from pleasant, is temporary. Above all, when chemotherapy is administered properly, it won't kill you. Radiation, on the other hand, can.

Remember we're dealing with energy produced from a radioactive source. Radioactivity is lethal for human beings, and societies throughout time have gone to great lengths to protect themselves from exposure. The harm that can result from radiation is well documented, and the fact that radiation constitutes one of the greatest risks for cancer development is without question. Why then, many would wonder, do we use radiation therapy as a form of cancer treatment? The answer to this question, of course, is that this therapy has the ability to change cells on a fundamental level. As such, radiation therapy can destroy or alter cancer cells and interfere with their ability to multiply and divide. In doing so, the cancerous tumor can be destroyed or reduced in size.

This is a remarkable feat, and many devoted and well-meaning specialists spend their professional lives administering this treatment to patients with cancer as well as other diseases and illnesses. Over the decades the process of giving and receiving radiation for cancer treatment has been refined and improved, and the process today is one that modern technology has made as safe as it knows how. And this, of course, is the problem.

Throughout the last century medical procedures have utilized radiation as a source of healing only to discover years later the harm created by these procedures. We still don't fully comprehend the nature and power of therapeutic radioactivity and its long-term effects upon the human body. Moreover, the method of directing the radiation to the affected body area, while it's the best we can do, remains clumsy and imprecise. At this time, it simply isn't possible to target only the diseased cells. Many cells in the surrounding tissues will be affected by the radiation as well. And, depending upon the location of the tumor, the ray may have to penetrate many layers of tissues and organs in order to hit the target area.

As the rays of radiation move through the body the matter in their path is caused to dissociate, or split, into ions. The distribution or extent of this ionization effect will, of course, depend upon the type of radiation being used and its penetrating power, the location of the radioactive source, and the nature of the material being irradiated. The level of cellular damage also will depend upon the stage of cell division at the time of exposure, the time span of the exposure and, of course, the strength and intensity of the particular rays.[116]

The electromagnetic high-energy waves of ionizing radiation such as x-rays and gamma rays, for example, penetrate matter deeply while ionizing radiation that dispenses particles such as alpha and beta particles only penetrates a few millimeters or a fraction of a millimeter respectively. All types, however, produce intense ionization along their paths that directly affects the living organisms with which they come into contact. The result is radiation that kills cells, retards their development and creates chromosomal anomalies and gene mutations.[117]

Clearly, the cells of the human body are extremely vulnerable to this effect. Indeed, tissues whose chemical composition contains elements with relatively high atomic weights are the most vulnerable. One of these elements is calcium and, therefore, tissues such as teeth and bones will be much more susceptible to ionization and will absorb greater amounts of radiation than the softer tissues of the body.

To further illuminate the extreme nature of radiation, let us examine the guidelines for hospital personnel in therapeutic settings whose job it is to care for patients undergoing the treatment. First, it's common knowledge that certain precautions must be taken when utilizing radiation in any form. Indeed, **radiation hygiene** is a term that refers to the art and science of protecting human beings from the adverse effects of radiation exposure.[118] Simple dental or medical x-rays, mammograms and CT scans are among the safest therapeutic uses of radiation and yet, even these procedures sometimes require the patient to wear protective shielding and always require technical personnel to vacate the room.

It's important to distinguish these forms of exposure, however, from the exposure one receives in radiation therapy. For the above x-ray procedures are used only to gain visual information for diagnostic purposes and the minimal risk they may present is greatly outweighed by the benefit they provide. Radiation therapy, on the other hand, harnesses the destructive properties of radiation and is used intentionally to target and destroy body cells.

Keeping this in mind, let's review the procedures for delivering external radiation treatment. As we know, this form of therapy utilizes a machine and is conducted in a specialized, temperature-controlled treatment room. When the machine is in use and is projecting a beam of radiation, the room is tightly sealed and the patient is left alone. All personnel including the radiologist and the radiation therapist conduct the procedure by remote control, observe through a window or on a monitor and communicate with the patient using an intercom. At no time does anyone enter the room until the treatment is concluded and the machine is turned off. The treatment is conducted in an extremely controlled and protected environment under close supervision and scrutiny.[119]

With internal radiation, the precautions for insuring safety are even more pronounced. When a patient receives an implant, the radiation not only affects tissues within the patient, it emits high-energy rays that travel outside the patient as well. Accordingly, implant patients are placed in private hospital rooms after the procedure is completed. The nurses and other care staff members are limited as to the amount of time they can spend in the patient's room. When in the room, they will work quickly and will communicate with the patient from the doorway or from outside the room whenever possible.[120]

Similarly, visitors will be given special instructions regarding safety procedures. Some, including children younger than eighteen and women who are pregnant, typically won't be allowed to visit the patient at all. Depending upon the dose of the implant, be it low dose or high dose, some visitors may be allowed to stay in the patient's room for a few hours while others may be limited to visits of half an hour or less.

Most will be advised to sit at least six feet from the patient and in some cases, a large lead shield will be placed beside the patient's bed to form a barrier between the patient and any visitor or hospital personnel. No one touches the patient, no one comes near the patient, and those who are allowed inside the room don't stay long. Clearly, everything possible is done to protect individuals from exposure to the adverse effects of the patient's radioactive implant.[121]

Further, in cases where the patient has received an injection of radioactive material through unsealed internal radiation therapy, one's body wastes, which now are radioactive, will be carefully collected and disposed. If such measures are taken to protect those around the patient from potential radiation damage, imagine for a moment what is taking place inside the patient. A radioactive implant is lying within the vulnerable tissues of her or his body, with every cell in the area absorbing radiation and dying or mutating as a result of the ionization process. The destruction of cancer cells is, of course, the goal of radiation therapy. Our concern, however, is for the healthy cells of the body destroyed or mutated in the process, as this will determine the extent and severity of radiation side effects. Many of the side effects associated with radiation therapy are the same ones associated with chemotherapy. Among these, alopecia, mouth and digestive tract disorders, fatigue and skin changes are the most common.[122]

Radiation, however, is a localized treatment and accordingly most of the side effects resulting from its use will be localized as well. Hair loss, for example, typically will occur only in the area of the body being treated. Mucositis and dry mouth normally will occur only if the patient's head and neck area have been treated. Similarly, problems with nausea, diarrhea, constipation, bladder irritation, general digestive distress and reproduction will result from treatment to the pelvic or abdominal area. The exceptions to this rule are fatigue and skin changes that can occur anywhere regardless of which body area is irradiated.[123]

In addition, the side effects from radiation can be acute in that they occur shortly after treatment begins and usually dissipate shortly after treatment ends. Others, however, can be chronic and as such, they may take several months or even years after the treatment is concluded to appear. These are particularly troublesome as these side effects can be significant in nature and permanent in duration. Indeed, many of the damaging and long-term side effects common to radiation therapy are so well documented that they're listed by name within the major dictionaries of the world.[124]

Localized Side Effects

The easiest way to catalogue the potential side effects from radiation therapy is to move through the major body parts and describe the effects most commonly associated with each. Starting at the top, radiation directed to cancers of the head and neck may result in alopecia. This condition may be temporary in duration or permanent, yet it's typically acute and occurs shortly after treatment begins. Once again, hair loss and hair regrowth will depend upon the type and the amount of radiation that the patient receives.

Radiation to this area of the body also may cause mucositis or dryness of the mouth and throat. One's sense of taste and smell may change, nausea may become common, and earaches may develop as the radiation causes the earwax within the ear canal to harden. Remember also that tissues high in calcium such as bones and teeth absorb more radiation. As a result, one's neck may become stiff and sore as well as one's jaw, a condition that may contribute to difficulties with chewing and swallowing.[125]

One's teeth also are susceptible to the effects of radiation and a condition known as **radiation caries** may develop. This term refers to tooth decay specifically triggered by directing ionizing radiation to the head. This decay results not only because the calcium rich tissues absorb greater levels of radiation, but because dry mouth, decreased salivation and changes in oral bacteria may occur as well. Treatment to the head also may cause **radiation cataracts**, which develop when the protein molecules within the lens of the eye undergo change as a result of the radiation. Further, the skin in the treated area typically will become red or tan, its texture may change and it may become irritated.[126]

For many of these problematic conditions, the care guidelines outlined in our discussion of chemotherapy side effects will apply here as well. Maintaining comfort and health regarding one's hair and scalp, mouth and throat, oral hygiene and diet basically remain the same. One will have to experiment, of course, to find the combination of suggestions that work best for her or him. And, as always, clear communication about any unusual or uncomfortable condition with one's physician is essential throughout the treatment process.

Radiation treatment to the breast tissue in women with breast cancer is one of the safest applications of this technology and one that quite possibly produces the least localized side effects for the patient. This is so because the breast is composed of soft tissue the chemical composition of which has a relatively low atomic weight. As we know, this means that the tissue will absorb a smaller dose of the radiation and the damaging effect will be less extreme. Further, there are no vital body organs within the breast that lie in the path of the radiation rays.

As a result, the patient's side effects from the therapy may be minimal and localized. Breast and nipple tenderness may occur, and the treated tissue may swell as a result of fluid buildup. The skin may change in color to red or tan, its texture may change and the pores may increase in size. In some cases, small but permanent red areas of dilated blood vessels known as **telangiectasias** may appear on the treated skin. The area also may become irritated and the tissue may become more or less sensitive to touch. Most of these conditions, however, are acute and will dissipate within a few weeks to several months after treatment is completed.[127]

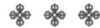

Headline:

Fight Cancer with Tropical Fruit

In its native Malaysia, the *Garcinia mangostana*, or as it's more commonly referred to, the mangosteen, has been called the "queen of tropical fruit." It's well known for the ice cream, juices and jams made from the meat of its particularly sweet, white flesh. It also occupies, however, an important place in the medical traditions of the people of southeast Asia where it has been used to treat infections, stomach and intestinal disorders and some sexually transmitted diseases.

As this headline states, this versatile fruit also is recognized today as a possible treatment for some types of cancer. Indeed, its rich purple peel is loaded with powerful antioxidant compounds known as xanthones. As a result, this is one claim that research may further substantiate and one fruit we should keep our eyes on.[128]

Radiation treatment to the chest area is somewhat more complicated than treatment to the breast. Commonly used in patients with lung cancer, this treatment will create immediate side effects that may include difficulty or pain in swallowing. The patient may experience a shortness of breath and an inability to breathe properly. An increase in mucous of the lung may develop and while this buildup may be kept to a minimum by drinking large amounts of fluids, a cough as well as a fever may develop. Once again, the skin covering the treated area may undergo many changes in color or sensitivity and may develop mild to severe irritation.[129]

Unfortunately, radiation treatment to the chest must penetrate the chest wall and the rib cage before it reaches the target area. As a result, some of these tissues as well as those of the lung also will undergo ionization. While the acute effects of radiation upon the lung and the skin are known, the chronic and long-term effects upon these and the additional tissues in the path of ionization aren't possible to predict.

Radiation therapy to the abdominal or pelvic area of the body is particularly troublesome. This is a major body cavity that encloses several vital organs including the stomach, liver, pancreas, bladder, intestinal tract and all the reproductive organs. These tissues are packed tightly within this cavity and radiation to any one of these organs may result in damage to any of the other surrounding healthy organs as well. Indeed, many of these vital organs and tissues may very well lie directly in the path of the radiation rays.

Treatment for colorectal cancer to the large intestine, for example, may cause ionization in tissues of the bladder and the liver. Treatment for cancer of the prostate may cause damage to the large intestine and the rectum. It simply isn't possible to treat one of these organs without affecting some of the nearby healthy organs in turn. As a result, radiation to this body area can cause all of the digestive disorders we have already discussed, including nausea, diarrhea, constipation and cramping. Affected organs such as the liver, kidneys, bladder or pancreas may lose their ability to function normally. Again, some of this unintended damage may be acute and short lived. That which is chronic, however, may not appear until years after treatment has been completed and unfortunately, may be permanent.[130]

Furthermore, we need to remember that the dense bone tissues of the body absorb more radiation than the soft tissues. When radiation is targeted to the abdominal and pelvic areas the hips become extremely vulnerable and their strength is compromised as they absorb the radiation. This can create or contribute to the condition known as **osteoporosis**, a disorder characterized by the deterioration of bone tissue and the loss of bone density.[131]

This condition increases the risk of bone fractures in older individuals and especially in postmenopausal women whose bodies have stopped producing estrogen. The hipbones are particularly vulnerable to osteoporosis as one ages and, of course, when pelvic radiation is added to the equation a woman's risk for developing the condition is increased. Yet, osteoporosis can occur in males as well, and particularly in those who have undergone any cancer treatment that decreases the production of androgens.

Men who have been treated for prostate cancer in ways that affect the production of male hormones, therefore, may be more likely to develop osteoporosis.[132] In addition, if these patients also have undergone radiation therapy to the pelvic area the likelihood of developing osteoporosis of the hips becomes even greater. Similarly, when radiation targets the arms or legs, the density of the bones may be compromised and, of course, the skin in the treated area may develop a variety of anomalies. Once again, the damage to the reproductive organs from radiation therapy may be significant and as such, this topic will be discussed separately.

A Few More Words About Skin

In all likelihood, every patient who undergoes radiation therapy will experience some change in the skin surrounding the treated area. At the very least, when the skin changes color to red or tan it creates a condition known as **radiation burn**. The skin also may become dry and as a result, it may begin to itch and develop a variety of other minor irritations.[133]

Radiation damage to the skin, however, also may be extreme. The skin may become blistered and develop open sores, a condition that often requires a significant amount of time to heal. Some types of radiation therapy may cause the skin to develop a **moist reaction** where the skin becomes wet and begins to ooze around the treated area.[134] Radiation therapy also can cause a severe inflammation of the skin in a condition known as **radiation dermatitis**. This form of dermatitis may be either acute or chronic and produces redness, blistering and sloughing of the skin in the treated area. Indeed, in the most severe cases this condition can progress to fibrosis and atrophy, and can cause scarring and changes in skin pigmentation.[135]

Accordingly, it's important to maintain proper skin care during the treatment period. This maintenance combines common sense with many of the suggestions mentioned in our section on chemotherapy. For example, the skin should be washed gently with mild soaps and lukewarm water. One should never rub the treated area, but rather should pat the area dry after bathing. Even though the skin may be dry, irritated or blistered, one should refrain from using lotions or creams, ointments, perfumes, deodorants or any other product on the area without consulting first with one's physician.

It also is advisable to avoid using anything that may further irritate the skin, such as heat and cold packs or electric razors. If the area is so badly burned that a bandage is required, one should learn the correct way to bandage the area from one's physician and should never place tape of any kind directly on the burn. Clothing that comes into contact with the area should be soft and loose fitting rather than binding. The area must be protected from the sun with proper clothing and perhaps a sunscreen if approved by one's physician. Finally, the condition of the skin during treatment must be monitored daily and as always, any change or complication must be communicated promptly to one's physician.[136]

Systemic Side Effects

Possibly the most common side effect of radiation therapy is fatigue, a problem that can occur with any type of radiation to any part of the body. This fatigue commonly is experienced in combination with a number of other side effects, which together are often referred to as **radiation sickness** or **radiation malaise**. This condition not only renders the patient severely exhausted physically, it also may produce mental fatigue and a general feeling of discomfort and confusion. It's been compared to severe motion or seasickness, or morning sickness in women.[137]

The cause of fatigue alone isn't clear as it may result from the disease itself or from the treatment. It also may be caused by pain, a lack of sleep, nausea or one's inability to eat properly during treatment. Similar to chemotherapy, however, radiation is known to affect the blood forming tissues of the body. As a result, if the treatment affects the white blood cells, the patient will become more vulnerable to infection. If the treatment affects the platelets the blood's ability to coagulate and clot will be interrupted. And, if the red blood cells are affected the tissues of the body may not receive the necessary oxygen to function properly.[138]

If this is the case, the muscles and tissues of the body may experience oxygen starvation and become sore and weak. This clearly will contribute to fatigue and, in fact, one's blood will be monitored regularly throughout the therapy to insure the patient's blood counts don't fall below an acceptable level. If the levels are found to be too low, the treatment may be changed or interrupted until the counts once again reach a medically acceptable level.

Fatigue is difficult to deal with, as there's no magic formula that will eliminate it completely. Indeed, one may experience days when getting off the couch for a glass of water requires a feat of gigantic proportions. By following the guidelines previously discussed in our section on chemotherapy, however, one can reduce the impact of fatigue on one's life and learn to manage activities on a day-by-day basis.

The Things No One Wants to Talk About

It's clear that radiation therapy has a place in the world's continuing battle against cancer. And in some cases, it can be used to destroy a malignancy without causing great harm to the patient. In other cases, however, the treatment can create medical problems the harmful nature of which may be much greater than the benefit it bestows. We have discussed several of these potential problems and many of them will be acute and temporary. Yet, some will be chronic, and the most sinister aspect of these chronic side effects is that they may not appear for decades after an individual has completed the treatment. These are the problems, the side effects, with which one must be most concerned for these can be severe, debilitating and permanent.

To understand the mechanics of such late side effects it's important to remember that radioactivity isn't a property that disappears when its source disappears. Similarly, the effect of radiation therapy doesn't stop when the machine is turned off or the implant is removed. It takes a long time for radioactivity to dissipate from the atmosphere or from the matter it has permeated.

Indeed, this process of dissipation is so slow that it's measured by a **half-life**, a term that defines the amount of time it takes for the presence of a radioactive element to diminish by fifty percent. Further, the term **effective half-life** specifically refers to the amount of time it takes for a radioactive element within an animal body to diminish by half. A rather complicated mathematical formula is required to determine how much time comprises an effective half-life, but dissipation only occurs as the radioactive element decays and is eliminated through the body's natural biological processes.[139]

Clearly, this may take considerable time to accomplish, and while any trace of radioactive material remains in the body, the tissues of the body remain vulnerable to damage, mutation and deterioration. Tissue damaged during treatment, therefore, may continue to disintegrate for years after treatment is completed and until the radioactivity is eliminated from the body. Eventually the damage will accumulate and present itself in some abnormal physicality forcing the patient to face yet another challenge.

Tissue that's been irradiated, either intentionally or unintentionally, differs fundamentally from normal body tissue in several ways. The cells that comprise the tissue may be mutated and their DNA may be damaged. These cells no longer multiply properly, receive nourishment properly or contribute to the body's health and sustenance effectively. Indeed, irradiated tissue is similar to tissue damaged by tobacco smoke in that it lacks the normal blood flow necessary to keep it healthy.

As a result, this tissue behaves differently from normal tissue and can be unpredictable. For example, it may be slow to heal if injured or it may not heal at all. Skin tissue in the previously treated area may suddenly "flare up" and become irritated, or begin to ooze or bleed. Internal tissues may begin to "break down" and cause difficulties in normal bodily functions.

To illustrate this point, let's discuss the potential damage that can occur when radiation is directed to the abdominal and pelvic area, one of the body's most vulnerable. With such irradiation, permanent kidney damage or permanent bladder cystitis and incontinence may develop. The liver or pancreas may suffer damage, which may render these organs incapable of performing their necessary metabolic and physiological processes. Long-term damage to the intestinal tract may include an inability to digest or eliminate properly which may force the patient to undergo a permanent colostomy.

Damage to the abdominal area also may lead to **tenesmus** in which one experiences persistent, painful, yet ineffectual spasms of the bladder or rectum.[140] **Intestinal tenesmus**, a condition characterized by the unpredictable spasms and painful inflammation commonly associated with irritable bowel syndrome and inflammatory bowel disease, also may occur.[141] Further, damage to the rectal area may result in recurring, permanent **proctitis**, a condition characterized by an extremely painful burning inflammation of the tissues and a repeated urge, yet often inability, to eliminate.[142]

Indeed, the damage that affects tissue unintentionally may occur in one of three ways. We already are familiar with two, the first being damage that occurs to tissues that lie directly in the path of the radiation as it moves through the body to the target area. The second is when tissues that surround the target area are affected by ionization as the effects spread out from the target area. But, there is a third way in which tissue that lies behind or beyond the target area can be damaged unintentionally as well.

In a phenomenon known as **overshooting** the radiation ray penetrates too deeply and passes into and through the target area to "hit" healthy tissue beyond the tumor site.[143] This phenomenon is a risk of radiation therapy regardless of the body area being treated. For example, while radiation to the breast tissue is one of the safest applications of the therapy, it isn't unheard of for the radiation to overshoot unintentionally through the breast tissue and chest wall to strike the lung as well.

The potential dangers of irradiated tissue are clearly recognized by the medical community itself. For example, many surgeons refuse to operate on tissue that has been irradiated due to the unpredictable nature of the tissue. It's hard enough to get healthy tissue to conform to a surgeon's wishes, and the unpredictability of irradiated tissue makes it a poor candidate for any surgery. There is concern that such tissue may not bind properly when sutured and wounds or incisions may not heal properly. Skin grafts taken from another body part may be required to close the wound or incision and yet, there's no guarantee that the irradiated tissue will accept a skin graft. And, of course, if sutures and skin grafts fail, an individual could be left with a large wound that never heals properly.

Some surgeons suggest that patients who have received under fifty grays or 5000 **rads**, **radiation absorbed doses,** may not encounter the same problems with irradiated tissue as those who receive over 5000 rads.[144] Other surgeons, however, refuse categorically to perform unnecessary surgery on any irradiated tissue or body part. This is an important point for patients who undergo cancer surgery and radiation therapy with the intention of having reconstructive surgery in the future. For such future surgeries may not be possible, or at least wise, due to the increased risk of complications. Patients who require necessary surgical procedures to body areas that have been exposed to radiation therapy in the past also may face the same troubling complications.

Additional long-term side effects from this therapy include a condition known as **radiation recall**, a phenomenon that can occur weeks, months and, in rare instances, even years after one has completed radiation therapy. The term refers to a variety of reactions that occur during a patient's radiation treatment and then recur later if and when the patient undergoes certain forms of chemotherapy. In fact, it appears that the chemotherapy anticancer drugs most associated with radiation recall reactions include **dactinomycin, doxorubicin, paclitaxel** or **taxol**, and **methotrexate**. These reactions typically appear in the form of red patches and irritation, or shedding and peeling of skin that was previously irradiated. Such skin also may develop blisters and moist reactions in which the skin becomes wet and begins to ooze.[145]

In addition to these skin reactions, however, one also may develop gastrointestinal and urinary reactions similar to those we've already described. **Radiation pneumonitis**, which is an inflammation of the lung, is yet another form of radiation recall that may occur. Indeed, it's theorized that any body organ that has previously been affected by radiation therapy could be subject to radiation recall and the development of numerous future adverse reactions.[146]

Finally, it's well documented that radiation therapy can lead to the development of future cancers. We know that patients who received radiation for ankylosing spondylitis develop more cancers of the lung, esophagus and bone. Similarly, thyroid cancer has been linked to children who underwent radiation treatment for anomalies of the head and neck. Moreover, radiation therapy can lead to the development of leukemia.[147]

As we know, leukemia is the broad term given to the systemic cancers that are characterized by anomalies of the blood cells and the blood forming tissues of the body. We also know that radiation therapy directly affects these same cells and tissues. In theory, therefore, it is possible that when these particular tissues are exposed to radiation they simply don't recover from the damage. They may remain more vulnerable to the cellular changes that present as leukemia in the future. Again, future cancers are additional long-term chronic side effects of radiation therapy that may take decades to appear.

Clearly, any discomfort a patient may experience during this treatment may be only the beginning of a long, unpredictable and difficult battle. Unfortunately, there's little one can do for many of the side effects resulting from radiation therapy. The recommended guidelines for short-term mouth, digestive tract and skin problems may help to temporarily alleviate one's discomfort in these areas. Yet, relief from chronic problems that affect the internal organs on a long-term or permanent basis may be extremely difficult to manage.

Some patients simply are more vulnerable to the side effects of radiation therapy than others. Known as **outliers**, these individuals experience reactions to radiation that lie outside the typical range, or bell curve, of reactions. Due to genetic factors, physical make-up or unique sensitivities these individuals can experience extreme side effects, which often are brought about by a minimum amount of radiation. Similar to an allergic reaction, side effects experienced by an outlier can be quite sudden and violent, and often require immediate hospitalization and observation. In such cases the treatment may be stopped, or if continued, will most likely be limited in duration and decreased in dosage.

Personal Note

In addition to the chemotherapy I received for my first diagnosis of colon cancer, I was scheduled to receive eight weeks of radiation therapy, one session each week. For the first three weeks I tolerated the treatment fairly well although my skin in the targeted area became significantly burned and terribly painful.

Halfway through the treatment, however, I became extremely ill. I was experiencing internal pain, I couldn't swallow anything, including the pain pills that had been prescribed, and the diarrhea was nonstop. When I collapsed in the hospital during a routine appointment I was admitted to emergency where I stayed for two weeks sustained by intravenous feeding tubes. I learned that the radiation had essentially "burned" the lining of my intestinal tract and I was aware of how close to death I had come.

When I recovered, I was told I was an outlier, the term used to describe an individual who lies outside the normal field of expectation, as one who performs outside the typical bell curve of academia. In this situation, it's a term used by medical practitioners to describe one who experiences an extremely adverse, unusual and even deadly reaction to radiation therapy. Unfortunately, there's no way of knowing if one is an outlier until the adverse, unusual or deadly reactions occur. Needless to say, I never completed the second half of my radiation treatment.

In any event, radiation therapy is a treatment that must be considered very carefully by each individual diagnosed with cancer. There are no hard and fast rules as to whom should receive the treatment and who should not. There appears to be a consensus among the medical community, however, that the younger a patient is, the more useful and necessary radiation may be. Patients in their twenties, thirties or forties, for example, are considered young to develop most types of cancers. In these cases, it is important to give the patient every opportunity and chance for survival as they may continue to live for several more decades. The use of radiation, therefore, is simply another tool to aid the patient in her or his battle with the disease.

In contrast, individuals who are diagnosed with cancer in their seventies or eighties should consider the use of radiation therapy carefully for the following reasons. First, older patients may have less strength and energy than their younger counterparts and their general health may not be as good. They may have additional health problems such as high blood pressure or cholesterol and they may take a variety of medications. Their ability to physically withstand some of the side effects associated with radiation may be compromised.

At the least, depending upon the type of cancer with which one is diagnosed, one's quality of life may suffer considerably and possibly for the remainder of one's years. Certainly when an older individual is diagnosed with a slow growing cancer such as some cancers of the prostate, radiation therapy may result in far more harm than good. Regardless of age, however, every patient must investigate all the benefits and potential risks associated with this therapy and must consult with not just one or two, but several, medical experts before committing to this form of treatment.

The Future of Radiation Therapy

The need for new and safer forms of radiation therapy is clearly recognized by specialists in the field of radiology throughout the world. And, the quest for harnessing the beneficial aspects of radiation while minimizing its risks to the human body continues in earnest. Several new methods of delivering radiation are in development although all may not be widely available. Among these is a technique known as **three dimensional conformal radiation therapy**. In this method a computer simulates an exact image of the tumor and the surrounding body tissues. Multiple radiation beams are then shaped and directed to the contour of the cancerous tissue. It's hoped that the use of such precisely focused beams will save the surrounding healthy tissue from damage.[148]

Similarly, **helical tomotherapy** utilizes high dose radiation sculpted to the exact shape of a tumor and dispensed through hundreds of pencil beams that rotate around the tumor. In another procedure known as **precision therapy** high dose radiation is delivered from several angles to a precise target area. It's similar to hyperfractionated radiation in that it delivers the radiation in fewer fractions, or doses, than conventional radiation therapy.

Several new techniques for irradiating tumors that are particularly difficult to reach, such as those of the head and brain, also are being developed. In **stereotactic radiosurgery** a linear accelerator or gamma rays are used to treat certain types of brain tumors. If a linear accelerator is used, the radiation is delivered in arcing paths around the patient's head. If gamma rays are used, the radiation is delivered in many precisely focused beams in a technique referred to as a **gamma knife**.

In this procedure the patient wears a helmet that focuses the gamma rays and aims them at the tumor from several different directions. This results in treatment that is bloodless, painless and without the typical danger of infection. Similar, but not as widely used, is a technique called the **cyberknife** which utilizes a miniature radiation machine and a robotic arm that delivers small doses of radiation from hundreds of angles while moving around the patient's head. Further, it's not necessary to use a frame to hold the patient's head still during this treatment because a computer adjusts for slight movements the patient may make.

A variation of the cyberknife is the **Peacock system**, which uses computer software to control the intensity of the radiation delivered in small beams as a machine rotates around the patient's head. A device known as a **particle accelerator** is now being used to deliver one massive dose of radiation to the tissue during surgery, which eliminates the need for weeks of special post-surgery hospital visits. Specialists hope that in the future they'll have the ability to remove a cancerous organ, administer radiation to the organ, and then replace it within the body.

The goal of these new techniques, of course, is to improve the effectiveness of radiation therapy in treating tumors while reducing damage to healthy tissues. Each attempts to focus the radiation and improve the precision of the therapy order to reduce the side effects and long-term harm that so many patients experience. And while promising, these techniques are not yet widely available and many will require further refinement before the goal is reached. The bottom line, however, is that medical experts and researchers are aware of the problems associated with radiation therapy and are continuing their efforts to improve the technology and make it safer for all cancer patients.

Personal Note

Fortunately, new options in the field of radiology are becoming available. One of these options is a new form of radiation treatment for small breast cancers known as a mammocyte. First, there are certain criteria that must be met before one qualifies for this form of radiation. The tumor must be singular and small, less than three centimeters. The tumor must be localized with clear margins and lymph nodes. And, once the tumor has been removed, there must be at least one centimeter of breast tissue between the now empty cavity and the chest wall and the skin of the breast.

When these criteria have been met, the mammocyte will be surgically implanted into the breast. Although it's sometimes implanted at the same time the lumpectomy is performed, it's more common for it to be implanted a few days or weeks after the initial surgery. This, of course, is done to allow a full examination of the post-surgery pathology and to make sure the tumor is localized and the mammocyte is the proper form of treatment.

Now, a mammocyte is a small inflatable balloon located on the end of a flexible, hollow rubber tube. The balloon is placed into the space previously occupied by the tumor and is then inflated. The hollow tube, which includes a valve attachment, extends outside the breast approximately four inches. Once the device has been implanted, the patient will undergo a CT scan to insure that the balloon is placed correctly and that the chest wall and skin are properly protected by surrounding tissue.

The radiation therapy itself typically takes five days, with two sessions each day. Each session will begin with a chest x-ray to make sure the balloon is still in the correct place and inflated properly, then the patient will be escorted to a room where she will lie comfortably on a table. A mobile radiation unit will be wheeled to the side of the table and a tube from the machine will be connected to the exposed valve on the patient's mammocyte.

Once this connection is made, a thin wire with a "bullet" of radioactive material at the end travels through the tube, into the valve and lodges in the balloon. This bullet stays in place, typically for five to eight minutes, until it automatically withdraws from the balloon and returns to its "home" in the mobile unit. A technician will then check the patient with a device similar to a Geiger counter to guarantee the bullet has, indeed, returned to its home. And, after the last treatment, the patient's radiologist will simply deflate the balloon, pull it out through the same small incision through which it was implanted, apply a small pressure dressing and send the patient home.

Although the mammocyte has only been in use for about ten years, research indicates that it's an excellent form of radiation treatment for small, localized breast cancers. It only treats the area around the tumor without harming additional, healthy tissue. It poses less risk of radiation exposure to the lung and results in little if any burning to the skin or fatigue. The cosmetic results are far superior to those of traditional beam radiation. Discomfort is minimal, although balloons that must be placed close to the nipple may be more uncomfortable as this area of the breast contains more nerve bundles.

Perhaps most importantly, the treatment is concluded in one week rather than the typical six and a half weeks of beam radiation. As one who previously had experienced the worst of beam radiation, I was thrilled to qualify for a mammocyte, a wonderful new option to traditional radiation treatment.

Special Problems–Reproduction

Where there is no hope, there
can be no endeavor.
Samuel Johnson

It's clear at this point that the difference between cancer that is localized and cancer that has metastasized is enormous. Cancer that has progressed will require much more treatment and follow up care than cancer that's diagnosed early. At the very least, most cancers will require some form of surgery, and many will require chemotherapy and/or radiation therapy as well. We have discussed many of the problems and side effects that are associated with all three of these treatments. All three also may produce significant changes in a patient's reproductive organs, so significant, in fact, that we'll now examine those problems separately in the following section. For, this is an extremely important issue for all men and women who have been diagnosed with cancer and wish to have children in the future.

For Women Only

Premature Menopause

Surgery, chemotherapy and radiation therapy all may result in **sterility,** the general term used to describe the inability to produce offspring. Obviously, surgery for certain cancers may involve the removal or partial removal of a woman's reproductive organs that may leave her unable to become pregnant. Other surgeries that have nothing to do with a woman's reproductive organs also may leave her incapable of having children. This occurs because any major surgery has a significant impact upon the entire body and recovery requires a great amount of energy. The body's immune system and restorative processes must work overtime to facilitate this healing process.

Sometimes, as a result, the body will shut down production in one area to garner the necessary energy to heal another. This may affect a woman's reproductive process, which in times of stress and crisis may be considered by the body to be non-essential. Accordingly, ovulation and menstruation may cease to preserve the body's limited energy and resources. While this cessation is often a temporary condition, it also may be permanent as a result of surgery. Known as **surgical menopause**, this phenomenon may occur in any woman of childbearing age depending upon many factors including the type of surgery performed, the body organs involved and the woman's overall health and strength.[149]

Chemotherapy as well may render a woman incapable of having children. As we know, chemotherapy utilizes many different drugs, some of which affect the normal cells in the body in a more profound way than others. Depending upon the ingredients in one's chemo-cocktail, the cells of a woman's reproductive system may be greatly impacted. The ovaries are particularly vulnerable to the toxic nature of chemotherapy drugs and ovulation may be impaired, her ability to conceive may be compromised or she may experience sterility or early chemotherapy induced menopause.[150]

Once again, the possibility of reproductive damage and its extent will depend upon many factors, including the type and strength of the anticancer drugs used in the therapy program. Furthermore, it's advisable for women who have undergone chemotherapy to wait at least one year before attempting to become pregnant. For even if it appears that the ability to ovulate or conceive hasn't been affected adversely by the chemotherapy, a risk of failed pregnancy and fetal malformations still exists. Indeed, this is a particular concern in cases where women have been treated with the drug cyclophosphamide in the course of chemotherapy.[151]

Similarly, the ovaries also are susceptible to the adverse effects of radiation, and it's this therapy that carries the greatest risk for sterility. Radiation for any cancer that directly affects a woman's reproductive organs such as the ovaries or the uterus will almost certainly result in sterility. Yet, a risk remains even if the reproductive organs are healthy and not affected directly by the cancer. Cancers located in the abdominal area such as those of the bladder, colon, kidney or liver, when treated with radiation, also present a great risk to a woman's fertility. For when radiation is used to treat these cancers there's always a chance the healthy tissues surrounding the treated area will be affected as well.

This means that a woman's reproductive organs will be extremely vulnerable to the adverse effects of the therapy. Not only may a woman experience sterility and the inability to ovulate and conceive, she may experience additional damage that once again may create premature menopause. Her fallopian tubes, ovaries and uterus may be "burned" by the radiation, rendering them non-functioning and essentially lifeless. It's necessary, therefore, for any woman diagnosed with cancer to be aware of the potential reproductive repercussions and the risks associated with her treatment. This is extremely important if a woman is of childbearing age and wishes to have children of her own in the future.[152]

Preserving Her Options

For many years, medical options generally referred to as **assisted reproductive technology** or **ART**, have existed for women who experience difficulties with fertility as well as those who face its loss.[153] For such women, the typical option for enhancing and preserving fertility has involved a two-step program respectively known as **ovulation induction** and **egg retrieval**. The first step, ovulation induction, refers to the use of medications to stimulate a woman's ovarian follicles to produce multiple eggs in a single cycle.[154]

These medications, commonly called fertility drugs, include a variety of different drugs such as **clomiphene citrate**, **gonadotropins**, **GnRh agonists** and **hCG** or **human chorionic gonadotropin**. For many women, clomiphene citrate is the first drug of choice for ovulation induction. It also is the easiest as it comes in pill form and is administered, one pill a day for five days, early in one's menstrual cycle. If, however, one fails to achieve adequate ovulation with this drug, gonadotropins typically will be used to stimulate the follicles into producing multiple eggs. These drugs are administered by injection, as are the GnRH agonists, all of which facilitate the body's production of high quality eggs in large numbers. A final injection of hCG will complete of the maturation process of the eggs and prepare them for retrieval.[155]

The injections of gonadtropins and the GnRH agonists typically begin early in a woman's menstrual cycle and are given on a daily basis for approximately one to two weeks. At the end of this period, a microscopic examination will be conducted to determine if the follicles have succeeded in producing multiple eggs. If they haven't, the entire cycle of injections usually is repeated. If, on the other hand, multiple eggs have been produced, a final injection of hCG will be administered and the process of ovulation induction will be complete.

Within one to two days following the final injection of hCG, the second step of the process known as **egg retrieval** may take place. This procedure is conducted in an operating room where the patient typically is given an intravenous sedative. In most cases, a probe is inserted into the vagina and alongside this probe the physician also inserts a needle. Directed by ultrasound visualization, the needle is guided into an ovary, then into each follicle within the ovary. The needle then collects, or aspirates, the egg from each producing follicle before it's redirected to the other ovary where the process is repeated.

Known as a **transvaginal aspiration,** or **TV collection**, a successful retrieval may yield as many as twelve or thirteen eggs from the ovaries, and when the twenty-minute procedure is over, the patient is free to go home. Although somewhat more complicated, the eggs also may be extracted through laparoscopic surgery in which an incision is made in the abdomen to gain access to the ovaries and aspirate the eggs.[156]

Once this two-part process to retrieve her eggs has been completed, however, a woman then must choose the method of preservation most appropriate for her. In years past, the options were limited and eggs removed from a woman's ovaries usually underwent **in vitro fertilization,** or **IVF**. In this procedure, the egg is fertilized with the sperm from a woman's spouse, significant other or designated donor and the resulting embryo is either placed within the woman's womb, or the embryos are frozen for future use.

The only option for women who are facing possible sterility as a result of cancer and its treatments is the latter. This option, however, places single women in the uncomfortable position of having to make important life-altering decisions concerning parentage quickly. Other women may be opposed to creating embryos that may never be used. Fortunately, advances in medical technology may provide an additional option these women in a procedure known simply as **egg freezing**.[157]

In this process, rather than exposing the retrieved eggs to in vitro fertilization, they're placed in a cryoprotective solution, then frozen in a tank of liquid nitrogen. While the process for freezing sperm has existed for many years, the process for freezing eggs wasn't a viable option until the mid 1990s. For unlike sperm, the egg is a large cell filled with fluid that can form damaging ice crystals when frozen. Additionally, the freezing process for eggs results in damage to the zona pellucida, the outer shell of the egg. It's this shell with which the sperm must bind to penetrate and fertilize the egg.

Today, however, new techniques are being developed to counter or eliminate these problems. A technique known as **vitrification**, for example, enables an egg to be flash frozen in a few seconds rather than hours, a process that prevents ice crystals from forming and reduces the egg's exposure to toxins found within the cryoprotective solutions. Similarly, another technique known as **intracytoplastic sperm injection,** or **ICSI,** allows the sperm to be injected directly into the egg's core, which makes the binding process irrelevant. The freezing process may still damage the shell, but the injected sperm retains its ability to fertilize the egg and create an embryo.[158]

Additionally, some researchers are injecting sugar solutions into the eggs and experimenting with improved freezing containers in the hope of providing better preservation. As a result, egg freezing is an exciting and viable option for preserving a woman's fertility until her health and personal circumstances permit her the opportunity to attempt pregnancy.[159] The risks and hardships associated with ovulation induction, egg retrieval and freezing must be analyzed as well. First, and most important, is the issue of time. When a woman has been diagnosed with cancer it's essential to embark on a treatment program as soon as possible. In most cases in which surgery is the primary form of treatment, the surgery takes place within days of diagnosis, or as soon as the necessary tests are completed and scheduling permits. If the cancer doesn't involve the reproductive organs, this necessary rush to surgery typically won't interfere with the process of saving a woman's eggs because it's chemotherapy and radiation that pose the greatest threat to a woman's fertility.

As we know, however, it's still possible for the surgery to affect her body in a way that creates surgical menopause. If this occurs, the shut down of her reproductive system and the resulting ovarian failure to produce eggs will render any egg saving procedure moot. Furthermore, if the cancer does affect the reproductive organs directly, the chances of saving eggs after surgery clearly may not be possible. Indeed, even if surgery were postponed in these cases in order to retrieve and save eggs, the nature of the disease may make ovulation or retrieval impossible.

While it's possible to undergo egg preservation prior to surgery, the process can be lengthy and surgery is rarely postponed once cancer has been diagnosed. Indeed, the entire process of ovulation induction, egg retrieval and possible freezing is time consuming and there's no guarantee that the process will be successful after one attempt. Success may only be experienced after a few, or several, attempts and the amount of time needed to accomplish the goal may stretch from a few weeks to several months.[160] This, unfortunately, is time that no cancer patient can afford to lose.

Assuming that surgery is performed, however, and a woman's reproductive system is still operating normally, time and timing continue to be issues. As stated, the most appropriate window of opportunity for undergoing an egg-saving process is after surgery and before chemotherapy or radiation. Typically, this is possible because the staging and grading process of the cancer in question may take several weeks. During this time a woman can begin the necessary injections needed to stimulate her ovaries to produce multiple eggs.

If the induction and retrieval process is successful on the first attempt, she'll be ready to begin additional cancer treatments within a few weeks. If the first attempt isn't successful, another cycle of injections and another attempt at aspiration will be necessary. In cases of typical infertility, this time-consuming process may not be an issue. In cases where the woman has cancer, however, the issue of time may become a matter of life and death.

The length of time she can wait before beginning chemotherapy and/or radiation is, of course, a question for her physician and attending medical experts. Clearly, the luxury of time doesn't exist for a woman diagnosed with cancer and the option of preserving her fertility, while possible, may not be feasible.

Second, the process of preserving eggs entails a certain amount of discomfort. The necessary ovulation induction medications typically are injected on a daily basis. These injections may be accompanied by oral medications as well and the full course of treatment may take several weeks. These medications delay the start of a woman's menstrual cycle to give the ovaries time to produce multiple eggs and often include a number of side effects. These might include headaches, blurred vision, mood swings and restlessness. They also may include hot flashes, fatigue and, of course, abdominal discomfort and bloating similar to the symptoms associated with pre-menstrual syndrome.[161]

Of a more serious nature, some of the ovulation induction medications also may increase a woman's risk for developing ovarian cysts and a rare condition known as **ovarian hyperstimulation syndrome,** or **OHSS**. This particular syndrome may induce nausea and vomiting, bloating and weight gain, breathing difficulties and severe chest and abdominal pain. It's a serious condition that will require immediate medical attention should it occur. Furthermore, when ovulation induction is used to treat women who have difficulty getting pregnant, it's important to avoid overstimulation of the ovaries. This is critical in preventing the overproduction of eggs and the occurrence of multiple births.[162]

When used to treat women who face chemotherapy or radiation, however, the goal of ovulation induction is to produce as many eggs as possible for retrieval and preservation. This more aggressive level of ovulation induction is referred to as **superovulation**, a delicate program that requires close supervision and, as a result, participating women also must subject themselves to regular monitoring through a series of blood tests and ultrasounds.[163]

Clearly, the complete process of ovulation induction, egg retrieval, in vitro fertilization and embryo or egg freezing is a complicated and exacting one. Accordingly, it also is an expensive process that may cost the patient several thousands of dollars for one cycle of medication, aspiration and in vitro fertilization or cryopreservation. If one cycle isn't successful in producing multiple eggs and the process is repeated, the cost, which isn't covered by insurance, will quickly escalate.

Furthermore, if a woman chooses egg preservation through freezing, it's important to note that while promising, it's a new option still considered experimental. For example, while the freezing process is improving, there remains great concern regarding the egg's ability to survive the thawing process. In 1994, only ten to twenty percent of frozen eggs survived the critical thawing process. In 2004, the survival rate increased to an average of seventy percent. And, in 2008 a new study estimated the survival rate of frozen eggs ranged from seventy to ninety-five percent depending upon the techniques used.[164]

Further, it's not known how long the eggs can be stored safely without being damaged. While it's been reported that pregnancies have resulted from fertilized embryos that have been frozen for as long as ten years, this longevity may not apply to the freezing of eggs. Even while the process of freezing and thawing eggs continues to improve, however, only a portion of these eggs will become viable embryos once fertilized. And, the success of implanting the viable embryos and actually producing a baby is far from certain.

While some reports in the year 2004 estimated that the number of worldwide pregnancies resulting from egg freezing was close to one hundred, others placed the figure closer to thirty. It's unclear, however, if these estimations included the thirteen live births reported in late 2004 from one study conducted in the United States. In 2006, this number was estimated to be about one hundred and twenty, while an estimate in 2008 put the number near five hundred. Of further importance, because so few pregnancies have resulted from the process, there isn't enough data available to determine if children born from frozen eggs experience a greater number of birth defects than those born from natural pregnancies or other birthing methods such as in vitro fertilization.[165]

One final alternative a woman may consider is the option of freezing not just her eggs, but also an entire ovary. **Ovarian tissue freezing** was developed specifically to preserve the fertility of women diagnosed with cancer and faced with chemotherapy or radiation treatments. All of a woman's eggs are found within one millimeter of the outer layer of the ovary. The follicles, as well, are located on the periphery of the ovary while the inside consists of tissue and blood vessels that have no specific function except to nourish the eggs.[166]

It's this structure that permits a complete ovary to be removed and allows the outer layer to be microsurgically dissected. The tissue is then exposed to a gradual computer controlled freezing process. In this way, the ovarian tissues are preserved until they can be transplanted back into the woman after she has recovered from the cancer and its necessary treatments. This procedure holds great promise for the future, although like egg freezing, it also is considered highly experimental. Indeed, as of 2004 only one successful pregnancy and live birth had been reported as a result of this particular procedure.[167]

Finally, it's important to remember that even if a woman does choose to undergo one of these fertility preserving procedures, the surgery, chemotherapy or radiation she undergoes may leave her in a state of premature menopause or may damage her reproductive organs making her incapable of carrying a child. If this should occur, no frozen egg, fertilized egg, frozen embryo or transplanted ovarian tissue will allow her to become pregnant and carry a child. Accordingly, it will be necessary for her to engage the services of a surrogate, yet another costly and time-consuming endeavor.

These are difficult issues for which there are no easy answers. It's fair to state, however, that if a woman has a male presence in her life, the safer decision is to choose in vitro fertilization and to freeze embryos rather than eggs. For embryo cryopreservation is a technique which has a solid track record and for which positive international statistics have been established.

Whichever process a woman chooses, however, her choice of a physician must be made just as carefully and should take into consideration her or his past success in freezing, thawing and fertilization procedures as well as resulting pregnancies and successful births. While the hope of preserving fertility is a most important factor for a woman faced with its loss, the decisions regarding her future must be reached quickly and must, unfortunately, be based upon the limited information available today.

Personal Note

After my diagnosis for colon cancer was confirmed, I underwent surgery within the week. My surgery involved an anterior resection in which the diseased part of the large intestine was removed via a large incision in the abdomen. One suspicious-looking ovary also was removed although that tissue ultimately was determined to be benign. Upon my recovery from the surgery and prior to the start of my chemotherapy, I was referred to a fertility specialist in an attempt to retrieve my eggs and preserve my ability to have a biologically related child.

I spent a few weeks undergoing the necessary injections, but when the time came for retrieval, the process proved unsuccessful. The specialist explained that my body had already gone into "ovarian failure," and my one remaining ovary was unable to produce any eggs. As a result of the surgery, ovulation had ceased, my periods had stopped and I was thrown into the premature condition known as "surgical menopause." In my case, however, even if the surgery hadn't created this condition of premature menopause, the chemotherapy I underwent might have.

Furthermore, my radiation treatments alone would most certainly have resulted in premature menopause and sterility as a result of the damage they caused to my reproductive organs. Even if egg retrieval after surgery had proved successful, therefore, I still wouldn't have been able to become pregnant and carry a fetus to term. The services of a surrogate would have been necessary.

Nothing in life is to be feared
It is only to be understood.
Marie Curie

Cancer and Pregnancy

Perhaps the most complicated situation a woman diagnosed with cancer can face is one in which her cancer diagnosis coincides with a pregnancy. Either situation requires specialized treatment and care, yet when both occur at the same time, the patient/physician relationship will be forced into new and challenging territory.

First and foremost, it's essential for every woman to know that cancer and pregnancy aren't necessarily mutually exclusive. Many women with cancer have experienced a simultaneous, full or partial term pregnancy and have given birth to mentally and physically healthy children. Yet, to understand the complexity of the situation, it's necessary to distinguish the disease from the treatments. To begin, if the cancer isn't one that directly affects the organs responsible for fetal protection and nourishment, such as the endometrium, there's little evidence the disease will harm the baby.

Breast cancer, for example, is the most common cancer among pregnant women, and while it's an extremely serious disease for the individual, it doesn't appear to create any additional health risk for a developing fetus. Indeed, it not only appears that many cancers aren't a direct health threat for a developing fetus, it also appears that with some cancers, such as breast cancer, the choice to terminate the pregnancy won't improve the mother's chances of surviving the disease either.[168]

In addition to breast cancer, the most common cancers that affect pregnant women include cervical cancer, melanoma and Hodgkin's lymphoma. Of these, cervical cancer and Hodgkin's lymphoma may be the most problematic, the former because of its location in the body and the latter because it's a systemic disease that affects the body's lymph system. In most cases, the concern regarding cancer and pregnancy is typically not one that arises from the disease, but rather from the drugs and treatments required to fight the disease.[169]

If cancer treatment requires surgery, there are many surgical procedures that can be performed without directly affecting a progressing pregnancy. It's vital, of course, for one's oncologist and physician to monitor closely all drugs and anesthesias that may be needed to insure surgical success. In cases, however, where treatment requires chemotherapy and/or radiation, the situation is quite different. For these two cancer treatments are the most common and the most likely to create specific difficulties in cases of pregnancies. As we know, chemotherapy is a treatment that utilizes many potent drugs known for their anticancer properties. We also know that chemotherapy is a systemic treatment the drugs of which work by attacking fast growing and dividing cells anywhere in the body. Such cells are found throughout the reproductive system and are certainly an issue in human pregnancy.

In pregnancy, this rapid cell growth begins when the female egg and the male sperm combine to become a one-cell embryo through the process of fertilization. Within a short twelve hours, however, this one cell will divide into two, each of which will divide into another two, and as the process continues, the numbers of these rapidly dividing cells will double every twelve hours. Within four or five days, the embryo will have grown from one to approximately five hundred cells and within seven days its size will double every twenty-four hours.[170]

Throughout the first twelve weeks of pregnancy the rate of fetal development and cell division continues to be swift. Indeed, the first trimester is considered by many health experts to be the most important period of growth as it's during this time that all of the major organs of the body are formed including the spinal cord, the heart, the intestines and abdomen, the lungs, the extremities, the head and facial features and the sex organs. It also is during this period of time, however, that the fast growing cells associated with fetal development are most vulnerable to the adverse effects of chemotherapy anticancer drugs.[171]

Accordingly, many health experts agree that, if possible, chemotherapy should be avoided during the first trimester of pregnancy. It does appear, however, that many anticancer drugs can be administered to a patient in chemotherapy during the second and third trimester without an increased risk of fetal malformations. In cases where immediate chemotherapy is advised and a woman is in her first trimester, it may be possible to begin treatment with extremely mild anticancer drugs, induce delivery prematurely at approximately thirty-two weeks, and then begin a high-dose regimen of chemotherapy.[172]

It's often the case, however, for chemotherapy and radiation therapy to be used in concert to treat many cancers. Unlike chemotherapy, radiation doesn't target fast growing cells of the body. It also differs in that it's not a systemic treatment, but rather a localized treatment that affects a limited area of the body. Radiation, however, has the ability to change the molecular structure of any cell with which it comes into contact. This change can damage the cell's DNA and hinder or prevent its ability to grow and develop normally. In addition, radiation is an imprecise procedure that can damage the body tissues surrounding a tumor as well as the tumor itself. If cancer, therefore, is diagnosed within the reproductive organs or any other organ within the abdominal cavity it may not be possible to undergo radiation for the cancer without adversely affecting a developing fetus.

If these organs aren't affected, however, and radiation is still recommended, a pregnant woman may be able to postpone the treatment until her second or third trimester, thus protecting the fetus during the earliest stage of development. It also may be possible to postpone the radiation until she delivers prematurely through labor induction or naturally after carrying her full term. Finally, if immediate radiation is recommended for cancers that don't directly affect the pregnancy and are not within the abdominal cavity, it still may be possible to protect the developing fetus from harm with proper shielding.[173]

Clearly, there's much to consider in this very complicated scenario. The important thing for women to remember, however, is that options do exist, and many women have battled cancer and delivered a completely healthy baby at the same time. The choice of treatment in such cases, as in all cancer cases, must be individualized. It must take into account all the typical considerations of a cancer diagnosis, as well as the mother's wishes and the length of time remaining in the pregnancy. The patient must acknowl-edge the significant demands she'll face as she battles the disease and strives to main-tain energy and strength for herself and her fetus.

In such a situation, of course, general guidelines cannot substitute for personalized medical advice that can only be provided by a team of health care professionals and only after a thorough consultation with the woman in question. It's been theorized that the incidence rate of cancers among pregnant women may increase because many women are postponing childbirth, and we know that the risk for cancer increases as we age. It doesn't appear that babies born to women who have had cancer in the past experi-ence an increased risk for developing anomalies. Furthermore, women with cancer who already have children may breastfeed unless they also are undergoing chemotherapy, the drugs of which can accumulate in the breast milk and be passed to the child.[174]

Finally, as mentioned, a woman who has undergone chemotherapy should wait at least a year before becoming pregnant to reduce the possibility of birth defects. Sexually active women who have been diagnosed with cancer and face treatment should take the steps necessary throughout their therapy to prevent pregnancy. Unfortunately, it remains a fact that women who have undergone extensive chemotherapy and radia-tion, and possibly bone marrow transplants, may experience more difficulties not only in becoming pregnant, but in giving birth to healthy children as well.[175]

One More Thing

As stated, radiation therapy is capable of causing great damage to the body's healthy tis-sues as well as to those diseased tissues specifically targeted. If the reproductive organs are affected either intentionally or unintentionally by this treatment, certain problems may arise. The vagina and cervix, for example, may become extremely dry and almost brittle. And, this condition is far more serious than the typical dryness and loss of tissue elasticity that may occur as a result of typical menopause.[176]

Accordingly, gynecological exams and sexual intercourse may become difficult, uncomfortable and even painful. While estrogen such as that used in hormone replace-ment therapy is helpful in restoring some normalcy to these tissues, even those affected by radiation, estrogen has been linked to endometrial cancer and, in cases of high dose or long-term use, possibly to breast cancer as well.[177] Moreover, the last thing any woman wants who has survived one cancer is to do anything that may put her at risk for developing another.

Once again, this is a tricky issue that requires evaluation, discussion and in most cases plain old fashioned trial and error. Sexually active women who don't want to risk the regular use of estrogen yet seek relief for vaginal dryness, for example, may choose to use one of the many natural substances or estrogen substitutes available in today's market. Fortunately, due to the increased awareness of the possible harm that may result from estrogen use, many new products are being researched and developed on a continuing basis. These products often are prescribed for the typical symptoms of menopause and may help alleviate similar symptoms, such as vaginal dryness, that result from radiation.

Of course, there are several other products as well, such as mineral oil or water-based lubricants that may help alleviate vaginal dryness and increase a woman's comfort during sexual intercourse. Petroleum jellies, however, should be avoided because they're dense and are difficult for the body to expel once they have entered the vaginal cavity. They also may increase a woman's risk for developing infections, as they don't allow the skin to breathe.

Further, a woman is not only more likely to develop general body infections during cancer treatment, her bladder and vaginal tissues are more susceptible to infection as a result of treatment induced menopause as well. Indeed, avoiding genital infections is important for all women, and as such, the use of petroleum jellies should be discouraged while the wearing of loose slacks or shorts, and cotton-paneled underwear should be encouraged.[178] Lastly, if intercourse remains painful, one should consult with her physician about using a vaginal dilator, a device used before sex to slowly expand and stretch the vaginal tissues to provide increased comfort during sex.[179]

For women who aren't sexually active, however, the issue isn't one of comfort during intercourse, but rather of general comfort and quality of life. Once again, natural products and hormone substitutes may be extremely helpful in reducing the symptoms of radiation, or for that matter, the menopausal symptoms that may result from other treatments, including surgery and chemotherapy. Further, while a woman may not be sexually active, she may still experience regular pelvic exams and PAP smears that are uncomfortable.

One solution to this problem may be the limited use of an estrogen containing cream that can be applied topically to the vagina and surrounding tissue. Using such a product for a few days to a week prior to an exam can greatly reduce the amount of dryness and discomfort and facilitate the entire procedure. While such creams do contain estrogen and the estrogen is absorbed into the tissue, their limited use creates such a small exposure for a woman that any resulting risk is extremely minimal.[180]

Another solution may be the use of an estrogen substitute that many women take to relieve some of the general symptoms of menopause such as mood swings, hot flashes and night sweats. As previously discussed, these substitutes are neither an estrogen nor a hormone and are known as selective estrogen receptor modulators, or SERMs. They're compounds that behave like estrogens in some tissues and like anti-estrogens in other tissues. They are helpful in reducing many of the uncomfortable symptoms of menopause and help build strong bones without negatively affecting the breast or uterine tissues.[181] As always, however, caution is required, and wrestling the octopus again becomes an issue as some of these products may actually increase some physical discomforts, such as vaginal dryness, while decreasing others.

Furthermore, it's not advisable for women, be they cancer patients or not, to use typical vaginal lubricants prior to an exam requiring microscopic analysis such as a PAP smear because their use may interfere with accurate test results. One may, however, ease the discomfort of a pelvic exam by using one of the new soft, inflatable speculums. Inserted like a tampon, these devices are gently inflated with a small hand-held pump once in position. Their flexibility results in greater comfort for the patient and, as they're disposable, there are no issues of hygiene or prior use about which one needs to be concerned.[182]

In the past, women typically have used some form of estrogen replacement to 1) protect the heart, 2) protect the bones and, 3) alleviate the symptoms associated with menopause. It's clear that as a woman enters menopause more cholesterol is found in the blood and this condition increases the risk of heart disease. It isn't clear, however, that estrogen in itself has a direct effect upon the heart that protects it from such disease. Some studies have found that estrogen appears to aid a woman's cardiovascular system by relaxing the blood vessels and preventing clotting. Conversely, others have found that estrogen appears to be linked to an increase in heart attacks and strokes.

Still others have found that estrogen in younger women makes nitric oxide, which protects the heart, while in older women estrogen makes a substance known as super-oxide, which damages these tissues. This, of course, appears to support the theory that the effect of estrogen upon the heart may depend upon the age of the woman in question. In any event, the beneficial effect estrogen may have upon these tissues remains a controversial and highly debated issue.[183]

The beneficial effect of estrogen upon the bones of the body, however, is much clearer. The value of estrogen in preventing and reducing the risk for osteoporosis is commonly recognized. Yet, estrogen taken for this reason alone is unnecessary as there are many over the counter products sold today that provide the calcium that many experts believe is required to protect the bones. Despite recent research that questions this particular benefit of calcium, most studies still support the claim that calcium, when taken regularly, remains helpful in this respect.[184]

In addition, one of the best defenses against osteoporosis is to incorporate weight-bearing exercises into one's daily health program. Similar to the muscles of the body, the bones must be used to keep them healthy. And, the way we use our bones is to apply pressure or weight to them through movement such as walking or exercises such as weight lifting. Further, such movement and exercise need not be strenuous. It's only important to move in a way that utilizes resistance and the simple law of gravity. Indeed, one of the biggest problems that affect astronauts of the world is the fact that they experience extended periods of time in weightlessness. This lack of gravity denies an individual the opportunity to "bear weight," and as a result, the bones of the body become more susceptible to deterioration and the effects of osteoporosis.[185]

Personal Note

I choose to take the non-estrogen supplement Evista due to my higher risk for breast cancer. Although it didn't prevent the occurrence of breast cancer it remains the right choice for me. After all, my maternal grandmother had breast cancer, I had fibrosis of the breasts and years ago, in the identical area of my breast tumor, I developed three benign cysts over a period of a few years. Each, of course, was harmless, and each was aspirated with a small needle.

It was an indication, however, that something "in there" (most likely an errant duct gland as my tumor was a ductal carcinoma) wasn't behaving properly and abnormalities were being created. If we remember our Cancer Blueprint, cells that behave improperly may contain compromised or damaged DNA and may become cancerous. This is no different from a nevi mole or significantly freckled skin. Both are an indication that the skin tissue isn't completely normal and as such, each could lead to serious skin diseases including cancer.

Indeed, in my case, my gynecologist told me that we should "keep an eye" on that area of my breast precisely because of my past benign cysts. Fortunately, I practice what I preach. I know the cancers for which I appear to have an increased risk, and I monitor for them diligently. The result is that instead of being blind-sided by my breast cancer, I met it head-on and took immediate action to eradicate the little bugger. As we all know, any cancer can strike anyone at any time. Yet, it's vital for us to know our risks and remain proactive, for even if our choices cannot prevent cancer, they can reduce aggravation and help mitigate the damage caused by cancer.

For Men Only

Cancer treatments may result in significant changes in sexuality and reproductive matters for men as well. It's important, for example, for sexually active men undergoing chemotherapy to use a condom during sexual intercourse as the anticancer drugs of the treatment may enter the sperm cells. A condom is recommended, because even without ejaculation, or in situations in which the couple in question practices penile withdrawal during sex, sperm can still escape and enter the female vaginal and uterine cavities. And, should a pregnancy result from these affected sperm, the increased risk of fetal malformations could be significant. Indeed, to be safe, condom use should continue for a few days to a few weeks, depending upon medical advice, following the last treatment.[186]

Clearly, other complications such as male sterility can result from cancer treatments as well. Obviously, surgery performed to remove any cancer of the male reproductive system, such as that of the testicles, or surgery for prostate cancer, may create sterility. Chemotherapy and radiation also carry a risk for this complication, especially radiation directed to any organ within the abdominal cavity. Accordingly, it also is advisable for men who wish to father children and have been diagnosed with cancer to preserve their sperm.

The procedure for preserving fertility is much easier for men than women and, indeed, the process of freezing sperm has been used for many years. Sperm cells are much smaller than eggs, and as a result, they're much more likely to survive a freezing and thawing process. Furthermore, it typically is much easier to obtain sperm as in most cases a man simply has to ejaculate into a receptacle provided by a physician. The sperm can then be used for in vitro fertilization to create an embryo for immediate implantation, to fertilize eggs for freezing, or to be frozen alone for future use.[187]

For some men, however, ejaculation of semen isn't possible. Fortunately, sperm retrieval is no longer limited to ejaculated semen and new technologies are providing greater options for these males as well. First, some men experience **azoospermia**, the lack of sperm resulting from an obstructive lesion, a failed vasectomy reversal or some other uncorrectable blockage. For these men, one method for removing sperm is **micro epididymal sperm aspiration,** or **MESA**. Microsurgery with a fine needle allows this procedure to collect sperm gathered near the blocked portion of the epididymis, the elongated, coiled duct that provides storage and passage for sperm from each testicle.[188]

A similar procedure known as **percutaneous epididymal sperm aspiration,** or **PESA,** also utilizes a small needle to penetrate the surface of the testicle and withdraw sperm near the epididymal blockage. Additionally, testicular tissue can be a source of sperm. Accordingly, **testicular sperm extraction,** or **TESE,** is another procedure whereby a small amount of testicular tissue is surgically removed, then cultivated for the presence of sperm.[189]

If the men undergoing these methods of sperm retrieval have a female presence in their life, the procedures typically will be scheduled to coincide with her ovulation. In this way, the sperm can immediately be combined with the female's retrieved egg through the process of in vitro fertilization. The resulting embryo can then be implanted in the female's womb or several embryos can be frozen for future use. Additionally, the sperm that is retrieved through MESA, PESA or TESE also can be used in **intracytoplasmic sperm injection** to fertilize a previously frozen egg.[190]

While cryopreservation for sperm is a common practice, only the sperm from MESA and PESA procedures can be frozen. The sperm gathered from TESE procedures, unfortunately, is not considered to be of a sufficient quality or quantity to be used in such a way. Furthermore, it's not recommended for men to undergo multiple MESA or PESA procedures as repeated surgeries could result in tissue scarring around the incision site.

Finally, as with most surgeries, side effects from each of these three procedures can occur. The most common, however, will include pain and swelling around the surgery site, and most patients, as a result, will be advised to avoid strenuous activity and to wear scrotal supports for several days following the procedure.[191]

In addition to MESA, PESA and TESE procedures, another method known as **electroejaculation** is sometimes used to retrieve sperm. This method can be a successful alternative for men who have normal testes, but cannot ejaculate due to a defect in the sympathetic nervous system. For example, this may include men who have experienced a spinal cord injury resulting in paralysis. In this procedure, the physician places a probe in the patient's rectum. The probe emits an electrical current that stimulates the nerve fibers within the male reproductive tract. And, this stimulation results in the emission of semen.[192]

This emission, however, won't be forceful and as a result the semen may be released into the bladder or through the urethra. This means that the semen may have to be retrieved from the urine. Anticipating this possibility, the patient typically will be given sodium bicarbonate tablets the day before the procedure. This will change the urine from an acidic to an alkaline composition and will protect the sperm from any toxic exposure normally associated with uric acids.

In addition to men who experience a failure of the sympathetic nervous system, this procedure also is an option for men who have already undergone prostate or testicular cancer surgery and later choose to preserve their sperm. For example, men who have had their testicles removed through an **orchiectomy** and wish to father children may be candidates for electroejaculation.[193]

Similarly, men who have undergone a **retroperitoneal lymph node dissection**, a surgery often performed to remove malignancies or lymphomas originating in the sexual or pelvic organs, may benefit from electroejaculation.[194] This procedure provides a second chance at fatherhood for many men, and what it lacks in technical delicacy, it makes up in opportunity, a second chance to retrieve viable sperm that can be used immediately for in vitro fertilization or saved for the future through cryopreservation.

Additional Therapies

Biological Therapy

In addition to the term biological, this type of therapy is known by many names including **biotherapy**, **biological response modifier**, or **BRM**, and **immunotherapy**. Simply defined, this treatment is used to restore, enhance or stimulate the ability of the immune system to fight disease and infection. The immune system naturally produces biological agents that aid the body in detecting and destroying foreign material such as cancer. These agents are known as **lymphokines** and among these the **interferons** and **interleukin-2** are the best known and most documented.[195]

Biological treatments boost the body's stores of these agents typically through injection, which may be administered alone or in conjunction with chemotherapy or radiation. Interferon, for example, has been found helpful in the treatment of colorectal and cervical cancer. Another agent, known as **interferon-alpha**, is useful in treating some cancers of the lymph system and the rare hairy cell leukemia.[196]

In the case of breast cancer, an antibody is used to slow or stop the growth of cells that have too much of the protein known as **human epidermal growth factor receptor-2,** or **HER-2**. By targeting these cells and blocking the production of HER-2 this antibody, known as Trastuzumab and marketed as Herceptin, enhances the body's ability to fight cancer in the breast tissue and helps prevent a recurrence of the disease.[197]

Similar to other treatments, however, biological therapy isn't without unintended side effects. The most common may include flu-like symptoms, such as muscle aches and weakness, chills or fevers. One also may experience nausea, vomiting or diarrhea and other digestive problems. In addition, the patient may develop problems with the skin including rashes or a tendency to bleed or bruise easily. While most of these complications are temporary in nature, some can be quite severe.

Furthermore, women who undergo treatment with HER-2 blocking antibodies risk heart damage that, in some cases, can lead to heart failure. These antibodies also can affect the lungs and create significant breathing problems. For these reasons, therefore, it's necessary for all women interested in therapy with such antibodies to undergo a complete exam of the heart and lungs before commencing treatment.[198]

Bone Marrow Transplant

As we know, the bone marrow is the soft spongy material located on the inside of our bones. It's responsible for producing stem cells, which in turn, become the red blood cells, the white blood cells and the platelets. When this tissue is healthy and functioning normally our bodies have the ability to fight off disease and infection and to stop bleeding when injured. Many diseases and conditions, including leukemia, lymphoma, Hodgkin's disease, non-Hodgkin's disease and multiple myeloma, however, can compromise the proper functioning of our bone marrow. Furthermore, high dose chemotherapy and radiation also can cripple the cells of the bone marrow and impair its ability to function properly.

In any event, when these cells imperative to the good health of the human body are threatened or damaged, they must be replaced through a procedure known as a bone marrow transplant. There are two types of transplants, the first of which is called an **allogeneic** bone marrow transplant. This is the more common of the two and requires a marrow donor. If the donor is an identical twin of the patient the transplant is further distinguished as a **syngeneic** transplant. In these cases, the patient is not at risk for a severe reaction to or rejection of the marrow because identical twins share the same genetic makeup.[199]

A donor also may be the patient's sibling or parent; however, compatibility isn't guaranteed and must be tested. This can be established by conducting a test for **human lymphocyte antigens** also known as an **HLA Test**. The HLAs are six proteins found on the surface of most of the body's cells, including the white blood cells, and the purpose of this test is to match as many of these proteins as possible.[200]

If two siblings in a family are tested, the chance of an HLA match between the donor and the patient is about twenty-five percent. If six are tested, however, the chance for a match increases to about seventy-five percent. Unrelated donors also may be compatible if their HLA system proves identical or nearly identical to that of the patient. To this end, several countries have begun bone marrow registries, which help locate HLA matched donors to unrelated patients.[201]

The second type of transplant, called an **autologous** bone marrow transplant, is one in which the patient makes the marrow donation her or himself. This type of transplant in which one uses one's own marrow presents no risk of rejection, or as it's also known, **graft versus host disease**. While bone marrow transplants often are procedures of a latter resort, some actually are performed as a preventive measure to help patients withstand high dose chemotherapy or to boost their immune systems in the fight against cancer.[202]

Bone marrow donation, however, is more complicated than simple blood donation. Typically, in either an allogeneic or an autologous transplant bone marrow is removed from the donor's pelvic bone while the donor is under a general anesthesia. The marrow is then injected into one of the patient's veins where it travels through the blood stream to the interior of the bones and begins producing new cells. In an allogeneic transplant this withdrawal and injection usually takes place within the same day. In an autologous transplant, the marrow may be frozen for months or years while the patient completes high dose chemotherapy or radiation and is ready for the injection.

In either case, when the injection does take place, the patient stays in a special ventilated hospital room with filtered air and receives intravenous antibiotics to minimize the risk of infection. Yet, unlike other organ transplants, those of the bone marrow do not compromise the future health of the donor. For unlike other organs such as the kidneys, the bone marrow replaces itself and, therefore, its temporary loss does not create the potential for future problems.[203]

Hormonal Therapy

For cancers that appear to be promoted in part by the production of and exposure to certain hormones within the body, **hormonal therapy** is a common form of treatment. Also known as **endocrine therapy**, this treatment fights disease with hormones obtained from the body's own endocrine glands or with substances that imitate the effect of these hormones. It's a therapy commonly used to treat cancers of the breast and prostate and often is used in conjunction with chemotherapy or radiation.[204]

For example, breast cancer in women has been linked, in part, to a woman's lifetime exposure to the female hormone estrogen. In response, breast cancer is often treated with Tamoxifen, a substance that works as an anti-estrogen agent in breast tissue. Tamoxifen doesn't prevent the body from producing estrogen, but it does prevent a cancer cell from using estrogen to grow. It hinders the development of breast cancer and is an effective form of treatment for pre and postmenopausal women alike.[205]

Women who haven't undergone a hysterectomy must remember, however, that while Tamoxifen acts as an anti-estrogen agent in the breast, it acts as an estrogen agent in the uterus and its use has been linked to the development of endometrial cancer. In addition, the use of Tamoxifen may cause vaginal irritation or discharge, nausea and even menopausal symptoms such as hot flashes. In some cases, women who have been diagnosed with breast cancer choose to have their ovaries removed to stop the body's production of all estrogen.[206]

For these women, the additional use of Tamoxifen is likely to create menopausal symptoms that are much more severe than those occurring from natural menopause. In contrast, the use of Tamoxifen in women of child bearing age may create irregular periods, and as a result, pregnancies that may occur more easily and unexpectedly. Although rare, Tamoxifen also may cause blood clots in a woman's legs and lungs and slightly increase her risk of stroke as well.[207]

While breast cancer in women is linked to the production of female hormones, prostate cancer is linked to the production of male hormones. Accordingly, hormonal therapy is a common treatment program for prostate cancer as well. It sometimes is used as a localized treatment to prevent cancer from returning after surgery or radiation. More typically, however, it's used in cases where the cancer has spread from the prostate to surrounding tissues and body parts.[208]

When used in this way, hormonal therapy for prostate cancer becomes a systemic treatment that affects cancer cells throughout the male body. The male hormones that promote the development of prostate cancer are known as androgens, and of these, testosterone is the most common. Prostate cancer cells need these hormones to grow and hormonal therapy prevents this from occurring by eliminating or reducing the hormones. There are several forms of hormonal therapy from which a patient may choose and the first, and most extreme, is the procedure known as an **orchiectomy**.[209]

Testosterone is produced in the testicles, and by surgically removing the testicles through this procedure the source of this cancer-promoting hormone is eliminated. The elimination of testosterone, however, also can be accomplished by monthly injections of drugs that prevent the testicles from producing testosterone. These drugs are called

leutenizing hormone-releasing hormone agonists, or **LH-RH.** Leutenizing hormone is a substance released by the pituitary gland and generally thought of in connection with female ovulation. In males, however, this hormone has the ability to stop the production of testosterone and the drugs, or releasers, which trigger this process include **leuprolide, goserelin** and **buserelin.**[210]

Even if testosterone production is eliminated, however, small amounts of male hormones are still produced by the adrenal glands. To deal with this situation, the patient may receive additional drugs known as **anti-androgens.** Similar to the anti-estrogen drug Tamoxifen, anti-androgens such as **flutamide** and **bicalutamide** don't stop the production of androgens but, rather, prevent cancer cells from using them to grow. Lastly, drugs including **ketoconazole** and **aminoglutethimide** work by preventing the adrenal glands from producing any androgens at all.[211]

If these different forms of drug-induced hormonal therapies are combined the treatment is called a **total androgen blockade.**[212] It's not clear if such a blockade is more effective than an orchiectomy alone, and the patient's decision regarding these forms of hormonal therapies must carefully be evaluated. Additionally, hormonal therapies may effectively control prostate cancer that has metastasized to other body parts for several years. These therapies won't, however, control the cancer forever. Eventually, prostate cancers gain the ability to grow with little or no male hormones, and when this occurs other forms of treatment will be necessary.

Similar to any other type of cancer treatment, hormonal therapy for prostate cancer has significant side effects. These effects will depend upon the form of therapy, yet they can be divided into two basic groups. The first are associated with the therapies that target the testicles and the production of testosterone. Men who undergo an orchiectomy or a program of LH-RH agonists often experience impotence and a loss of sexual desire. They also may experience symptoms similar to female menopause, such as hot flashes and weight gain. The lack of testosterone may lead to memory loss, depression and confusion.[213] Furthermore, when both an orchiectomy and an LH-RH program are combined, LH-RH agonists may worsen any symptoms the patient already may be experiencing. This phenomenon is called a **flare** and is temporary in nature. To prevent it from occurring, however, the patient may be given an anti-androgen in the early phase of LH-RH therapy.[214]

The second group of side effects is associated with the therapies that target the effect and production of other male androgens. Anti-androgens, for example, can cause diarrhea, nausea and vomiting. They also can cause breast tenderness and even breast growth. Men treated long-term with ketoconazole to block the production of androgens may develop liver problems, and men treated with aminoglutethimide may develop skin rashes. Indeed, a total androgen block may create more side effects than any other single form of hormonal therapy.[215]

Similar to the loss of estrogen in women, any form of therapy that decreases the level of male androgens may result in bone weakness or osteoporosis, especially in older men.[216] These complications, of course, will vary from patient to patient and while many will be temporary, some will be permanent. All cancer treatments carry risks and benefits that must be carefully weighed, yet those that may alter one's basic sexual image of oneself may be more difficult to adjust to and may require additional thought and consideration.

Photodynamic Therapy or Photochemotherapy

More commonly known today as **photodynamic therapy,** or **PDT**, this treatment begins by injecting the patient with a special cancer-fighting chemical. Cells throughout the body then absorb this chemical, yet while it quickly leaves normal cells it remains in cancer cells for a longer period of time. The area in which the tumor has been found is then exposed to a laser light, which enhances the chemical's ability to destroy the cancer cells. PDT may be the treatment of choice for certain cancers where the tumors are small or where other treatments are simply not appropriate for the patient.[217]

For example, in lung cancer cases where surgery is not advisable, PDT may be used to alleviate the symptoms associated with the disease. It may be used to treat blocked airways that impair the patient's ability to breathe properly, or it may be used to control or eliminate bleeding that occurs as a result of the disease. The typical side effects of this therapy will include skin and eye sensitivity to light for a period of several weeks following treatment.

Accordingly, it's advisable for patients to avoid direct sunlight, and even bright indoor light, for a minimum period of six weeks. If this isn't practical, however, the patient must protect her or himself with protective clothing including hats and sunglasses. It's also possible that the skin exposed to the laser light may become swollen, red and even blistered. These side effects, however, are temporary and also may include shortness of breath, coughing or difficulty in swallowing.[218]

It's important to remember that chemotherapy generally, or photochemotherapy specifically, may use a variety of drugs in the treatment. In our section on medical treatments and conditions that contribute to the development of cancer, we discussed a specific form of photochemotherapy known as PUVA, a treatment for skin disorders such as psoriasis that uses a family of drugs known as methoxysporalens, which is sometimes spelled "psoralens." It also may use coal tar ointments to treat the problem skin before applying ultraviolet A light.[219]

Both methoxysporalens and coal tar ointments have been linked to the development of skin cancers in patients who have been exposed to either one.[220] These concerns, however, don't apply to photodynamic therapy in general which utilizes anticancer drugs that haven't been associated with the development of future cancers. Every patient should be aware of the type of drug to which she or he is being exposed, and every patient should question the safety of such drugs until a satisfactory answer is supplied.

Headline:

Female Nonsmokers More Likely to Develop Lung Cancer Than Male Nonsmokers

The untimely death of medical activist Dana Reeve forced the public and medical profession to re-examine the small, yet significant, risk that nonsmokers face from lung cancer. It's true that more female nonsmokers develop the disease than male nonsmokers. The whole truth, however, is that this disparity does not appear to imply there is a greater risk inherent in being female. Rather, it appears the disparity exists simply because there are far more women over sixty who have never smoked than there are men.

Indeed, in the United States census data indicates that there are approximately 16.2 million women in this category compared to approximately 6.4 million men. Clearly, when there are more individuals in a particular group, the chance of developing many diseases becomes greater as well. Even though there are nearly two and a half times more women than men over sixty who have never smoked, and more of these women develop lung cancer more often than their male counterparts, it's the males over sixty who have never smoked who share the higher death rates from lung cancer.[221]

Part 2:
Basic Medical Know How

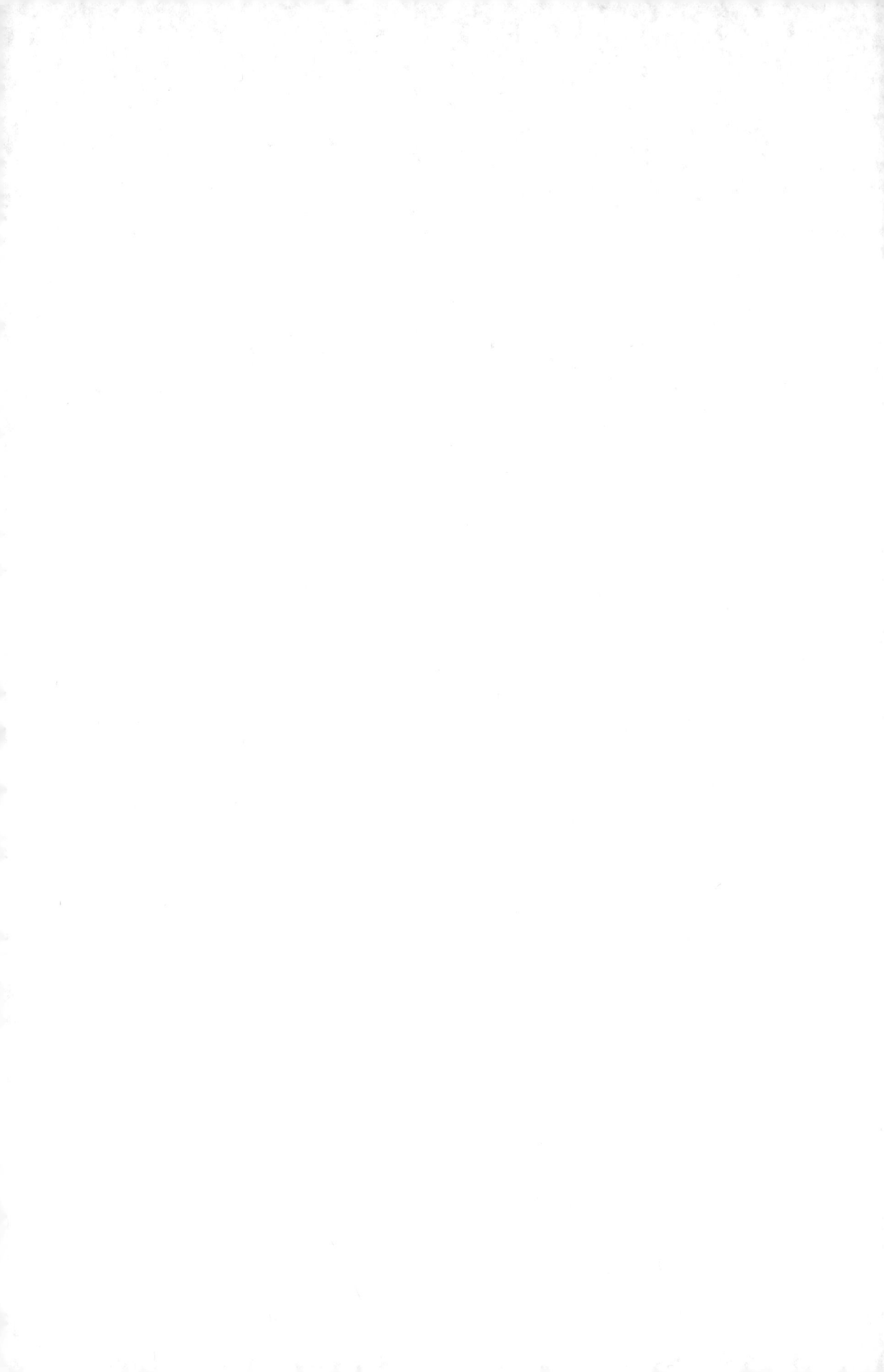

Chapter 2:
What Makes a Good Technician?

Real knowledge is to know the extent of one's ignorance.
Confucius

The ease with which any treatment or procedure is conducted and the comfort afforded the patient greatly depend upon the medical personnel in attendance. The attending technician has the ability to reduce the stress and apprehension associated with medical tests and to make the experience, if not quite pleasant, at least harmless. And, there's a world of difference between a caring and helpful technician and, well, a technician.

There are many things that every technician should incorporate into her or his job, and the overall goal should be to anticipate the patient's fears and insecurities and take the necessary steps to reduce both. A good technician, for example, will always introduce her or himself to the patient and fully describe the procedure the patient is about to undergo. She or he will always review the paperwork with the patient to make sure it's accurate and that the patient, and the procedure, match the name and instructions on the chart. She or he will encourage the patient to ask questions and share any concerns about the procedure. If possible, she or he will maintain communication during the procedure and explain each step as it's conducted.

A good technician takes the initiative to insure the patient's comfort in small ways such as providing two hospital gowns instead of one, a gown to cover the front and another to cover the back. A good x-ray technician will have a blanket nearby to prevent the patient from becoming too cold while waiting in the treatment room. A good mammography technician often will cover the steel plates of the machine with towels or heating pads to warm them before use. Some technicians hold the patient's hand, some place cool compresses on the patient's forehead and some simply provide a calming presence when needed.

A good technician understands her or his limitations and doesn't hesitate to summon additional help if necessary. A good technician will always step aside when another can do a particular job better. If, for example, one technician is having difficulty finding a vein to draw blood or insert an IV, another should promptly be called. Clearly, some technicians have great technical skills while others have great people skills. The trick, of course, is to find a technician who excels at both.

Medical technicians, however, are like any other professional in that their ability to perform their job well involves a learning process. Problems or patient discomfort regarding medical procedures don't always result from indifference or lack of care, but from a lack of knowledge. Some technicians are new on the job and simply inexperienced. In addition, there's a pecking order among medical personnel and assignments that can be a little messy typically are given to junior technicians while other more desirable assignments are saved for those with more seniority.

For example, the simulation process of external radiation often involves working with patients who already are ill with cancer treatment side effects. These patients may not be able to control their bowels, bladders or their nausea. Accidents occur, and it's the job of the technician in charge to oversee these situations and clean up if necessary. Clearly, many technicians don't want these assignments, and as a result, they often are delegated to new personnel who have no choice in the matter.

When this occurs, the inexperienced technician may not know how to handle the situation, may be embarrassed to discuss the patient's condition or simply may not know what to expect. This, of course, is a loss for the patient because it's precisely these sensitive situations that most require the presence of an experienced and understanding technician. Should this be the case, the patient will have to assume responsibility for her or his own comfort and will have to initiate communication if the attending technician appears to lack the experience or knowledge to do so.

Overall, however, a good technician has the ability to make any patient feel comfortable in situations that are anything but. A good technician brings a balance of medical knowledge and personal sensitivity to the job. A good technician exercises good communication skills and is proactive in the care of the patient. A good technician can make all the difference in the world for a patient by turning a situation that's uncomfortable and frightening into one that is reassuring, protective and informative.

Chapter 3:
What Makes a Good Doctor?

Obviously, many of the qualities that make a good technician also make a good doctor. Once again, a good doctor must combine the technical qualities of the profession with excellent people skills, or what often is called a "good bedside manner." A good doctor anticipates the fear of the patient and understands the impact a diagnosis of cancer makes on an individual and the individual's life. A good doctor will encourage the patient to ask as many questions as possible about the illness and the appropriate treatments, and if the doctor will be conducting a significant procedure her or himself, she or he will call the patient the night before to explain the procedure fully and assuage any doubts the patient may have.

The doctor should always provide adequate time so that the patient never feels rushed when discussing important issues. A good doctor will explain and answer all questions in terms the patient understands and will explain more than once if necessary. She or he should be available to the patient as much as scheduling permits and certainly whenever the patient's medical condition requires attention. This also means the doctor should make sure the patient is able to make personal contact in case of emergency, or at least know where to go and who to call if the doctor is unavoidably unavailable.

In addition to the illness, a good doctor should be willing to discuss the costs associated with the medical care and the facility in which the patient will receive this care. The patient shouldn't have to wait excessively long periods of time to see the doctor, and although emergencies may occur, lateness in seeing the patient shouldn't be a habit.

A good doctor will support a patient's decision to seek a second, third or fourth opinion and will willingly compare notes. In the best of situations, the doctor will encourage the patient to participate in the decisions regarding treatment and health care and promote a true team effort with doctor and patient working in concert to reach a common goal. For like a good technician, a good doctor can make an enormous difference in the life of a cancer patient by guiding the individual through this difficult period of time with knowledge, compassion and sensitivity.

The Quarterback Doctor

We've discussed the qualities a patient should look for and expect in her or his doctor in any medical situation. With cancer patients, however, we need to go one step further. For treating cancer is not only a team effort that involves the physician and patient, it's a process that involves many health care specialists whose expertise becomes essential at different stages of the patient's treatment. In most cancer cases, with the exception of early skin cancers, this team will include an oncologist and, in addition, may include a surgeon, a radiologist, a radiation oncologist, radiation therapists and technicians, nurses, a dietician, a nutritionist, a gynecologist, a fertility specialist, a pain management advisor, a plastic or cosmetic surgeon, a physical therapist, a psychiatrist or psychologist, alternative medical practitioners, and perhaps a social worker or family services representative.

The health care team for one cancer patient can be enormous, and a multitude of decisions concerning the patient's treatment and welfare will have to be made on a daily basis. Decisions regarding which therapies will be necessary, how often the therapies should be administered, which physicians should be consulted, what drugs should be used, which facilities offer the best specialized care, and what patient concerns need to be addressed immediately is an ongoing and complicated process. Accordingly, it's essential for every patient to have one primary "go to" physician who can oversee the entire operation and coordinate every aspect of the patient's treatment.

Appropriately, we'll call this indispensable physician the **quarterback doctor**. This is the individual who will lead the entire team, call all the shots, oversee each play and take full responsibility for every diagnostic and therapeutic effort made on the patient's behalf. One's quarterback doctor may be the patient's personal family physician, the patient's primary oncologist or another trusted physician. The choice will be up to the patient, yet one must choose a physician fully qualified to advise the patient on the entire treatment and recovery process. The physician as well must be willing to accept the role and to commit to the patient's long-term recovery and continuing care.

This is the individual whom the cancer patient will come to rely upon more than any other medical caregiver on the team. This is the individual who will communicate with the patient on a continued and perhaps daily basis throughout the patient's diagnosis, treatment and rehabilitation. This is the individual who will coordinate the medications, handle additional doctor referrals, juggle multiple medical appointments and organize the patient's treatment schedule.

She or he will assemble a medical team and arrange the meetings and conference calls that may be necessary among the various members. She or he will make sure that each member of the team is aware of every other member and that each knows what the others are doing for the patient at any given time. It's the quarterback doctor who will keep track of the records, test results, x-rays, CT scans and lab work and will make them available to the other team members whenever required. And, it's the quarterback doctor who will keep the ball rolling when fatigue, or illness, or pain prevents the patient from actively engaging in her or his own recovery process.

What Makes a Good Doctor?

Clearly, this is an extremely important relationship that requires thoughtful and thorough consideration on the part of the patient. If the patient becomes disenchanted with her or his choice after the treatment process has begun, starting over with a new physician may be difficult and stressful. Obviously, anything that makes this already trying situation more so should be avoided if at all possible.

On the other hand, the quarterback doctor that is chosen wisely will be an indispensable partner for the patient and the patient's family. She or he will be a true professional asset who will assume responsibility for the technical organization and business aspects of the patient's recovery process while the patient is simply allowed to recover.

Personal Note

In my case, my quarterback doctor was my oncologist. His knowledge, compassion, ability to manage and willingness to help were instrumental in my recovery and survival. The process would have been so much more difficult without him. Thank you, Michael.

Chapter 4:
What Makes a Good Patient?

The ease of a patient's recovery is dependent only in part upon the skill and accessibility of the medical team with which one is surrounded. Technicians, nurses, physicians, and even one's quarterback doctor, can only help the patient to the extent the patient allows. For just as the patient has the right to certain expectations regarding the medical professionals tending her or his case, these professionals also have the right to certain expectations regarding the patient.

Etiquette

First and foremost, perhaps, the patient needs to remember that each technician, each nurse and each physician or specialist responsible for the patient is responsible for many other patients as well. These professionals are extremely busy, and most do their best to accommodate and care for several cancer patients each and every day. It's essential for each patient, therefore, to be aware and considerate of the rights of other patients as well as the medical personnel.

For example, when a patient has an appointment, the patient must be on time for that appointment. It only takes one patient, late for one appointment, to make any physician run late for the rest of the day. And, of course, when the physician is kept waiting, the physician's staff is kept waiting and the remainder of the physician's patients are kept waiting.

While every patient should expect promptness from the physician, a good patient, out of consideration for the physician and other patients, should be prompt in return. If it isn't possible to make an appointment or to arrive on time, a good patient will always notify the physician and the appropriate staff as soon as possible.

A good patient will communicate clearly with the medical personnel and make her or his doubts, fears and needs about the medical treatment known, and a good patient will separate her or his demands and expectations that are reasonable from those that are not, and will eliminate the latter. A good patient will make sure the physician has a complete medical history and all the information necessary for proper treatment.

This, of course, includes any risk information that may be related to the patient's cancer, such as genetic factors and family medical history, workplace situations or lifestyle and personal habits. Without such information, the physician cannot provide the best and most appropriate care. A good patient also makes sure that she or he understands everything the physician says and requests explanations if anything is unclear.

And, a good patient always follows the physician's instructions and directions regarding the patient's treatment.

On the other hand, if the patient refuses recommended treatment or fails to follow medical instructions for whatever reason, a good patient will realize that she or he is responsible for this decision and the consequences that may result. A good patient also realizes that the financial obligations incurred as a result of her or his medical care are a responsibility the patient must address and resolve in a timely fashion.

A good patient is responsible for following all the facility's policies and procedures and showing appreciation for the professionals involved in the complicated treatment process. When any member of this team has performed a job well, be it a major miracle or a small kindness, a good patient acknowledges the effort. A simple "thank you" is a common courtesy often overlooked in the rush and confusion of medical situations. This simple phrase can go a long way in forging a positive and mutually rewarding relationship between the patient and her or his caregivers.

Empowerment

Clearly, the technicians and physicians as well as the entire medical team are vital and necessary components of the treatment and recovery process. Yet, as important as each of these professionals is, none is as important as the patient her or himself. And as much as each of these professionals may care for the patient, or as much as one's family and friends may care for the patient, no one will care as much as the patient.

For, it's the patient's life that's in question and the patient's health that's at stake. It's the patient who stands to win or lose the most. Accordingly, it's the patient who must assume primary responsibility for every aspect of her or his illness and recovery. Through acceptance, communication and confidence, a good patient can develop the tools that will empower her or him and insure a "hands on" recovery process in which the patient is the primary participant.

Acceptance

The empowerment process, of course, begins the instant an individual suspects that something is wrong. It may begin with a skin discoloration, a small lump, a change in bowel habits, unexplained fatigue, weight loss or any of the symptoms we've already discussed. It may begin with something less obvious, a feeling or an instinct that something isn't quite right or that one's body isn't functioning in quite its typical way. As we know, no two human bodies are exactly the same, and what is typical or normal for one may be atypical or abnormal for another.

Indeed, most initial suspicions arise purely by accident in the course of one's routine activities, such as exercising, dressing or bathing. It's this first moment of recognition, however, that's the most important part of the empowerment process. It's in this moment that the individual must acknowledge the possible existence of a problem and must take the appropriate action.

It also is in this first moment that the individual may face her or his greatest obstacle to taking appropriate action – denial. Denial is a natural human mechanism that allows an individual to avoid emotional conflict and anxiety by refusing to acknowledge the thoughts or feelings the individual finds intolerable. Moreover, denial is difficult to overcome because it's largely an unconscious mechanism and, as a result, one may not even be aware of its presence.

In contrast, acceptance requires one to make a conscious choice based upon solid knowledge and information. To begin, one must have a complete understanding of one's own Risk Profile. One must know the cancers for which she or he may be at risk. One must know what cancers run in her or his family and what genetic qualities make one more likely to develop certain cancers. One must know what cancers may be associated with one's workplace or with one's lifestyle. One must understand cancer risk analysis and know how to limit or avoid potential problems. One must undergo regular cancer screening procedures and know the baseline results that indicate personal normalcy. One must be familiar with one's own body and the way it works, and one must conduct thorough self-exams. And, one must understand and be able to recognize the symptoms commonly associated with cancer.

It's through this pro-active approach to cancer prevention that one's awareness about the disease will increase. As one's awareness is increased, the vague notion of cancer is transformed from a shadowy image into a concrete reality that must be acknowledged. It pushes the idea of cancer from a repressed subconscious thought to the forefront of our conscious mind. Once this is accomplished, it's easier for an individual to recognize a potential problem and once a problem is recognized, it's easier for an individual to make a conscious decision to act. And, once an individual takes action, help can be obtained and the false safety of denial can be avoided.

Communication

Overcoming denial, however, is only the first step in the empowerment process. Once a potential problem is recognized, it's essential for the individual to clearly and promptly communicate that recognition to the appropriate professionals. There was a time when most patients simply accepted the advice of a physician completely and without question. Indeed, there was a time when most patients were content to let their physicians make all the decisions and to simply follow instructions. Clearly, this isn't the way that medical situations are best handled today.

Today, the best medical treatment is the result of a continuous dialogue between the physician and the patient. A good patient is one who actively participates in her or his entire treatment process. It's up to the patient to describe in detail the symptoms she or he is experiencing, when the symptoms began, what makes them worse and what makes better. It's up to the patient to follow up with telephone calls, doctor appointments and the scheduling of tests and procedures. The patient must choose the quarterback doctor, choose a treatment facility and inform family, friends and employers of the situation.

Indeed, of all the responsibilities the patient will be required to assume and all the tasks she or he must undertake, the ability to communication clearly will prove most valuable. Good communication is essential in conveying one's wishes, describing one's discomfort or concern and questioning anything that's unclear. Indeed, a good patient will continue to ask questions until each and every one has been answered to the patient's satisfaction, and a good patient will always feel free to consult additional physicians if necessary.

Further, if any problem should arise in one's relationship with one's doctor, it's the patient's responsibility to communicate her or his concern, ask for explanations and request certain changes. If this direct approach fails to produce the desired results, the patient must find another doctor. For just as there are doctors who will fail to meet the patient's expectations, there are those who will far exceed those same expectations.

Confidence

Empowerment also demands that the patient have confidence in oneself, one's abilities and one's judgment. The patient must trust in her or his knowledge of one's body and in one's ability to recognize physical problems. The patient must have confidence in one's instincts and feelings and know that seeking professional advice and confirmation is right and necessary. Moreover, in seeking professional help, the patient must never allow her or himself to be bullied or intimidated by any member of the medical profession.

This is a crucial point in that many individuals have a tendency to disregard their own beliefs or feelings when in the presence of a physician. Doctors, more than any other professional, are often considered by others to be infallible individuals whose word or opinion should never be questioned. They're often seen as all knowing, all wise individuals who are superior beings incapable of making a mistake. This, of course, is a misconception that can create an uncomfortable and in some cases, a harmful situation for the patient. And, this is something the good patient must strive to overcome.

In overcoming this medical myth, one needs to remember that a doctor, like everyone else, is simply a human being. As a human being, a doctor like everyone else can be rude, wrong, tired, confused and very capable of making mistakes. While the field of medicine is a highly trained profession, the patient may need to be reminded that, like any other profession, every class has someone who graduates last. Like any other profession, fifty percent of each year's graduates are in the bottom half of the class.

Of course, academics remain an important factor one must consider when engaging the services of any professional. Yet, academic excellence isn't the whole story and certainly isn't enough to guarantee a good doctor. There are many different factors that must come together to make a good doctor, including experience, dedication, sensitivity, compassion and intuition. One who may excel in academic technicalities may completely lack the ability to relate to patients on a personal level and to engage successfully in the all-important "bedside manner."

Unfortunately, every professional training program graduates individuals who probably should never have entered the program in the first place and who will never really be qualified to perform the job for which they've been trained. Whether we're speaking about attorneys, plumbers, accountants, teachers or doctors, this is a truth every individual must keep in mind. While every professional can make mistakes, those made in the medical arena of life and death can be irreversible and devastating.

Accordingly, whenever a patient begins to feel uncomfortable with a doctor, or believes she or he is being ignored or not taken seriously by the doctor, it's crucial for the patient to stand her or his ground. One must remain confident in one's own judgment. One must trust in oneself. A doctor may ultimately disagree with the patient's concerns, but the patient should never allow her or himself to be dismissed without receiving the doctor's full attention in the form of a complete consultation or a thorough examination, either of which may confirm or refute the patient's concerns.

Personal Note

The first time I began to suspect that something was wrong with me, I visited a physician who specialized in gastroenterology. I described my symptoms which included abdominal bloating, a feeling of fullness even after using the bathroom and a persistent fatigue. The specialist, however, dismissed my complaints, and when I actually asked if I could have cancer, the specialist laughed and replied, "Of course not! You're too young!"

I continued to insist something was wrong and the specialist, clearly tired of wasting time and deciding to humor me, finally agreed to conduct a seigmoidoscopy. The reluctant specialist, however, had a complete change of mood when the test revealed a large polyp in my intestinal tract. This specialist, who had openly considered me to be a hypochondriac, couldn't look me in the eye as the news was delivered. After saying, "Sorry. You have an abnormal growth, and you must contact a surgeon immediately," the specialist went down the hall, into an office and closed the door.

I didn't realize until later what the specialist obviously realized then, that if I had relied upon this person and had ignored my own judgment, it might have cost me my life. I also was fortunate in that my growth was located in the two-thirds of the descending colon and, therefore, detectable through a seigmoidoscopy. And, while many anomalies can be removed during this procedure mine was too advanced and, as it turned out, malignant.

Another aspect of patient confidence, however, is the ability to recognize one's lack of confidence and one's own limitations. Confidence regarding medical issues may be a trait that develops over a period of time, and some patients may not believe themselves capable of managing the treatment and recovery process in the beginning stages. Initially, some patients may feel too exhausted, too confused or too frightened to take charge. They may be distracted and unable to concentrate or listen carefully.

If this is the case, it's important for the patient to enlist the help of a trusted friend or family member to assist whenever necessary. The patient, for example, may need someone with her or him when undergoing the required diagnostic tests or when the results of those tests are delivered. The patient may need someone to help prepare a list of questions before meeting with a doctor and someone to take notes during the appointments or, with the doctor's permission, record the sessions. The patient may need someone to help schedule appointments, organize paperwork and file important telephone numbers and addresses.

Ultimately, the patient simply may need someone to take charge of the process and protect the patient's rights until the patient feels confident enough to manage these tasks on one's own. Knowing when to ask for help is an important part of being a good patient. Even if confidence is lacking, the patient should never be in the position of blindly following medical advice without a trusted individual helping the patient to carefully analyze all the options and possibilities presented.

Entitlement

Acceptance and communication, however, only constitute a part of the empowerment process. In addition to these responsibilities the patient also has a number of personal and legal rights of which she or he must be aware and take steps to protect. We already have touched upon many of the personal rights to which every patient is entitled in the above sections. For example, every patient has the right to participate in her or his plan of treatment and the decisions regarding the appropriate medical care. This, of course, also includes the patient's right to refuse treatment and leave the hospital or treatment facility at any time, even if this goes against the advice of one's physician.

Similarly, every patient has the right to refuse access to student physicians and interns who are not directly involved with the patient, but are simply trying to further their education. Every patient has the right to receive care that's considerate, respectful and provided within a safe environment. Every patient also has the right to expect a reasonable response to any reasonable request she or he may make for service during the course of treatment. Every patient has the right to receive complete information regarding her or his cancer, the available treatments and one's prognosis in language that the patient fully comprehends.

To this end, a critical aspect of every patient's treatment and recovery process should include the maintenance of a **medical diary**. Be it a tablet, a notebook or a computer file, this diary should include notes on every step of one's treatment, the name of every medication and the date of every procedure. It not only will help the patient to remember and organize her or his own questions, it will be essential when dealing with financial and insurance matters down the road.

In addition, every patient should be advised of the **grievance process** of the facility in which she or he receives treatment. This knowledge will prove useful if anything occurs during the course of treatment that's perceived by the patient to be harmful to or disrespectful of her or his rights. Concerns regarding the quality of care or disagreements with the administration of facility policies all may need to be communicated through a specific procedure.

Usually, this procedure will include 1) a verbal notification to the contact person in charge of grievances for the facility, 2) the preparation of a written notice detailing the problem or grievance, 3) an internal investigation of the grievance and, 4) the preparation of a written reply to the patient outlining the steps of the investigation taken on her or his behalf, the final determination of the grievance and the date the investigation was completed.[222] It also is important for every patient to understand that the information contained within her or his medical record and the results of every test procedure, down to each x-ray, blood test, urine analysis and body temperature reading, is property that belongs to the patient as much as it does to the health care facility.

Knowing this, the patient has the right to request copies of any or all of the information in her or his medical file and to be provided with this information within forty-eight hours of making the request. Moreover, every patient has the right to examine and receive a full explanation of all the charges that appear on the patient's bill regardless of the manner or source of payment.[223]

In addition, there are a number of important legal rights that affect every patient and apply to every medical facility and health care provider. We'll divide these rights into two basic groups, including those that pertain to the patient's **decision-making power** and those that pertain to the patient's **expectation of privacy**. First, every patient possesses the ultimate control to decide what is and what is not done to their bodies or minds while under professional medical care. The patient makes the final decision as to what tests, procedures, therapies and drugs will or will not be administered during her or his course of treatment.

This is the rule, yet like every rule, this rule has its exceptions. For example, the patient's decision-making power regarding medical treatment only exists as long as the patient is of "sound mind." The patient must be **legally competent,** which means the patient must have the ability to understand the nature and effect of the acts in which the patient is engaged.[224] Conversely, one who's deemed incompetent lacks the ability to make or carry out important decisions regarding one's affairs. Each patient, however, is presumed to be competent and capable of controlling her or his medical treatment until proven otherwise.

Indeed, the question of competency regarding an adult cancer patient typically won't be an issue unless the patient also is affected by additional medical conditions such as mental retardation, another debilitating illness, injury or senility that interferes with one's decision making ability. In cancer cases where the patient is a minor, however, it's typically the parent or guardian who retains the legal power to make final decisions regarding the minor's health care. Further, there are situations in which the patient, although competent, may lose this right of self-determination.[225]

This may occur, for example, if the patient's life is endangered due to the patient's refusal to undergo specifically recommended care. This right also may be lost if another person who is dependent upon the patient faces harm due to the patient's refusal of treatment.[226] Of course, depending upon the state, national or provincial laws that govern the individuals and the facilities in question, this patient right will vary. The fundamental issue of patient control over her or his own body, however, remains fairly constant throughout the world's medical communities.

Ideally, of course, the medical providers, the patient and the patient's family will all come to an agreement concerning the patient's care and course of medical treatment. When an agreement is reached, consent from the patient or the patient's legal guardian is required before any medical procedure can be performed. This consent is often communicated verbally although it also may be obtained through a signed **informed consent agreement**. In the latter, **informed consent** simply means that the patient and/or the patient's family have been given complete information regarding the risks and benefits of the treatment and that the information was clearly understood before consent was given.[227]

It's possible, however, for a cancer patient to encounter an emergency situation in which she or he is too ill, unconscious or otherwise incapacitated and unable to give consent for immediate treatment. In such cases, treatment still may be given based upon a legal term known as **implied consent**. If this is the case, it's presumed under the law that the patient would have given consent if able and, therefore, the consent is deemed given and the treatment may take place.[228]

Sometimes patients wish to plan in advance of a possible emergency and record their treatment choices in writing. This may occur in situations where the patient has a number of medical problems in addition to the cancer, where the patient wants to avoid burdening others with making decisions on the patient's behalf or where the patient has no family close by to rely upon. Through a variety of legal documents known as **advanced directives,** a patient can clearly communicate specific information about the types of medical care or life-sustaining measures that the patient does or does not want provided.[229]

Indeed, some patients use an advanced directive to simply state one's beliefs or personal values that may become issues during the course of treatment. Among these directives are a **Designation of Health Care Surrogate**, a **Durable Power of Attorney for Health Care** and a **Health Care Living Will**. While each document will vary in structure, all are similar in that each names the person or persons authorized to make the health care decisions on the patient's behalf should the patient, for any reason, be unable to make such decisions on her or his own.[230]

These documents also will vary depending upon the state, country or province in which the patient resides and a document that is legal in one location may not be legal in another. It's necessary, therefore, for any patient interested in preparing an advanced directive to consult first with her or his health care provider. Both the physician and the facility will have experience with these documents and will be able to advise the patient accordingly. Further, many of these directives can be prepared by the patient her or himself by following simple procedures or by filling out a printed form.

As a result, it's not necessary for the patient to hire an attorney to prepare the document. Consulting an attorney may be helpful, however, in answering questions concerning the status and validity of such a document in the region in which the patient and health care provider reside. Once the document is prepared, the patient should make sure that her or his physician and facility, the individuals designated in the document and trusted family members all read the document and retain copies.

In any case, an advanced directive is one way to assure the patient she or he will be treated precisely as she or he desires throughout the course of treatment.

Moreover, a written document communicating one's wishes is always preferable to an oral communication and, in some instances, is the only method that has legal status. Wishes and directives communicated verbally can be difficult to prove and, therefore, difficult to enforce. A written document, however, will insure both in practical and legal terms that one's wishes will be carried out as requested. In the event of an unexpected health complication or medical emergency, the patient won't have to rely upon the judgment of another person to handle the situation or burden another person with this important decision making.

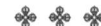

Headline:

Patient Dies after Receiving Organs
From Incompatible Blood Type Donor

Unfortunately, this headline is true. It also is true that hospital errors occur more commonly than one might expect. In this particular case, the patient received a heart and lung transplant after waiting for a year. No one, however, including the attending physicians, surgeons or nurses, noticed that the transplant organs contained type A blood and the patient's blood was type O.

Once again, no one can afford to withdraw from her or his medical treatment and trust others to do the right thing. Each patient must take an active role in each step of treatment to help insure personal safety. One must read one's own medical chart and make sure the information contained within it is correct. One must make sure the name is correct on the chart, the diagnosis is correct, the blood type is correct and one's allergies or other special considerations are listed.

The patient, or the patient's designated advocate, must carefully examine all medications the patient receives. And, before undergoing any surgery, one must make sure one's name is correct on one's wrist tag and the right organ or area to be operated upon has been properly identified. This is an issue the importance of which cannot be over emphasized.[231]

Privacy Issues

Protecting the privacy of patients has been an essential element of the physician's ethical code of conduct since the Hippocratic Oath was created in the fourth century B.C.[232] Yet, in today's world there are many entities in addition to one's physician who have become necessary parts of each and every patient's treatment and recovery. Insuring prompt and effective health care for a patient has become an enormous undertaking in which many health care practices and communications play an essential role. Further, the nature of these practices and communications and the medical surroundings in which most patients receive their health care combine to create an environment in which the protection of the patient's health information and privacy may be compromised.

In many parts of the world, whenever a patient is admitted to a health care facility, an enormous amount of private information may be requested in addition to the basic information regarding one's physical health. For example, one's medical record may include information about one's family, family history or family relationships, the number of one's dependents, their names and ages, the number of pregnancies and one's marital status.

The record may include information on one's past or present substance abuse, sexual history and behavior and one's mental health. One's education, employment history, place of residence and contact numbers, emergency contact numbers, driver's license, insurance coverage and one's social security or personal identification number may be included. Unfortunately, while much of this information may be necessary to establish the guidelines for one's medical treatment, its misuse can prove very harmful. For instance, such information may be used to negatively influence one's employment and educational opportunities, one's credit and financial status, one's ability to obtain health insurance and the rates one must pay once health insurance is obtained. The knowledge that other individuals, most of them strangers, have access to information that details the most intimate aspects of one's life can create discomfort, humiliation and a sense of personal invasion. Clearly, this potential for such breaches to occur has forced many of the world's medical and legal communities to join forces and implement laws designed to minimize this threat and insure reasonable safeguards.

The laws governing privacy issues will, of course, vary depending upon the location of the health care facility. It's the facility, not the individual patient, that's required to implement and follow the guidelines provided by the state, provincial and national governments in question. In most countries, the confidentiality of medical records was for many decades protected by the family physician who sealed the records in a file cabinet and simply refused access to any unauthorized personnel. In the information age of today, however, medical records are faxed, e-mailed and dispersed throughout a network of computer systems that connect a plethora of health care providers, treatment facilities, insurance companies and financial institutions to one another.[233]

Further, many of these individuals and organizations, such as government program officials, insurance representatives, attorneys and employers, aren't governed by the codes of medical ethics, as are those in the medical professions. This confidential information, therefore, becomes easily accessible to a number of different entities from a number of different sources. While it's customary for all health care providers and facilities to make reasonable efforts to protect this highly sensitive information, safeguards may not be present once this information is in the hands of others.

The various governmental systems designed to protect an individual's health information typically are complex and incomplete. In the United States, for example, the regulatory guidelines for protecting this information was for many years outlined in a fragmented framework of state laws that left significant gaps in the rules of patient confidentiality. Some protections were limited to specific groups, such as school children or government employees. Some only applied to certain types of medical information such as that related to substance abuse or to certain medical conditions such as HIV and AIDS. Some protections overlapped one another while others fell short of comprehensive and complete coverage.[234]

As the uses and requests of medical information multiplied, however, the United States Congress recognized the need to adopt a national standard, which addressed the privacy rights of all medical patients. The result of this recognition was the **Health Insurance Portability and Accountability Act of 1996**, also known as the **HIPAA Privacy Rule**, the first federally regulated guideline for protecting patient confidentiality.[235]

The Rule, which came into effect in April 2003, was designed to save health care facilities and businesses money by encouraging electronic transactions. Yet, the Rule also set forth new guidelines to protect the privacy and security of that transferred electronic information and guaranteed patients new rights regarding the misuse and disclosure of their health records. Essentially, the Rule provides a "federal floor" that insures a minimum amount of protection for all patients and allows existing state laws that may offer even more protection to stay in effect.[236] Like many legal documents, the Rule is rather cumbersome and complicated. Yet, we'll attempt to simplify its provisions so that a bare bones understanding of its policies will be possible.

First, the fundamental premise of the Rule states that 1) certain uses and disclosures of personal medical information is permissible and that, 2) certain incidental uses and disclosures that occur as a result or by-product of a permissible use or disclosure are also permissible if, 3) the individual or facility has exercised "reasonable safeguards" and "minimum necessary standards" with respect to the primary use or disclosure. In other words, accidents happen. Private information must be used or disclosed responsibly and appropriately to be lawful, and if this is done, any misuse of that information that occurs unintentionally or by accident may be lawful as well.[237]

First, let's explain what is meant by the term "reasonable safeguards." This term is a variation of the well-known **reasonable standard**, a flexible legal term used in a number of different contexts. It can apply to an individual or an industry, and essentially means that the person or business in question generally will be deemed to have acted lawfully if the entity behaved the way any other reasonable person or business in similar circumstances would have behaved.[238]

In this case, the term implies that any physician's office, hospital, facility or other "covered entity" must behave reasonably and exercise common sense in conducting business. Of course, the standard will vary from one entity to another depending upon many factors such as the size of the facility in question, the amount of money it has available to provide security measures and train personnel, and the nature of the entity's business. In exercising this common sense, the entity must understand its own circumstances and needs as well as those of the patient.[239]

It also must acknowledge the sensitivity of the information it possesses and the risk any misuse of this information may present for a patient. For instance, the practice of isolating or locking records rooms and file cabinets may be considered a reasonable safeguard. The use of additional security measures such as access passwords for computers and records that maintain personal health information may be considered reasonable. Training personnel to speak quietly in waiting rooms, hallways and elevators when discussing a patient may be considered reasonable. [240]

Similarly, signs and interoffice memorandums reminding employees to avoid using the patient's name whenever possible and avoid leaving patient files unattended may be considered reasonable. Furthermore, some facilities require a "code word" from all telephone inquiries regarding a patient, even if the inquiry comes from a patient's family members. These are all examples of appropriate physical, technical and administrative safeguards that health care and information specialists should provide to comply with the new Privacy Rule.

To fully comply, however, these entities also need to implement the "minimum necessary standard" procedures and policies to **limit the amount of health information** used or disclosed for specific purposes. These minimum necessary standards also must **limit the number of individuals** who have access to protected health information. For instance, if an insurance carrier requires financial information about a patient and the necessary information can be obtained from one page of a patient's file, it may not be lawful under the Rule for the carrier to receive the patient's entire file.[241]

Similarly, if an employee who answers telephones or conducts elevator maintenance within a facility has access to patient medical records that have nothing to do with the employee's job, the access is inappropriate and possibly unlawful under the Rule. In fact, if it appears that an employee has routine and unimpeded access to patient medical records when access isn't necessary to the employee's job, the facility clearly isn't applying the minimum necessary standard, and this disclosure of information would be unlawful under the Rule.

Further, if another employee should accidentally overhear this first unauthorized employee discussing this private information that, too, would be an unlawful disclosure under the Rule. On the other hand, the Rule doesn't apply to disclosures among health care providers who need to share medical information for purposes of treating the patient. In these cases a physician, for instance, isn't required to limit the amount of information disclosed when discussing a patient's medical record with another physician or specialist.

Under the Rule, the covered entity has the responsibility of protecting every patient's private medical information from misuse. Further, the ways in which the entity must fulfill this responsibility are fairly clearly outlined under the Rule, and some of these include the requirement that the entity provide patients with a clear written explanation of how the entity may use and disclose the patient's private information.[242] This explains why those of us who have been to a physician's office, hospital, clinic or other facility in the United States within the last few years have been given a lengthy typed form at the beginning of our appointment.

It's this form that outlines the situations in which the entity may lawfully use and disclose the patient's private health information. The entity, however, still cannot use the information without first obtaining the patient's consent to do so. This, of course, is why every patient is asked to sign the form. Now, in the instance the entity wants to use a patient's private information in some way that has nothing to do with the patient's health care, the entity must obtain an additional and separate authorization from the patient before acting.[243]

In general, the entity also will have to adopt a written policy that states how protected information will be used within the entity, who within the entity has access to the information and when the information may be disclosed to others outside the entity. In addition, when this information is disclosed, the entity must take steps to insure that these other entities and business associates take precautions to protect the information as well. Under the Rule, the entity also is charged with training its employees in privacy procedures and appointing one individual to make sure the procedures are followed.[244]

In return, the patient has a number of specific rights of which she or he should be aware. While we have already touched upon a few of these rights in our previous discussions, others may be new. First, under the Rule, the patient has the right to inspect and copy the entity's privacy policies as well as any information held by the entity that pertains to the patient's health care. If an entity's privacy policies are amended in any way, the patient has the right to request a copy of those amendments. If any disclosures of the patient's private information for purposes other than treatment, health care issues and payment have been made by the entity, the patient has a right to obtain an accounting of those disclosures.[245]

In addition to the privacy policies of the patient's primary physician or facility, the patient also has the right to receive a **Notice of Privacy Practices** from every other entity in the health care system with which the primary entity does business. Further, the patient has the right to request that confidential communications regarding her or his health be transmitted or mailed to any telephone number or address she or he chooses.[246]

Indeed, the patient has the right to request restrictions on the use and disclosure of private information, although the entity isn't required to follow the restrictions and retains the right to make the final decision. Under the Rule the patient has the right to file a formal complaint with the U.S. Secretary of Health and Human Services as well as the entity if the patient disagrees with the entity's privacy policies or if the entity violates any provision of the Rule.[247]

While these privacy issues will apply to all cancer patients, some cancer patients will be faced with additional privacy concerns. For example, some individuals with cancer may have developed the disease, at least in part, as a result of substance abuse, AIDS or a genetic predisposition. In these situations, the policies designed to protect one's private health information under the Rule may not apply.

In some situations, the use and disclosure of a patient's private information may be exempt from the Rule's protection or it may be governed by a different law. In the United States, the **Public Health Service Act** protects information related to substance abuse and chemical dependency treatment. This Act takes precedence over the Privacy Rule as well as various state laws even if the state laws provide greater protection than the Act. The Act requires that the disclosure of information regarding one's substance abuse or chemical dependency may only take place with the individual's signed authorization.[248]

The exception applies to information exchanged among different entities of the United States Armed Services and in many cases any entity that's federally conducted or funded such as the Medicaid program. Under these circumstances, the transfer of information revealing one's history of substance abuse or chemical dependency doesn't require the individual's signed authorization.[249]

The disclosure of personal health information that contains one's HIV or AIDS status again will vary depending upon the state, province or country in which one resides. In the United States, state law rather than federal law controls information relating to one's HIV or AIDS status. Similarly, state law typically controls the disclosure of private health information in situations where a patient is diagnosed with an HIV or AIDS-related cancer. The protections these laws provide vary greatly, however, with some states prohibiting the release of HIV/AIDS related information without the written consent of the patient.[250]

Some states allow disclosure of this information to certain individuals, such as school officials and law enforcement authorities. Other states designate HIV/AIDS-related information as "super confidential," which imposes specific burdens upon entities and gives patients a large amount of control over any disclosure. Some states limit disclosure of this information to entities defined by law as having a "need to know" which pertains to personnel within the entity itself. In contrast, some states grant "broad discretion" to health facilities giving them the right to subjectively assess the need for protecting third parties, public health and disease surveillance and investigation.[251]

In health situations that involve a communicable disease, it's always difficult to balance the individual's right to privacy with the need to control or prevent the spread of the disease. In such cases, it has long been customary for the disease to be reported to public health authorities directly responsible for this task such as state and local health departments, the Food and Drug Administration and the Centers for Disease Control and Prevention.

Indeed, the Rule does address this issue and permits an entity to disclose private health information without patient consent to public health authorities for the purpose of disease control and prevention. In general, however, covered entities are required to comply with both the Rule and the state law, if possible. In many instances where the Rule and the state law are in conflict, the entity must comply with the Rule.[252]

In situations where the state law agrees with the Rule, but offers more protection and in situations that involve the reporting of disease, public health surveillance and public health investigation or intervention state law rules. It's essential, therefore, for any cancer patient affected with HIV, AIDS or another communicable disease to become familiar with the privacy laws of the state in which her or his health care provider is located.

For many cancer patients, their illness and genetic background are intimately intertwined. As we know, some of the most common cancers are largely influenced by an individual's heredity. Under the Rule, genetic information is generally considered to be protected health information.[253] Genetic information, however, is sensitive in nature, and the potential harm that might result from its misuse could be significant. Recognizing this, the United States Congress introduced special legislation for the protection of this information in 1997. The result of this legislation was the **Genetics Nondiscrimination Act**, passed by the Senate Committee on Health, Education, Labor and Pensions in 2003.

This Act provides basic protections for genetic information such as prohibiting its use in employment decisions. It also prohibits health insurance plans from denying enrollment or charging higher premiums based upon an individual's or family member's genetic information. In addition, these basic genetic-related provisions combined with those found in the Rule and the various measures that as of 2004 had been passed by 43 states, provide solid protection for all patients and their genetic information.[254]

So what can a patient do to protect her or his medical history and private health information? The most important thing one can do is to protect one's national or governmental personal identification card or number. This protection is essential, for it's this data that is often the key to an individual's entire file of personal history and medical information. In the United States, this identification is one's social security number, and it's common for financial institutions, employers and educational facilities as well as medical and dental entities to ask for this number on a variety of forms and applications. While this information is necessary in many cases, it may not be necessary in others. Accordingly, one must carefully consider the need for sharing this information before doing so.

In medical situations, for example, requesting one's social security number may be necessary to coordinate one's files from different physicians or facilities, to access information regarding one's past treatment or test results, or to organize payment and insurance matters. If, however, one is simply meeting a physician for a consultation, seeking a second opinion or getting a flu shot or a cavity filled, it clearly may not be necessary for the provider to have one's social security information.

Further, if a small medical procedure is covered by a cash payment rather than the patient's insurance carrier, there is no need for the provider to have access to one's social security information. If the patient is unsure of the need for this information, she or he simply should ask the provider why the information is being requested, how it is going to be used and if it's absolutely necessary to the provider. Indeed, this information is so sensitive that insurance companies are no longer permitted to print it on a member's medical insurance identification card. While a bill passed in 2005 called for the existing system of social security cards in the United States to be replaced by a new system of national identification cards in the year 2008, no action has yet been taken.

The final decision about what information and how much information is going to be divulged to a second or third party is up to the individual. In addition to one's personal identification number, a provider may make requests for other personal information. It's advisable, therefore, for every patient to read carefully the forms with which she or he's presented and to be selective when sharing that personal information.

It's necessary to supply accurate information and answer every question that directly impacts one's illness and treatment. It is not necessary, however, to answer questions that are personal in nature and have no bearing upon one's illness or treatment. And, once again, if the patient is unsure of the necessity of certain information, she or he should question the provider about their requests and act accordingly.

Moreover, it's important for every patient to know if her or his private medical information can be accessed by anyone from outside the physician's office or the facility. If the answer to this question is "yes," the patient should then substantiate the need for this access and know how this additional entity is going to use this information. It also is important for an individual to periodically review one's medical records just as one periodically reviews one's credit reports.

Every individual should be familiar with her or his medical records and the information contained within. In addition, every individual should ask medical providers to notify her or him in the event these records are requested from the provider by another entity. Similarly, if an insurance company or another health care provider requests these records, the individual may ask to view the records before the transfer of information takes place.

As we know, the provider may not be required by law to get consent from the individual before this transference of information occurs. Notification of the transfer will alert the individual to the request and allow the individual to know the specifics of the request and the full content of the record that has been requested. The individual also should request notification in the event her or his medical information is ever subpoenaed for a legal proceeding.

> *Whatsoever things I see or hear concerning the life of men, in my attend-*
> *ance on the sick or even apart therefrom, which ought not be noised*
> *abroad, I will keep silence thereon, counting such things to be as sacred*
> *secrets.*
>
> *Oath of Hippocrates*[255]

Finally, there's one last protection afforded every patient, derived from the Hippocratic Oath itself. Commonly known as the **Physician/Patient Privilege** in the United States, this is a long recognized ethical principle of the medical community in which communications between a physician and a patient remain confidential and private. This, of course, also means that the patient's physician holds a patient's medical records in confidence. Further, this principle is a legal doctrine that prevents a physician from testifying in court about comments a patient may have made while seeking medical advice or treatment from the physician.[256]

Similarly, a physician is prohibited from revealing this confidential information to a third party or entity unless the law requires it. We know, for instance, that certain medical conditions that involve communicable diseases may be reported to specific health authorities to insure public safety. Additionally, communications in which a patient confides information about her or his participation in a future crime may be an exception to this privilege. Overall, however, the privilege functions as a necessary tool intended to allow individuals to be open and honest with their physicians to facilitate efficient and proper care. It's a privilege that the medical community and the American Academy of Family Physicians honor as they continue to oppose all efforts to eliminate or erode its integrity.[257]

It also is a privilege that belongs to the patient. In other words, only the patient can make the decision to disregard the privilege and allow the physician to share and divulge confidential communications. This means that the physician doesn't even have the right to tell one's spouse, significant other, family member or friend about the patient's diagnosis, condition or prognosis without the patient's consent. In this simple, yet time honored way, the patient again is afforded another opportunity to limit and control the manner in which her or his personal information and private medical records are used and disclosed.[258]

Part 3:
Pain Management

A universally accepted nursing diagnosis defines pain as "an unpleasant sensory and emotional experience arising from actual or potential tissue damage." Physical pain is a sensation with which every individual has had experience at one time or another. Contrary to common belief, however, pain is typically not a symptom of cancer in its early stages. Indeed, the lack of pain is one of the reasons that early cancer diagnosis can be problematic. Many individuals wrongly believe that as long as nothing hurts, nothing is wrong.

This is a misconception in the field of cancer, for often an individual with the disease won't experience pain unless the cancer grows and becomes widespread. In these instances, pain may result as the tumor begins to interfere with body organs, muscle functioning or nerve pathways. The pain also may result from poor circulation and blocked blood vessels, bone fractures or infections caused by the tumor. In general, the more advanced the cancer, the more likely the individual is to experience pain.

Similarly, the more advanced the cancer, the more likely the individual will experience periods of severe pain. If we add to this the emotional responses of depression or anxiety, the pain can become even worse. On the other hand, many individuals diagnosed with cancer, and certainly those who are diagnosed early, may not experience pain at all from the disease itself. Even those who do will most likely experience pain that's mild or moderate and far less intense than pain that often results from nerve disorders and some forms of arthritis. In fact, it's more likely that pain experienced by cancer patients will be the result of cancer treatments and their side effects rather than from the disease itself.

We become aware of pain when the body's nerve endings detect damage in certain tissues and parts of the body. Once this damage is detected, the nerves transmit a warning through the nerve pathways from the body part to the brain. The brain then interprets the signal from the nerves, recognizes that damage is occurring in the body and produces the sensation of pain in the damaged area. Pain can be acute or chronic. Acute pain is characterized by a sudden onset and a limited duration that may last for a few days, weeks or months. This type of pain also is typically localized and the affected area is usually easy to identify. Further, acute pain is generally easy to correct and the likelihood of a complete recovery from the pain is good.[259]

In contrast, chronic pain may develop slowly and increase in intensity over time. Chronic pain may last for several months, years or even permanently. This pain is less likely to be localized and may appear to affect the body in a number of areas and in a number of different ways. As a result, the sensation of chronic pain may change, which makes it more difficult for the patient to describe and more difficult for the physician to identify and evaluate. The sensory pattern of chronic pain also varies as the pain itself may be continuous or intermittent, and the intensity of the pain may increase, decrease or remain constant. Unfortunately, while chronic pain can be controlled, complete relief may not be possible in some cases.[260]

The most insidious aspect of pain, of course, is that it has the ability to greatly compromise one's quality of life. Physically, pain can drain an individual of energy and can aggravate a cancer patient's already existing condition of fatigue and exhaustion. One may become more susceptible to developing other illnesses and infections, and one's ability to withstand the continuing cancer treatments may decrease. One's ability to work, drive, exercise, run errands and engage in everyday activities becomes diminished. One's ability to appreciate family, friends and life's other simple pleasures may be greatly affected. As a result, one may begin to feel detached from the world and this, of course, may contribute to feelings of sadness, hopelessness and isolation.

Further, pain can interfere with one's ability to sleep well or eat properly, and problems in these areas can directly affect one's physical strength and the body's ability to fight the cancer and withstand the necessary treatments. Clearly, therefore, managing pain is a vital component of a cancer patient's overall treatment. The only person who knows when pain becomes an issue is the patient her or himself and as such, the responsibility for recognizing the pain and communicating its existence belongs to the patient.

Once again, good communication becomes an essential part of the cancer patient's treatment and recovery process. As soon as one becomes aware of any pain whatsoever one must communicate this fact immediately. One should never feel embarrassed to admit that pain is occurring and one should never think she or he would be perceived as a complainer or malingerer for voicing concerns about pain.

Nor should one wait until the pain becomes significant before seeking help. Pain is a real subjective sensation, and the most important part of effective pain management is to arrest the pain before it intensifies and, if possible, even before it begins. For once pain takes hold and becomes severe, it's much more difficult to manage and control.

The ideal person in whom the patient should confide the experience of pain is, of course, one's quarterback doctor. For, remember, it is one's quarterback doc who knows all the details of one's progress, the problems one has encountered, the side effects one is experiencing, the results of relevant tests and every other doctor involved in treating the patient. It's this doctor who oversees every aspect of the patient's treatment and this doctor who will be best qualified to evaluate the pain and enlist the help of others if necessary.

This evaluation, however, will be based upon the patient's ability to explain and describe the pain in detail. Moreover, any evaluation will only be as accurate as the information the patient provides. It's important, therefore, for one to identify the location of the pain and the intensity of the pain. In describing the intensity it may be helpful for the patient to use a common **pain assessment scale**, which utilizes numbers from 0 to 10 — with 0 designating no pain at all and 10 designating the worst pain possible.[261]

One also must determine if the pain is constant or intermittent. If the pain is inter-mittent, one must know when it occurs, how often it occurs and how long it lasts. One must determine if the pain began quickly or developed over time. One must determine the quality of the pain and if it's a dull and aching pain, a burning sensation, throbbing pain, or sharp and piercing. One must share anything in one's daily life that appears to make the pain worse or better, such as a specific food or drink, certain exercises or activ-ity, body movements or even perhaps a particular time of day.

In addition, one must discuss the ways in which this pain in interfering with one's life. One must focus upon the effect the pain is having upon everyday activities, inter-personal relationships and the ability to be intimate with one's mate, the ability to con-centrate and think clearly, sleep habits and appetite. It's important to be as honest as possible throughout this process, yet if it's too difficult for the patient to focus clearly upon these topics, the following suggestions may be helpful.

If, for example, verbal skills fail, the patient should write down every thought she or he has regarding the pain. Every aspect should be listed on paper and if this approach is too difficult for the patient, she or he should engage a family member or friend to take notes. Turning one's mental observations into tangible words on paper is a valuable exercise that can help the patient focus on and verbalize the pain. In turn, verbalization helps move the sensory experience of pain to the forefront of objective awareness. For the patient, this facilitates the entire process of pain recognition, pain assessment and effective communication of the existence of pain to another.

Clearly, this process of effectively communicating one's pain is absolutely necessary if one's quarterback doctor is to accurately evaluate the pain. A proper evaluation of the pain will insure the proper choice of treatment for the pain. A proper evaluation also will help the quarterback determine if she or he can handle the situation or if a pain special-ist or pain management team should be engaged on the patient's behalf.

We've already discussed the ways in which surgery, chemotherapy and radiation can be used in specific ways to reduce and treat certain types of cancer pain. This discus-sion, however, will focus on the additional treatments widely used in cancer programs, which include a variety of drug and non-drug approaches. First, drugs and medications have long formed the foundation of traditional cancer related pain treatment. In part, this is due to the relief that drugs provide which is typically fast, efficient and long last-ing. In addition, drugs are fairly easy to administer and in most cases pose little threat of creating serious side effects.

If drugs appear to be the correct choice of treatment, the pain first will be typed according to its intensity and will be classified as mild, mild to moderate or moderate to severe. Based upon this classification, one or a combination of drugs will be chosen and for the most part, these drugs will fall into one of two categories, **non-narcotics** and

narcotics. The non-narcotics typically will be used to treat pain considered mild and the narcotics will be used to treat pain that ranges from moderate to severe.[262]

The most common of the non-narcotic pain medications include NSAIDS, or non-steroidal anti-inflammatory drugs such as ibuprofen, aspirin and naproxen. Another common non-narcotic is the pain-relieving analgesic acetaminophen, which in itself has no anti-inflammatory properties, but may be used in combination with other medicinal products. These medications can be taken by mouth, and while some are available over the counter, others remain available by prescription only. The patient must remember, however, that even non-prescription medications can be misused, can interfere with other treatments and can cause unintended side effects.

It's important, therefore, for the patient to consult with her or his physician before using any non-prescription drug for pain relief even if that medication is only aspirin. Unfortunately, even aspirin can create severe gastrointestinal problems for some patients and acetaminophen can produce liver damage. Further, while a new category of NSAIDS known as the COX-2 inhibitors, which includes the drugs Celebrex and Vioxx, appears to produce fewer side effects and have a minimal negative impact on the gastrointestinal tract in particular, these drugs aren't without their own problems, and significant side effects can occur in some individuals.[263]

Accordingly, the use of any non-narcotic drug to relieve cancer-related pain must be monitored carefully. Further, one should never underestimate the relief that aspirin, muscle relaxers and other non-narcotic medications can provide for pain. Indeed, the non-narcotics can be quite effective and in some cases can provide the same pain relief as many of the more powerful narcotic medications.

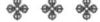

Headline:

Drugs Used to Treat Inflammation May Help Prevent Lung Cancer

According to recent studies, this statement appears to be true. COX-2 is an enzyme already known to play a role in inflammatory conditions such as arthritis. This enzyme, however, also is involved in the development of many cancers. It's responsible for the overproduction of prostaglandins, which are the substances that cause inflammation. In the 1990s, the presence of the COX-2 enzyme was detected in lung cancer cells. This makes sense in light of the fact that smoking creates significant inflammation within the airways, and if we apply our Cancer Blueprint, such chronic inflammation, over time may set the stage for cancer.

Drugs that contain COX-2 inhibitors, by definition, inhibit the enzyme that causes or contributes to inflammation. True, these drugs have been used primarily to treat arthritis and other common forms of inflammation, and recently they have come under fire for unintended side effects. The anti-inflammatory nature of the COX-2 inhibitors, however, still holds promise for treating and reducing inflammation of the lungs due to smoking and, therefore, may help prevent lung cancer.[264]

If the pain in question is moderate or severe, it usually will require a stronger medication that stems from the family of narcotics. The most common of these medications belong to a class of drugs known as the **opioids**, or as they're more commonly known, the **opiates**. An opiate is derived from opium. Indeed, it's derived from the juice produced from the unripe seedpods of the *papaver somniferum* species of poppy indigenous to the Near East. The opiates, which include codeine, morphine, tincture of opium and meperidine or Demerol, are effective painkillers that act directly upon the central nervous system and alter one's perception of pain.[265]

The opiates also can be combined with acetaminophen to produce Percocet or with aspirin to produce Percodan, two commonly prescribed medications for pain. Although most of these medications are administered orally or by injection, some can be given rectally in suppository form. In addition, some such as the narcotic fentanyl are available in a patch that can be placed directly on the skin. This patch is approximately the size of a credit card and only needs to be changed about every three days. Finally, some of these medications come in a form that can be absorbed transmucously by placing the drug under the tongue and allowing it to melt into the tissues. When the intensity of one's pain requires the use of narcotics, the dosage usually begins at a low level and then is increased until the patient experiences satisfactory relief.[266]

Further, the dosage of the narcotic will increase proportionally if and as the pain increases in intensity. It also is important to maintain a constant level of the narcotic in one's system to provide a consistent level of relief and prevent sudden surges in the pain. Remember, proper pain management requires the drug, whatever it may be, to be administered on a regular and continual basis.

Pain relief won't be effective if the patient stops taking the medication as soon as the pain decreases and doesn't resume taking it until the pain returns. The point of pain control is to achieve a certain level of comfort, then maintain that level. For pain is very difficult to control once it takes hold, and every patient should continue with their prescribed drug use until one's physician or pain manager advises otherwise.

Not all narcotics are opiates, but all opiates are narcotics, and all narcotics are strong pain-relieving drugs. Unfortunately, the stronger the drug, the greater is the potential for side effects. And of all the potential side effects associated with the use of narcotics, the most common is perhaps constipation. Indeed, constipation will affect nearly every patient who uses narcotics for pain relief, including cancer patients who already may be suffering gastrointestinal difficulty due to chemotherapy or radiation treatments.[267]

If these patients are experiencing diarrhea, the use of narcotics for pain may help stabilize the condition. If, however, these patients are experiencing constipation, the use of narcotics to relieve pain will only make the situation worse. And, constipation itself can develop into an extremely uncomfortable and painful condition. Accordingly, before a patient embarks on a pain relief program that utilizes opiates or any other narcotic, her or his physician should place the patient on a special bowel regimen as well. To prevent constipation from developing this regimen should begin as soon as the patient begins taking the medication.

In addition, patients taking narcotics should drink plenty of water and other fluids and, if necessary, make dietary changes in order to restore or preserve gastrointestinal balance. Once again, with the help of one's physician or pain manager, the patient must be aware of every side effect she or he already is experiencing from the cancer and its treatments, and must determine how the use of narcotics will further impact those existing conditions.

It also is common for some individuals to experience nausea when taking narcotics for pain relief.[268] Sometimes, the nausea only occurs in the first few days or weeks of taking the medication and disappears over time. Sometimes, the nausea only occurs when the patient is taking a particular type of narcotic. The opiate morphine, for example, may cause nausea in some patients whereas codeine, Demerol or tincture of opium may not. In these cases, simple experimentation will reveal a narcotic that not only controls pain, but agrees with one's digestive tract as well.

If it's determined, however, that a particular narcotic is necessary for a patient, regardless of the nausea it may create, there are excellent antiemetics that can alleviate the problem. Among these are Zofran and Kytirl, two medications that are effective in battling nausea and that may be taken in combination with the nausea-producing narcotic.[269] On the other hand, while some narcotics such as Demerol may not produce nausea, they can produce mouth sores, which is problematic for patients already experiencing mucositis from chemotherapy.

In addition, most narcotics produce mental fatigue and sleepiness in patients, especially in the first few days of use. Typically, sleepiness is a temporary side effect that will dissipate over time. If it continues, however, the patient's physician or pain manager may switch the narcotic in question to another or may choose to treat the sleepiness in some other way. It also is possible in some cases for larger doses of pain-relieving narcotics to create confusion or even delirium. It's also possible for one using narcotics to experience respiratory difficulty in which one's breathing can become labored and shallow. This side effect, however, is rare when narcotics are taken properly as prescribed and this issue usually is not a concern for patients seeking relief from their cancer related pain.[270]

Chapter 5:
The Truth about Narcotics

The narcotic family of drugs are powerful substances that when misused can result in a compulsive and uncontrollable psychological dependence upon the drug in question. When this occurs, an individual develops a physical and emotional craving for the drug known as **addiction**. In these cases, one takes the drug to fulfill certain psychological needs, not in order to relieve physical pain. In contrast, when narcotics are used under proper medical guidance the chances of a patient becoming addicted to the drug are extremely small.[271]

Indeed, a 1990 study of patients who used opiates to relieve their cancer related pain indicated that only seven out of 24,000 became addicted to their medication.[272] In a medical setting, narcotics are taken for physical pain and, accordingly, their dosage and strength are carefully monitored. It's true that as the patient continues to take the narcotic, her or his body will begin to adapt to the drug's presence. This adaptation is a natural occurrence and is referred to as **physical dependence**.[273]

This dependence, however, is temporary, for as the patient's pain subsides the amount of narcotic prescribed by one's physician to treat the pain also will be reduced. By slowly decreasing the amount of drug in the patient's system in this way, addiction and the physical side effects associated with it, such as cramps or nausea, can be avoided. It also is true that when a patient begins a regimen of narcotics for pain relief the dosage may need to be gradually increased over time to provide a constant level of relief.

Known as **tolerance,** this expected development occurs as the human body becomes accustomed to a drug or medication. As this occurs, the patient's body over time will require a larger dose of the drug in question to get the same level of pain relief that a smaller dose provided initially. Once again, however, one's physician can manage this development easily by gradually reducing the amount of the drug until it's no longer needed.[274]

It also is important for patients experiencing cancer-related pain to understand that the use of narcotics generally won't interfere with their mental or cognitive abilities. While narcotics may have this effect when used in non-medical situations without professional supervision, it typically isn't a problem for cancer patients treating their pain. Experts with a complete knowledge of opiates and their use are available to assist every individual requiring their help. And these experts will work with each patient on an individual basis to provide complete pain relief while insuring one's clarity of mind.

The goal of pain management is to control one's physical discomfort without harming one's ability to work, interact with others and live a productive life. Moreover, no patient should be reluctant to enlist the aid of narcotics to battle their cancer related pain. Opiates in particular are the most effective medications available for fighting this type of pain, and any fears or prejudices one or one's family or friends may have concerning their use must be put aside. For, pain is a disabling and unnecessary experience that can impede one's recovery process and greatly interfere with one's quality of life.

Chapter 6:
The Schedule of Drugs

Narcotics have long been a cornerstone of pain relief therapy throughout the world. Not all narcotics, however, are recognized by the world's legal systems as appropriate or valuable medicinal tools. Indeed, some of these drugs are considered too dangerous by certain governmental agencies to be approved for any medicinal use whatsoever. The determination as to whether or not a drug may be used for medicinal purposes typically is based upon a particular scheme of classification.

One scheme, for example, may attempt to classify drugs according to their chemical structures. While this type of classification may prove useful for medicinal chemists intent on drug research and study, it doesn't provide a meaningful classification for those interested in the effects of those drugs upon the human body. This is because some drugs that belong to the same chemical class, such as morphine and heroin, produce similar effects while other drugs with the same chemical structure, such as apomorphine and nalorphine, produce different effects.[275]

In reverse, some drugs that differ in chemical structure such as amphetamines and cocaine have a similar biological effect upon the human body. As a result, another scheme of drug classification focuses on the psychopharmacological perspective of the drug or the effect the drug has on human behavior and normal and abnormal mental functioning.[276]

In the United States, the legal use of certain drugs for medicinal purposes was determined in 1970 by the **Controlled Substances Act**, which divided chemical substances into five different classifications. In this scheme, the classifications are determined by the drug's potential for misuse and abuse and the drug's potential level for addiction. This classification is listed in a document known as the **DEA Schedule of Drugs** and, appropriately, it is the Drug Enforcement Administration which is charged with regulating and enforcing this scheme of drug scheduling.[277]

From the top, **Schedule I** drugs are those that have a *high* abuse liability and no approved medical use in the United States. These drugs are available for research only and the research may only take place after being approved by the Food and Drug Administration and after the research facility has received a license to handle the drugs. These substances aren't sold at pharmacies, and physicians cannot prescribe them. They're provided only by manufacturers under federal contracts and require special record keeping procedures and greater storage security. Examples of these drugs include heroin, peyote, mescaline, lysergic acid diethylamide or LSD, and marijuana and its active ingredient tetrahydrocannabinol, or THC.

Schedule II drugs also have a *high* abuse liability, yet have been approved for medicinal use in the United States. As such, physicians can prescribe these drugs and pharmacies can dispense them although no refills are allowed. The possession of these drugs also requires physicians and pharmacies to maintain stringent record keeping and storage procedures, though not as stringent as the Schedule I drugs. Examples of Schedule II drugs include codeine, morphine, opium, cocaine, meperidine methadone and methamphetamine.

Schedule III drugs have an abuse liability considered *moderately high*, are approved for medicinal use in the United States and can be issued by telephone or a written pre-scription. These drugs may have five refills over six months and include Tylenol with codeine, paregoric and anabolic steroids. **Schedule IV** drugs have a *moderate* abuse liability, also are approved for medicinal use in the United States and can be obtained with a prescription either telephoned in or written.

Similar to Schedule III, these drugs also are allowed five refills over six months and include diazepam, chloral hydrate, methohexital and phenobarbital. The last group of drugs under **Schedule V** have a *low* potential for abuse, are approved for medicinal use in the United States, can be obtained without a prescription and include drugs such as Robitussin A-C which contains a trace amount of codeine.[278]

Quite frankly, it's extremely difficult for entities to reach a consensual agreement concerning the perceived addiction level or liability of most drugs, and accordingly, drugs on the DEA Schedule are continually being reclassified. In general, however, science is in agreement regarding drugs that appear to produce the highest abuse liability, which includes the opiates and the psychomotor stimulants such as methamphetamine and cocaine. Science also generally agrees upon those drugs that appear to present a relatively low abuse liability such as aspirin and other over the counter medications.

This, however, leaves many substances and drugs the abuse and addiction issues of which remain controversial, substances such as caffeine and nicotine and, of course, a variety of drugs, including marijuana. Although marijuana and its active ingredient THC have been classified as Schedule I drugs with no medicinal value by the DEA, research continues in an effort to identify and isolate the potential medicinal values of both.

The Marijuana Controversy

Marijuana, or cannabis, is an herb derived from the flowering tops of hemp plants, although all parts of the plant contain psychoactive or psychomotor substances. For centuries, can-nabis has been used by different cultures and societies for a variety of medicinal reasons but primarily to treat chronic pain. In the United States, cannabis was used on the battlefields during the Civil War as an analgesic or pain-relieving drug.[279]

Cannabis, however, isn't effective against severe pain, and its use was eventually replaced by morphine, a much more powerful substance that acted faster in relieving pain. Indeed, the use of morphine at the time was commonplace and, unfortunately, its use lacked the safeguards and professional expertise that dictate its medicinal use today. As a result, numerous individuals developed a condition known as "soldier's disease," or as it's currently known, an addiction to morphine.[280]

Nevertheless, the medicinal use of cannabis continued in the United States throughout the first several decades of the twentieth century. In 1937, however, the United States passed several anti-marijuana laws, the first of which was known as the **Marijuana Tax Act**. This Act apparently made it extremely difficult for physicians to prescribe cannabis for medicinal purposes, and accordingly, physicians simply stopped using it. Finally, in 1941 cannabis was dropped from the United States' official encyclopedia of accepted medicinal substances and drugs known as the *Pharmacopoeia*.[281]

Scientific research continued to examine the beneficial attributes of marijuana in clinical applications. In the 1980s, for example, the National Cancer Institute approached the Drug Enforcement Administration with its promising research results regarding marijuana's active ingredient THC and the substance's ability to relieve nausea and vomiting in cancer patients undergoing chemotherapy.[282] Additional research indicates that marijuana and THC prove helpful in treating glaucoma by reducing the intraocular pressure in the eyes, in treating epilepsy and in relieving the pain of muscle spasms associated with multiple sclerosis, paraplegia and quadriplegia.[283]

The DEA, in turn, is aware of this research and recognizes the important implications presented by the use of marijuana and THC in certain medical situations. The majority of prejudice surrounding marijuana or THC, therefore, isn't really an issue of whether or not the substances possess acceptable medicinal value. It appears, rather, that the prejudice and controversy surrounding this issue are more significantly related to the manner in which these medicinal substances are delivered.

Indeed, a decision handed down in 2005 by the United States Supreme Court didn't address the issue of whether or not marijuana is good medicine. The decision only ruled that federal law would overrule state law in questions regarding the medical use of marijuana. In 2009, however, the United States Justice Department reversed its policy and stated that federal law would now defer to state laws governing this issue.[284] Although state laws continue to change, as of 2010 fourteen states including Alaska, California, Colorado, Hawaii, Maine, Michigan, Montana, Nevada, New Jersey, New Mexico, Oregon, Rhode Island, Vermont and Washington had enacted effective laws allowing legalized patient use of medical marijuana with a doctor's consent.[285]

Marijuana typically is smoked. We already have discussed in length the harm associated with tobacco use and the smoking of cigarettes and cigars in particular. When marijuana is smoked, an individual is exposed to more than four hundred different chemicals, which include most of the hazardous chemicals found in tobacco. Indeed, the level of tar in a marijuana cigarette is four times greater than the level of tar found in a tobacco cigarette. Smoking marijuana for one health problem, therefore, may only create an entirely new array of health problems for an individual based upon the harmful chemicals and carcinogens that are byproducts of smoking itself.[286]

Smoking, in general, is a poor way to deliver medicine for any condition. Further, it's difficult to provide safe and properly regulated doses of medicine when it's in a "smoked" form. Opium, for example, is a drug that has proven itself medically beneficial in a variety of different forms. Scientists have extracted the active ingredients from opium to produce a number of pharmaceutical products, including morphine, codeine, oxycodone and hydrocodone.[287]

The smoking of opium itself, however, has never been endorsed as a medically accepted method of delivering the drug. Similarly, neither the scientific or medical communities within many parts of the world, including the United States, have found sufficient data to conclude that smoking marijuana is the most efficient way to administer the drug and deliver its medicinal properties.[288]

Of the many studies designed to determine the medicinal value of smoked marijuana, perhaps the most comprehensive was conducted by the Institute of Medicine in the United States. This Institute, an organization chartered by the National Academy of Sciences, released its 1999 research results that concluded smoked marijuana for medicinal purposes couldn't be recommended. It further concluded, however, that marijuana could be dissected, just like opium, and its active ingredients could be identified, isolated and developed into a number of pharmaceuticals that weren't dependent upon smoking to be delivered.[289]

Further, while the Federal Drug Administration hasn't approved the smoking of marijuana in medical applications, it has approved the use of its active ingredient THC in a scientifically regulated form. This form, developed by scientists in concert with the DEA, is found in a pharmaceutical product, marketed as **Marinol**. Known as the "medical marijuana," Marinol is widely available through prescription. At present, it comes in a pill form that's taken orally although research continues to investigate patches or inhalants as alternative methods of delivery.[290]

Marinol is used to treat pain in a variety of situations, glaucoma, chemotherapy-related nausea, convulsions in the epileptic and in AIDS patients to improve appetite. It's true that Marinol is a synthetic rather than natural product. It's also true that smoked marijuana is about three times more powerful than any form of marijuana that is taken orally. For the time being, however, Marinol is an excellent way to deliver some of the beneficial properties of marijuana without creating any of the additional problems associated with smoking.[291]

It's a compromise of personal anecdote and scientific evaluation that allows patients to benefit from some of the medicinal properties of cannabis while providing science with the impetus to continue its research on the substance. It also is a compromise that may perhaps encourage the DEA to re-evaluate its classification of cannabis, moving it from a Schedule I substance with no apparent medical application, to a Schedule II substance recognized and approved, like opium, for its medicinal applications.

Nerve Blocks

One additional application of drugs in the battle against pain includes a procedure known as a **nerve block**. Also called **conduction anesthesia**, this procedure involves the injection of an anesthetic medication into the affected area of the body, which blocks the nerve pathways that carry pain impulses to the brain. Bupivacaine or lidocaine, either used alone or in combination with corticosteroids, are the most commonly used medications in a nerve block procedure.[292]

Typically, a temporary block will be performed first in which the medication of choice is injected into the patient to test its effectiveness. If the drug proves successful in relieving pain, a permanent block may then be administered. Although this second type of block isn't really permanent, it can last up to six months. There are some risks associated with nerve blocks, but for individuals who cannot tolerate the side effects associated with narcotics or other pain relievers, a nerve block may be an effective choice. Indeed, there are certain form of cancers, including that of the pancreas for which a nerve block has become quite commonplace.[293]

Radiofrequency Ablation

This procedure itself doesn't require or depend upon drugs to be an effective pain reliever. It does, however, require that the patient be sedated during the procedure and as such it will be discussed in this section. **Radiofrequency** is defined as a high frequency, alternating electromagnetic current, and **ablation** is defined as the process of eroding, removing or melting. In radiofrequency ablation, a radiologist uses a special needle to deliver the electromagnetic current to a specific body part or tissue to destroy harmful cells.[294]

This procedure is commonly used to treat abnormal conditions of the heart such as arrhythmias, atrial flutters and idiopathic ventricular tachycardia. Today, it also can be used to destroy cancer cells to reduce the size of a tumor when surgery or other treatments aren't feasible. As a result, any tumor-related pain also could be reduced. In addition, radiofrequency ablation produces few side effects, provides pain relief that can last for several months and can be repeated whenever necessary.[295]

Chapter 7:
Drug Free Pain Relievers

Physiatric Techniques

Transcutaneous Electrical Nerve Stimulation

Also known as **TENS, transcutaneous electrical nerve stimulation** is a method of pain control that utilizes a low voltage application of electric impulses to the nerve endings. The impulses are transmitted to the body through electrodes placed on the skin and attached to a battery-powered stimulator by flexible wires. TENS generates electric impulses similar to those of the body, but have the ability to block the transmission of pain signals to the brain in the area to which they're applied.[296]

The procedure creates a tingling sensation that can be adjusted in intensity in accordance with each individual's personal level of comfort. TENS is a completely non-invasive procedure and has no known side effects. Further, the equipment and portable power source are reasonably priced and can be used in the privacy of one's home after receiving instruction in its use from a health care professional.

Percutaneous Electrical Nerve Stimulation

This procedure, also known as **PENS**, is similar to TENS in that it also produces a low level electrical impulse that has the ability to block the transmission of pain signals to the brain. It differs from TENS, however, in that it doesn't utilize electrodes placed on the skin to transmit the impulse. Rather, PENS uses needles inserted into the soft tissue around the bones. Clearly, it's an invasive procedure that may or may not require a local anesthesia, yet it can be effective in relieving bone pain associated with certain cancers.[297]

Orthotics

Orthotics refers to the design and use of external appliances to support a particular body part or to promote a specific body motion. When bones or muscles are weakened as a result of cancer or cancer treatments, pain can result. Orthotic devices such as splints or neck collars can be used to effectively support or immobilize areas of the body affected by pain and, in some cases, can provide significant relief.[298]

Therapeutic Exercise

Therapeutic exercise is that which is planned and prescribed by a physical therapist to regain normal body functioning or to attain a specific physical benefit. Such exercise may include simple range of motion movements or exercises that stretch, strengthen and condition certain body areas. Therapeutic exercise also may involve the use of body or limb wraps or pressure stockings to facilitate the benefits of the physical movements. Indeed, commitment to a regular program of these exercises can repair weakened muscles, improve cardiovascular and respiratory function and increase joint flexibility. In turn, when weakened or damaged body parts related to cancer begin to function normally as a result of such a program, any cancer-related pain also can be reduced.[299]

Massage

Massage, of course, is the manipulation of the body's soft tissues through a combination of rubbing, tapping, stroking or kneading. It's a simple activity that can be performed with bare hands or with the help of a mechanical device such as a vibrator. It also can be performed by a trained massage therapist in a clinical or office setting or a family member or friend in the privacy of one's own home.

While uncomplicated and straightforward, massage shouldn't be underestimated, as it's an effective tool in the field of pain management. Massage can increase blood circulation, improve muscle tone, relieve tension and relax the patient. While massage of inflamed or excessively sensitive areas of the body typically is avoided, massage of the back, neck, feet and hands can be useful in managing and reducing cancer-related pain.[300]

Skin Stimulation

Stimulating the nerve endings in the skin also can lessen or block the sensation of pain. Indeed, the application of pressure to the skin through massage is one form of skin stimulation. In addition, however, stimulating the skin in other ways through a temperature change, friction or the application of certain substances such as menthol also excites the nerve endings and reduces one's perception of pain.

Of these, the most common form of skin stimulation may be the use of simple hot and cold packs. Heat can relieve spasms, relax muscles and help increase the blood circulation of the body. Heat can be extremely useful in reducing pain, although it shouldn't be applied to tumor sites or to areas of the body that have undergone radiation.[301]

Cold, on the other hand, can reduce inflammation and significantly relieve pain in the nerve endings. The cold pack itself, however, shouldn't be applied directly to the skin, but rather, should be contained or wrapped within a cloth. For maximum benefit, the application of either heat or cold shouldn't exceed twenty minutes and their use should be alternated with rest periods of about twenty minutes.

Cognitive/Behavioral Modification Techniques

Hypnosis

Among the most common of the behavioral modification techniques, **hypnosis** is defined as an artificially induced mental state that resembles sleep characterized by an increased susceptibility to suggestion. This state is usually induced through a monotonous repetition of a word, phrase or gesture as the patient relaxes. Once the hypnotic mental state is achieved and the patient is deeply relaxed, she or he is given a specific suggestion.

When used for pain relief, the patient will be asked to experience the sensation of pain in a different way. As a result, the pain itself may not actually be reduced, but the patient's perception of the pain is altered in such a way that the pain appears to be reduced. In this way, hypnosis can be an effective non-drug and non-invasive technique in the battle against pain. Further, it isn't necessary to consult an expert hypnotist to utilize this technique, as it's possible to learn the process of self-hypnosis from a variety of audiotapes designed for home use.[302]

Biofeedback

This technique is a process that provides a patient with either auditory or visual information about the physiological functions of her or his body. These body functions may include the patient's blood pressure, brain wave activity, skin resistance or muscle tension, and special instruments connected to the patient provide the information. As the patient becomes more aware of these physiological systems the patient also becomes more aware of the ways in which the body's stresses influence these systems.

Through a process of trial and error, the patient learns to consciously control these body systems previously considered involuntary and the effect stress has upon them. Thus, tension and anxiety can be reduced so that the patient can better cope with her or his cancer related pain. In addition, biofeedback is another technique that can be practiced at home with personalized portable biofeedback equipment.[303]

Relaxation/Contemplation/Meditation

These techniques share a common goal, to provide physical and mental comfort and reduce tension and discomfort. While contemplative and meditative techniques have been a part of many of the world's religious and cultural practices for centuries, psychotherapeutic relaxation therapy wasn't used to treat hypertensive patients until the scientist Edmund Jacobson introduced it in the 1920s. Relaxation therapy can take many forms. The most common, however, may be the method known as **progressive muscle relaxation**.[304]

In this technique, one learns to focus on individual muscles and muscle groups. Lying down, the patient tries to tense a specific muscle for five to ten seconds until the muscle can be easily identified. As the muscle tension is released, tensing and releasing another muscle or muscle group repeat the procedure. In this way, a patient becomes familiar with the various muscles in her or his body and develops the ability to relax each muscle, one at a time. When cancer patients use this technique to focus upon those muscles involved with their cancer related pain, progressive muscle relaxation is a valuable tool that can improve sleep, reduce anxiety, increase energy and allow additional pain relief methods to work more effectively.

Of the contemplative techniques, visualization and distraction are two of the most common. **Visualization**, also called **guided imagery** or **visual imagery**, is a method in which relaxation is effectively increased and one's stress resulting from real life situations is decreased. This technique works by combining positive experiences with imagined or actual negative situations to reduce one's trauma and desensitize the individual to the negativity. For example, when used to treat pain, the patient may imagine the pain as a bright, searing fire, then visualize the pain disappearing as cool, clear water is poured on the fire, putting it out. Or the patient may imagine the pain as a deep, red color that disappears as a brilliant, white light displaces it.[305]

Once again, visualization is a technique that can be learned from widely available audiotapes and used in the privacy of one's own home. In a similar vein, **distraction** is a technique that can reduce or prevent the perception of pain by focusing one's attention on sensations that are completely unrelated to pain. In this method, a patient may choose to concentrate on pleasant things such as listening to music until the sensation of pain diminishes. Although the technique is simple, distraction can prove a powerful tool that provides temporary relief for even the most significant type of pain.[306]

Finally, **meditation** is a technique that enables an individual to eliminate environmental stimuli as she or he maintains an easy mental focus. This focus may be one's pattern of breathing, a repeated mantra or word, a phrase or prayer, or a sound or image. There is a wide variety of meditation techniques, including **Zen**, **Transcendental Meditation** and **yoga**, yet all are similar in that each is used to clear the consciousness of stressful outside influences and increase one's peace of mind.

Ideally, meditation should be practiced in a quiet environment where interruptions can be prevented. Unlike the preconceived and inaccurate images many individuals have of the meditative techniques, one doesn't need to twist oneself into strange postures or positions to practice and benefit from meditation. Nor does one enter a trance or hypnotic state of mind while practicing a meditative technique. Rather, one typically sits comfortably in a chair or bed and with eyes closed engages in the technique of their choice for twenty or thirty minutes.

Practiced once or twice a day, such techniques allow one's physiological responses to slow down and relax while one's mental awareness is increased. Although audiotapes may be available for some meditative techniques, many require an instructor who will teach the individual how to direct her or his attention inward and to focus and relax at the same time. Once instructed in the process, however, an individual easily can continue to practice the technique on one's own wherever and whenever surroundings permit.[307]

According to research, the great benefit of the meditative techniques is that as the mind develops the ability to disregard external stress and stimuli it creates a state of mental and physical relaxation within the individual. This, of course, results in less tension and less anxiety for the individual, which can facilitate the healing process and reduce pain.

Alternative or Complementary Medicine

In addition to the several non-drug approaches we've already mentioned, there exist other medical practices used widely for the relief of pain. These practices are often referred to as "non-traditional" practices and typically are used in one of two ways. If a non-traditional practice is used alone without engaging the additional use of any of the recommended traditional treatments, the approach is referred to as **alternative medicine**. If a non-traditional practice is used in conjunction with other forms of recommended traditional medical treatments, the approach is referred to as **complementary medicine**.[308]

We must clarify, however, that some practices the Western world considers "non-traditional" often form the foundation of tradition in other parts of the world. Furthermore, many of these practices are gaining favor throughout the world and are now used commonly in conjunction with the recommended traditional Western treatments. Among these is a practice known as **acupuncture**, a technique of traditional Chinese medicine used for centuries in the Far East.[309]

It's based upon the theory that the body's energy, also called **chi** or **qi**, flows along pathways known as meridians. Practitioners believe that when the energy along these pathways is blocked or unbalanced, illness or pain will result. To relieve a blockage or restore balance, thin or hollow needles are inserted into the skin at specific points along the meridians. Acupuncture, for example, is often used by cancer patients to relieve the pain and uncomfortable side effects produced by the standard treatments of chemotherapy and radiation. Researchers theorize that the pain reduction attributed to acupuncture may result from biological mechanisms such as the stimulation of the hypothalamus and pituitary gland, or changes in the body's neurotransmitters, hormones or immune system.

This is a slightly invasive procedure, yet it's virtually painless and requires no anesthesia or sedative. The technique does require, however, that a patient receive treatment from a certified acupuncturist licensed by the proper regulatory boards in the state or country in which one resides. The technique also requires that the acupuncturist use sterilized or disposable needles throughout the process to prevent cross contamination and the unintentional spread of illness or disease.[310]

Moxibustion is another well-known Chinese medicinal technique that produces analgesia or a reduction in pain, or alters the functioning of an individual's body systems in some other way. It involves the burning of mugwort, a small, spongy herb, wormwood or another slow burning combustible substance. The material to be burned, called moxa, is either formed into a cone and placed directly upon the skin or is rolled into a stick shape that's lit and held over the treatment area for several minutes.[311]

More commonly, however, the moxa is placed upon the end of a needle during acupuncture and ignited which allows the heat to generate into the needlepoint and the surrounding skin tissue. This method is the most common form of moxibustion application and, in fact, the actual Chinese character for acupuncture when translated literally means "acupuncture-moxibustion." As the moxa continues to burn, the patient experiences a pleasant warm sensation that flows from the needle, penetrates deeply into the tissue and provides a welcome relief from many types of cancer related pain.[312]

Although there is no separate licensing or accreditation required for one to practice moxibustion, the treatment is usually taught within the context of a traditional Chinese medical degree program or as part of a recognized acupuncture training program. In addition, one must remember that burning moxa produces a fair amount of smoke and odor. Accordingly, patients who wish to use moxibustion, yet suffer from respiratory problems, should request that their practitioner use smokeless moxa sticks in place of the other more common forms of moxa.

Other methods of pain relief and management include **acupressure**, **Tai Chi**, **Qi Gong** and a variety of **herbal remedies**.[313] The first, acupressure, is another ancient Chinese method of healing similar to acupuncture, but uses the application of pressure to specific meridian points to relieve pain rather than the insertion of needles. Clearly, acupressure like acupuncture, requires an individual interested in its use to find a practitioner certified in the technique.

Practiced primarily for its health and medicinal benefits, Tai Chi is a Chinese martial art that helps one reduce stress and tension by engaging in a series of slow and flowing physical movements. Similar to acupuncture and acupressure, these precisely executed movements are believed to encourage the proper flow of the body's energy or chi thereby maintaining health and reducing pain. Qi Gong, known literally as "energy cultivation," is another Chinese practice that also uses a series of physical exercises to improve health and reduce pain by facilitating the flow of chi throughout the body. Obviously, one must be mobile and physically capable of performing the movements and exercises involved in Tai Chi and Qi Gong to benefit from the techniques. And both require initial instruction from a certified teacher before one is able to engage in either activity on one's own.[314]

Lastly, the use of specific herbs and herbal remedies has been reported by many cancer patients to be helpful in reducing their disease related pain. Yerba mate tea, for example, has been found to ease the neuropathic pain sometimes associated with chemotherapy and an herb known as valeriana officinalis appears to facilitate rest and sleep as it decreases pain. Once again, however, any patient who wishes to use herbs in her or his nutritional health program should always consult an expert in the field before making dietary changes that include the use of herbs or supplements.[315]

Another non-traditional treatment is the practice of **chiropractic medicine**. Although evidence suggests chiropractic dates to the time of ancient Egypt, it wasn't re-introduced to the "modern" world until the late nineteenth century. Chiropractic training differs from the training of licensed medical practitioners in that it requires two years of science-based undergraduate work and a minimum of four years of training at an accredited chiropractic college. Somewhat similar to acupressure, practitioners of chiropractic believe that illness and pain occur when certain nerve pathways along the spine develop blockages.[316]

Unlike the common stereotype, chiropractic rarely involves the strong-armed manipulation and "cracking" of one's bones. Rather, a typical treatment may include the application of pressure to certain body areas and muscles, careful positioning of the limbs and head, or certain exercises all of which are designed to realign and balance the skeletal structure. In this way, practitioners believe harmful blockages that interfere with the proper functioning of the body will be dislodged and pain, in particular, will be relieved.

Biodynamic craniosacral therapy is another non-invasive technique used by practitioners to alleviate pain and promote good mental and physical health. It is based upon the theory that the human cranial sutures are designed to express small degrees of motion. This subtle motion is believed to facilitate the inter-related workings of the body's tissues and fluids including the cerebrospinal fluid, the sacrum, the central nervous system and the surrounding membranes. This, in turn, is believed to enhance the body's own self-healing and self-regulating abilities.[317]

While this motion or rhythm occurs naturally, the practitioner of craniosacral therapy seeks to insure that this rhythm is not interrupted or blocked. Through touch and subtle palpatory skills the practitioner identifies areas of the body in which this rhythm is lacking and gently encourages the conditions that will reinstate it. Once rhythm is restored and balance is achieved, it is believed that health and well-being will follow.

Originating in India, **Ayurveda** is a natural system of medicine recognized for more than three thousand years. Translated literally, it means "knowledge of life" and is founded upon the belief that disease and pain are due to stress or imbalance within the individual's consciousness. Ayurveda encompasses a holistic approach to treatment that combines natural therapies and certain lifestyle changes in an effort to establish a balance between the mind, the body and the environment.[318]

Typically, an individual will undergo a physical purification process of fasting, followed by a special diet, herbal remedies, yoga, meditation and massage therapy. In India, Ayurveda is considered a traditional form of medical care for which practitioners receive institutionalized training and must be state recognized. Ayurveda practitioners aren't licensed, however, in many parts of the Western world, including the United States. Nevertheless, it remains a practice that continues to grow in popularity and appears to provide positive results when used in a complementary fashion with standard medical treatments for relieving pain.

A Word to the Wise

We've discussed many of the ways in which cancer patients can relieve their pain, either pain that results from the disease itself or from the treatments associated with the disease. Some of these pain-reducing methods involve the use of drugs, both non-narcotic and narcotic. Some involve invasive procedures that utilize needles or injections, while others are completely non-invasive. Some use mental techniques to relax the patient and reduce the pain whereas others utilize physical techniques. Some methods will work effectively for some cancer patients while different methods may be required for others.

The method of choice and its effectiveness for a particular individual will depend upon many factors, including the cause of the pain, the location of the pain, the type of pain and the individual's overall health. We must emphasize again that each patient is unique. Each human physiology differs and no two individuals will respond to medical treatments and therapy in exactly the same way. It remains, however, that all of the methods we've discussed have been reported at one time or another by a variety of cancer patients to be helpful in managing some forms of cancer-related pain.

Many of these methods are used by cancer patients not only to combat pain but to increase energy, reduce nausea, maintain mental clarity and facilitate the much needed rest and relaxation essential to every patient's recovery process. Nevertheless, it's most important to remember that all of these methods, be they drug or non-drug, invasive or non-invasive, mental or physical, should be used in conjunction with the primary cancer treatments, not in place of them.

None of the pain relief or health maintaining methods we've discussed has been shown scientifically to reduce tumors or cure cancer in and of itself. Only the primary treatments, including surgery, chemotherapy and radiation, are known to assault cancer directly. Accordingly, no cancer patient should depend upon or expect any therapy or treatment considered alternative or complementary to be a primary treatment in their fight against cancer. When possible, these methods must be paired with the standard traditional medical methods and techniques to insure the safety and well being of the patient.

Further, alternative and complementary cancer treatments must be distinguished from unproven treatments for which no scientific support exists. Simply put, there are no miracle drugs or herbs, no wonder cures or amazing devices that have been shown scientifically to reduce tumors or eliminate cancer. We all have heard at least one variation of the story about the friend of a neighbor's great aunt's employer's son who was "cured" of cancer by drinking a special herb tea, wearing metal amulets and bracelets or by lying in thermal hot springs and mud baths.

For many years, a "natural" drug known as laetrile was rumored to be one such miracle cure for cancer. Made from the residue of apricot pits and promoted as vitamin B-17, it was used to eliminate a vitamin deficiency that the drug's proponents believed caused cancer in the first place. This belief, however, and the drug's beneficial properties in fighting cancer have never been scientifically substantiated.[319] Similarly, a device known as an oscilloclast was promoted for years as a cure for cancer. This device was said to emit sympathetic vibrations that were absorbed from the air into the ointment-covered tissues of a patient's body.[320]

This isn't to say that none of these methods have ever worked. To repeat, each human is a unique being that varies greatly in its physical composition and response mechanisms. We live in an ever-changing world in which it's possible that one or some of these methods may have been, or may have coincidentally appeared to have been, medically beneficial for someone, somewhere, at some time. Medically accepted cancer drugs and treatments, however, are those that have proven their benefit for many decades, in numerous case studies, conducted on hundreds of thousands of cancer patients, by scientists and researchers from a variety of hospitals and clinics throughout the world.

It's always tempting for one in need to seek "wonder" cures when faced with a diagnosis of cancer. It's also fairly common for one in need to claim the existence of a "conspiracy" when a rumored wonder cure isn't easily available to the individual. This, of course, is an unfounded and inaccurate conclusion. It's true that new experimental drugs are always being developed. It's true that until these drugs attain government approval and insurance coverage recognition their use may be limited and prohibitively expensive. Yet, none of the world's medical establishments, the world's governments or the world's drug and research facilities have conspired to prevent or hide a cure for cancer for the purpose of financial gain.

The financial impact created by cancer upon all aspects of societies throughout the world is enormous. In the United States alone, the total financial cost of this disease, including the direct health expenditures for individuals and institutions, the cost to society of lost productivity due to illness and the huge loss of productivity due to unnecessary and premature death is quickly approaching $200 billion annually.[321] If a wonder drug, or a miracle cure or an amazing device known to "cure" cancer existed, the medical and governmental entities of the world would not only make it available, they would rejoice in the opportunity to do so.

Last, as always, the use of any drug, mental technique, physical technique or exercise, or any herb or supplement must be preceded by a thorough and complete consultation with one's quarterback doctor and medical support team. To their credit, many cancer centers in the United States and around the world today have already incorporated the non-traditional approaches to cancer treatment into their existing therapy programs. It's unfortunate, however, that while many of these methods are becoming increasingly common tools in the traditional battle against cancer, most still are not covered by traditional health care plans.

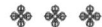

Headline:

Cancer Risk Greater on the Graveyard Shift

Yes, it appears that women who work the night shift may have a greater risk for developing breast cancer than women who do not. This sounds strange, so let's take it one analytical step at a time. First, scientists have wondered for years if individuals who work at night are more likely to develop cancer because of their extended exposure to light. We know that extended exposure to sunlight increases one's risk for developing certain cancers due to ultraviolet radiation. Apparently, however, extended exposure to daylight or bright lights also inhibits the body's ability to produce melatonin.

Now, melatonin is a hormone secreted by the brain and, as many of us know, it is nicknamed the sleep hormone because it flows primarily while one is sleeping. Many scientists today, however, also believe that melatonin is instrumental in suppressing the growth of new cancer cells. Indeed, recent studies conducted in the United States have found that melatonin appears to serve as an anticancer signal to the development of human breast cancer cells and that the cells stop proliferating when the hormone is present.[322]

In theory, therefore, women whose brains produce greater levels of melatonin decrease their risk for developing breast cancer while women whose brains produce lower levels of melatonin increase their risk for developing breast cancer. If exposure to bright light suppresses melatonin, and a decrease in melatonin increases one's risk for breast cancer, then it follows women who work at night and are exposed to bright light produce less melatonin and increase their risk for the disease. This is exactly what these particular studies found. In fact, female night shift employees who had measurably low levels of melatonin in their systems were found to be significantly more likely to develop breast cancer than female employees who were awake during the day and slept at night.

Additional research also suggests that melatonin may improve survival in advanced cancer patients and protect healthy body cells from the negative effects of chemotherapy and radiation. As with any research, however, these results must lend themselves to replication before the role of melatonin in breast cancer prevention and cancer survival can firmly be established. These findings must be put in context with prior research, and in the meantime, women should heed the common sense advice dispensed for years by the medical community, to make sure they "get plenty of sleep."[323]

Part 4:
From Patient to Survivor:
The Big Transition

He conquers who endures.
Persius

Surviving cancer is no longer a matter of beating the odds. Indeed, today the odds of beating cancer are with us. The line, however, that delineates the point at which one's life as a cancer patient ends and one's life as a cancer survivor begins remains unclear. Many of the physical and emotional issues that face a cancer patient during treatment and recovery continue long after the therapies, the hospital visits and the constant contact with one's medical care team come to an end.

Medically, a cancer survivor is an individual who shows no evidence of the disease five years after completing treatment. This determination, of course, forms the basis for the cancer survival statistics discussed earlier. We'll refer to a survivor, however, as an individual diagnosed with cancer, treated for cancer and successfully completing the appropriate treatments. Completing treatment and winning the physical battle against cancer is, unfortunately, only one part of the overall war.

Many challenges remain for the individual such as coping with the long-term side effects of treatment, lingering pain, dietary concerns, medical follow-up, maintaining one's health and numerous emotional issues that may require an individual to re-define her or his role in the world of family, friends and work. We'll now discuss some of these new challenges and, more importantly, discuss the ways in which they can be managed and, hopefully, overcome.

Chapter 8:
Survivorship: Physical Concerns

Reviewing One's Risk Profile

Perhaps the single, greatest concern experienced by a cancer survivor is the possibility that the disease will recur. Indeed, this concern isn't without foundation as cancer, similar to many other diseases, can recur years after one has been treated for and recovered from an initial occurrence. One who has experienced colon cancer, for example, is clearly susceptible to this particular form of the disease and retains an increased risk for developing it again at some future point in one's lifetime. Yet, the same individual may have an increased risk for developing other forms of cancer as well.

Accordingly, it's essential to long-term health care for every cancer survivor to thoroughly review her or his Risk Profile and be completely familiar with the cancers indicated. Once again, one's Risk Profile may not be foolproof as it may indicate an increased risk for some cancers that never materialize and it may omit others that do. It is, however, a good place to start and is an effective tool that will empower each individual with the ability to actively participate in her or his own cancer prevention program. It will force an individual to focus on potential problems as well as to take control and alter aspects of her or his lifestyle to insure better long-term health.

Don't Forget Your Buddies

In reviewing one's potential cancer risks, however, it's important to remember that there are two different aspects upon which one must focus attention. The first, of course, is the **initial primary cancer** of which the individual has already been diagnosed and treated. For those who have survived colon cancer, breast cancer or any other cancer, this first diagnosis is referred to as the initial primary cancer. This first cancer is certainly one for which the individual must take all precautions and preventative measures to avoid a recurrence.

The second point of attention must be directed toward any form of cancer that appears to be *related* to the initial primary cancer. For our purposes, we'll refer to these as **buddy cancers** — cancers that quite often appear simultaneously with or some time after the appearance of the initial primary cancer. This phenomenon occurs typically when 1) factors not clearly understood appear to influence the development of different cancers in similar ways, 2) certain cancers share the same known risk factors or when, 3) certain cancers spread to other specific body parts.

In the first case, for example, we know that colon cancer in women that appears to be hereditary has been linked to the future development of endometrial cancer. These two cancers don't share an abundance of known risk factors and the reasons for their buddy relationship are not clear. Further, the increased risk for endometrial cancer only appears to exist when the initial primary colon cancer is greatly influenced by heredity rather than other possible risk factors.

In the second case, we know that women who develop breast cancer have an increased risk for developing melanoma as well as endometrial and ovarian cancer. All of these cancers once again are buddy cancers of the initial primary breast cancer. In this relationship, the link between breast cancer and melanoma is similar to that between genetically influenced colon cancer in women and endometrial cancer. The cancers do not share significant known risk factors, yet women who experience breast cancer appear to have an increased risk for developing a future melanoma. The reasons for this particular buddy relationship are not clearly understood.

In contrast, the link between breast cancer and endometrial and ovarian cancer appears to be one of shared known risk factors, which in part, may be traced to heredity and the BRCA-1 and BRCA-2 genes. In any event, when the buddy relationship is defined by one cancer that creates an increased risk for another as seen in these first two cases, whether the factors for that increase are completely understood or not, the buddy cancer as well as the initial primary cancer should be addressed in one's Risk Profile as previously illustrated.

In the third case, some cancers are known to spread from one particular type of body tissue to another. In theory, of course, virtually any cancer can spread to almost any body part once the cancer metastasizes, and those body parts that lie in close proximity to the initial cancer are particularly vulnerable. There are certain cancers, however, that have a tendency to spread to specific body parts once they metastasize. This buddy relationship is distinguished from the first two cases in that this one does not necessarily mean that one's risk for developing another cancer in addition to the primary cancer appears to increase. It simply means that *if* the primary cancer does metastasize it's more likely to spread to some body parts than others.[324]

It appears, for example, that breast cancer that hasn't been detected early and has metastasized often spreads and creates new cancers in the tissues of the brain, liver, bone or lung. Indeed, a breast cancer tumor may contain specific genes that indicate the disease may not only have a greater tendency to spread, but may have a greater tendency to spread to the bones or the lungs in particular. Colon cancers also have a tendency to spread to the liver, an organ that shares several major blood vessels with the colon. Some metastasized colon cancers have a tendency to spread to the tissues of the lung where the malignant cells multiply and present as a new cancer.

In contrast, the cells from many other cancers can travel easily through the tissues of the brain, liver, bone or lung without lodging in the tissues and creating new cancers. Ovarian cancer cells, for example, rarely spread to the tissues of the lung once the cancer has metastasized. The reasons why some cancer cells proliferate in some body tissues and other cancer cells appear to pass harmlessly through are not fully understood. It appears that certain types of cancer cells prefer certain body tissues and, in turn, that certain body tissues are susceptible to certain cancer cells.[325]

In theory, researchers believe that different cancers carry different "keys" and different tissues have different genetic "locks." As a result, a cancer cell can only gain entry into a body tissue if the cell's key and the tissue's lock match. In any of the above cases, however, one who has experienced one type of cancer must guard not only against the recurrence of that initial cancer, but also against the occurrence of any known buddy cancers as well. And, as cancer research is continuous and ever changing, those cancers known to have a buddy relationship with another today may change or expand as new research becomes available.[326]

Having the most current information on the cancers that pertain to one, therefore, is an ongoing task that can best be accomplished through the continued and collaborative efforts of both the survivor and her or his oncologist. One must always ask questions. One must always be informed. One must always arm oneself with all the knowledge and information available at any given time.

Proper Medical Follow-Up Care

Checkups

As important as the proper medical care is for the cancer patient, proper medical care is just as important for the cancer survivor. Indeed, follow-up medical care for one who has survived cancer will begin shortly after the individual has completed her or his last course of cancer treatment and usually will continue throughout the individual's life. Regular checkups are an essential part of one's follow-up program and are typically conducted by one's oncologist. The survivor usually is required to return to the medical facility or office every three months for perhaps the first year. If no problems or concerns develop during this time, additional checkups may be scheduled once every six months unless, of course, the survivor chooses to return more often.

Follow-up medical care is vital because one's post-cancer physical body may be quite different from one's pre-cancer physical body. Clearly, if surgery was a part of the required treatment, the appearance of one's body will be altered in some way. But the way one's organs and body function, the levels of proteins, glucose and cholesterol, the blood counts, the ability to handle stress, the changes in energy and strength also may be different. It's important, therefore, to establish new baseline guides that indicate what the new physical "normalcy" for the survivor may be.

It's from these new guidelines that every post-cancer checkup will be measured. In this way, any change in one's health, regardless of how small it may be, will be noticed and documented. Under the supervision of one's oncologist, these checkups will be similar to one's pre-cancer checkups and may include a urinalysis, the recording of one's weight, blood pressure and temperature as well as an examination of one's eyes, ears, nose and throat. With a stethoscope, one's heart rate may be monitored and recorded as well as any abnormal sounds in one's lungs or abdomen. One's field of vision, balance, coordination and reflexes may be tested and, of course, the sites of cancer treatment will be examined.[327]

In addition, one's abdomen may be palpitated to check for any unusual enlargements of the spleen, liver or other organ, and one's neck, groin or armpits may be examined for swollen lymph nodes. This routine will change slightly, of course, depending upon the individual's personal history and needs. One aspect of a post-cancer checkup that remains fairly constant for all survivors, however, is the blood testing that typically will be conducted during each and every visit.

Post-Cancer Blood Tests

Blood tests are used commonly to help physicians diagnose an illness, monitor an illness or rule out an illness. They can be extremely helpful, for instance, in detecting infections and anemia as well as the possible presence of a number of different cancers. In some tests, a few drops of blood may be all that is required. If so, one's fingertip is usually "pricked" with a needle and the drawn blood is placed in a small vessel called a **capillary pipette**. If, however, the test requires more than a few drops, the blood will be drawn from a vein with a thin needle, then placed in a sterile syringe or several vials known as **vacuum containers**. The number of vials used in the procedure will depend upon the number of different tests to be conducted.[328]

Of the many possible tests, the **Complete Blood Cell Count** is the most common. This test, also known as a **CBC**, is actually a standard series of tests that together determine one's overall state of health. This series includes the 1) hematocrit test, which measures the level of red blood cells for anemia, 2) the hemoglobin test, which measures the grams of red cell pigment in the sample, 3) the platelet count, which measures the level of platelets and the blood's ability to properly clot and, 4) the white blood count, which obviously measures the level of white blood cells for the presence of infection. These measurements, of course, are especially important to the cancer survivor whose blood counts may have been significantly altered during one's course of treatment with chemotherapy or radiation.[329]

In addition to the CBC, the **blood chemistry group** of tests may be performed. These tests may include an analysis of one's glucose, liver and kidney functions as well as one's level of albumin, a major blood protein. They also may examine the body's levels of electrolytes including potassium, phosphorus, sodium and chloride. A **lipid blood test** may be performed to measure the level of fats, including triglycerides and both total cholesterol and high-density lipoprotein or HDL cholesterol, all of which pertain to one's risk for coronary heart disease.

Coagulation tests such as the **partial thromboplastin time**, or **PTT**, and the **prothrombin time**, or **PT**, are useful in identifying blood clotting and liver diseases. Other tests can measure one's levels of enzymes that may indicate damage to the liver or pancreas. Still others can be used to measure certain body hormones that may relate to a number of thyroid disorders.[330]

Now we come to the blood tests specifically designed to reveal the possible presence of malignant tumors within the body. As we've already discussed, these tests are known as tumor markers or biomarkers and may be used to monitor individuals who have already survived cancer as well as a preventative screening measure for individuals who have a high risk for developing certain cancers. Once again, a tumor marker is defined as any substance, typically a protein, within the body that may be related to or associated with the presence of cancer.

We know, for example, the proteins known as CA 15.3, CA 27.29, CA-125 and Tru-Quant are linked to the development of both breast and ovarian cancer. We also know that HE4 is a protein that may indicate the presence of ovarian cancer. In addition, **carcinoembryonic antigen,** or **CEA,** is a protein normally produced in a fetus during the first two trimesters of pregnancy. It also is produced, however, by adenocarcinomas of the digestive tract including those of the stomach, pancreas, liver, colon and rectum. Elevated levels of CEA also may indicate the presence of breast and ovarian cancer, as well as lung cancer.[331]

Alpha fetoprotein or **AFP** is another protein produced by a developing fetus. The level of production, however, gradually decreases as the fetus develops and after birth the level of AFP stabilizes as the child reaches the age of twelve months. An elevated level of this protein in an older individual, therefore, isn't normal and may indicate the presence of liver cancer. And, of course, prostate-specific antigen, or PSA, may indicate the presence of prostate cancer in men with elevated levels of the substance. While they're helpful, it's important to remember that tumor marker blood tests aren't infallible. A marker test that indicates elevated levels of these proteins associated with cancer doesn't "prove" that the disease exists.[332]

Elevated levels of these tumor markers may indicate a non-malignant disorder of the body tissue in question rather than a malignant one. Similarly, a marker test that produces normal results doesn't completely rule out the existence of cancer. An early stage cancer may exist. These tests are more accurate in detecting cancers that are more advanced. Regardless of their limitations, however, new tumor markers are being discovered every year, and tumor marker blood tests are an essential part of a cancer survivor's follow-up medical care program. Similar to their role in the overall program of early cancer detection, their value must not be underestimated.

Post-Cancer Screening Tests

The importance of undergoing appropriate and regular cancer screening tests for the cancer survivor is another follow-up step that cannot be underestimated. As important as these procedures are for individuals actively engaged in the process of cancer prevention and early detection, they're equally important for survivors monitoring their health for a cancer recurrence. For a survivor has moved from the world of theory in which certain cancers may occur according to one's Risk Profile, to a world in which cancer has become a reality. A survivor knows without a doubt that she or he is susceptible to a particular cancer. Accordingly, a survivor must become even more vigilant in the process of cancer prevention and early detection than she or he was before the initial diagnosis.

Not surprisingly, the screening procedures for specific cancers are the same for individuals whether they've experienced cancer or not. Most colon cancer survivors, for example, must expect to undergo regular colonoscopies following the release from their initial cancer treatment program. In fact, the recommended scheduling of this procedure will most likely increase to once a year for the first few years following one's release. If no anomalies are detected during this time, one's oncologist may change the screening schedule and suggest the individual undergo a colonoscopy every other year or every third year. Similarly, if one has survived breast cancer, undergoing a mammogram as well as an ultrasound once or twice every year may be advised.

In any event, post-cancer screening will remain more frequent for one who has already experienced the cancer than for one who has not. In most cases, this increase will continue throughout the survivor's lifetime.

It's not enough, however, for one to thoroughly understand one's initial primary cancer and to take all the steps and precautions necessary to prevent or signal its recurrence. As we already have discussed, one also must have full knowledge of the buddy cancers with which it is associated and must take the necessary steps to prevent the occurrence of these as well. For example, women who have experienced colon cancer that appears to have been genetically influenced should 1) undergo regular colonoscopies **and,** 2) maintain vigilance to prevent or monitor the development of endometrial cancer.

All individuals who have experienced colon cancer, whether it appeared to be genetically influenced or not, should 1) undergo regular colonoscopies **and**, 2) receive regular chest x-rays to monitor the health of the lungs **and**, 3) monitor the health of the liver through physical exams or occasional CT scans or MRIs. Women who have experienced breast cancer should 1) commit to regular mammograms **and**, 2) undergo regular blood tumor marker testing for breast and ovarian cancer **and**, 3) receive an annual full body skin check for melanoma **and**, 4) monitor the health of the uterus for endometrial cancer **and**, 5) if the breast cancer was advanced, monitor the health of one's brain tissue, liver, bones and lungs.

Further, individuals who received radiation therapy as a part of their cancer treatment, especially those who received radiation to the limbs or the abdominal and pelvic areas, should consider having a bone density test conducted within the first year of survival, then regularly thereafter. Buddy cancers that result from the spread of an initial primary cancer typically will develop within the first five years following one's release from the initial cancer treatment program.[333] Accordingly, the scheduling for post-cancer screening procedures will not only vary according to the individual and the recommendations of her or his oncologist, but may change with each passing year as well.

In this way, tissue anomalies such as colon polyps can be detected early and can be removed before the anomaly becomes cancerous. If a cancer recurs, or if a new one develops, it will be caught in an early stage and will be treated immediately. Damage to bones can be identified and treated appropriately to prevent future problems and osteoporosis. Indeed, due to this intensive program of post-cancer screening, most cancer survivors reduce their personal risk for developing certain cancers to a level that is lower than that shared by individuals in the general population and increase their chances for surviving a subsequent cancer to a level greater than those in the general population.

Life Considerations

With cancer survival comes a second chance for life and a renewed responsibility to care for and maintain that life. It's essential, therefore, for every survivor who has completed treatment to adopt and practice a complete program of health care that may include several lifestyle changes. For example, if one smoked or used tobacco at the time their cancer was diagnosed, now might be a good time to stop. If one never or rarely exercised at the time their cancer was diagnosed, now might be a good time to start. If one drank alcohol heavily at the time their cancer was diagnosed, now might be a good time to slow down.

In addition, diet will become extremely important in one's overall maintenance program. If one hasn't already done so, now might be a good time to consult a nutritionist. Post-cancer dietary dos and don'ts can be complicated and may vary tremendously depending upon the type of cancer one has survived. Once again, we're reminded of our octopus. One who has survived colon cancer, for instance, may want to avoid or reduce the amount of roughage she or he consumes. Foods such as nuts, popcorn, grains and many fruits and vegetables may be too difficult for a resectioned colon, especially in the first few months following treatment, to digest properly.

Yet, many of these foods provide essential nutrients and vitamins necessary for healing and maintaining healthy body tissues. Further, as we already have discussed, many of these nutrients and vitamins cannot be supplied by substituting supplements for many of these foods. Proteins also are important to the healing process, yet the digestion of proteins can be hard on the kidneys and, for one who has survived kidney cancer, the consumption of proteins may be problematic. Individuals who consider themselves overweight may want to increase their intake of fruits and vegetables while individuals who are vegetarian may need to find new ways to balance their fruit and vegetable intake with varied sources of protein in order to promote healing. Women in particular may wish to avoid caffeine, a bitter alkaloid that may aggravate the symptoms of cancer treatment induced menopause.

Moreover, chemotherapy can leave numerous chemicals in the body tissues that may take years to dissipate, and radiation can weaken and destroy body tissues permanently. Many of the organs involved with digestion may be affected and their ability to perform their jobs efficiently may be compromised. Selecting food more carefully and consuming more organic or natural foods that may reduce the amount of ingested drugs, chemicals and pesticides often becomes an important objective for many cancer survivors who wish to reduce the amount of ingested unnecessary additives and ease the work load of the digestive tract.

What Exactly Is Organic?

This deceptively simple question, unfortunately, has no simple answer. First, the term "organic" is only used in English speaking countries whereas in other countries the proper term is typically "bio," "oko" or "eco." Technically, organic is defined as "pertaining to or derived from living organisms" and when discussing foods, organic refers to the methods used to produce the foods rather than to the foods themselves. In general, organic usually refers to those foods that have been produced without pesticides, artificial fertilizers, preservatives, hormones or antibiotics. In addition, organic farming typically utilizes methods such as crop rotation, rotational grazing, intercropping, plant and animal waste recycling, tilling and natural mineral soil additives to promote biological diversity and ecological balance.[334]

Often, foods grown in these ways will be labeled "certified" organic. The standards and definitions for what constitutes "organic" may vary from one country to another yet, in the United States, the National Organic Standards Board states that this certification can only be given after produce has been grown for three years without the application of synthetic pesticides or chemicals. At this time, the entire farm, including its equipment and processing facilities, are inspected by an independent agency that is unaffiliated with the farmer, the processor or the vendor. If the inspection process finds that the above standards have been met, the agency will then issue a certificate certifying the farm's produce as "organic."[335]

Livestock as well can be certified organic if the animals have been raised on grains and other products that have been grown according to certified organic standards for a minimum of one year. In legislation passed in the United States in 2002, the **National Organic Program** further clarified the standards for organic foods, stating that raw or processed foods such as fruit juice or tomato sauce that contain ninety-five percent organic ingredients can be labeled organic. Processed foods that contain between seventy and ninety-five percent organic ingredients must have labels that read "made with certain organic ingredients." And, processed foods that have an organic content of less than seventy percent must have labels that specify the organic ingredients individually.[336]

These are only guidelines, however, and many products are marketed either intentionally or unintentionally with inaccurate and misleading labels. Products labeled organic may fall far short of one's expectations and the organic content of certain foods cannot always be guaranteed or substantiated. To further complicate matters, the guidelines that define organic are constantly in flux. For example, in April of 2004 the National Organic Program and the United States Department of Agriculture announced that growth hormones, animal drugs and antibiotics would be allowed on organic farms. As a result, calves and cows treated with antibiotics and other drugs can produce milk labeled organic as long as a year passes between the time of treatment and the time of milk production.

This is in contrast to the prior interpretation in which most organic dairies removed a treated cow from the herd permanently. The department also stated that livestock on organic farms could be fed tainted, non-organic fishmeal that frequently contains **bioaccumulators** such as PCBs and mercury that can become concentrated and stored in the tissues of the animal. Furthermore, the USDA stated it would no longer monitor organic labels on non-food products and that seafood, as well as pet food and body care products, could be labeled organic without adhering to any specified regulations at all. Due to widespread opposition these proposed changes haven't yet been enacted, however, the standards for organic food products remain a somewhat confused and nebulous issue.[337]

Additional drawbacks to organic food products include the fact that they can be scarce in some regions and even when availability isn't a problem, the cost of purchasing these foods can be. Typically, organic foods are more expensive because the methods required for their production are more expensive for the grower. Organic produce is grown without synthetic pesticides or chemicals. As a result, the task of keeping crops healthy is more difficult and more labor intensive. In most cases, additional workers also are required to replace the mechanization commonly found in conventional farming.

Furthermore, because organic produce requires the use of natural fertilizers and pest control efforts the crop yields often aren't as large as those grown in non-organic conditions.[338]

It's important to note, however, that even if foods are raised according to current organic guidelines it doesn't mean that the product necessarily will taste better. Taste is dependent upon freshness, and freshness is determined by the distance and time involved in shipping the product to market. In addition, certified organically grown produce isn't really healthier than produce grown in non-organic conditions in that the nutritional content of an orange, for example, will remain the same regardless of the way in which it was grown.[339]

Organic foods, however, may be safer for consumption. Meats and dairy products are free from growth hormones, antibiotics and fishmeal supplements and produce is free from pesticides and chemicals. These products also should be free of genetic engineering, ionizing radiation and fertilizers made of sewage sludge. Of course, one can wash produce before eating it; however, certain residues such as pesticides can be located within the produce as well as on the surface.[340]

Accordingly, even proper rinsing with warm or hot water and some form of soap may not remove pesticides or chemicals completely from produce before it's consumed. And while we're on the subject, products developed specifically to wash fruits and vegetables haven't been found to be more effective in cleaning produce than regular soap and water. They may, however, be more effective in removing the wax coating so often applied to produce to make it look more attractive.[341]

It's not clear how much of a threat is posed by the pesticides found in conventionally farmed produce or how much safer organically grown produce may be, and there are many proponents on both sides of the fence. Organic foods may not necessarily offer more health, but they may perhaps offer less harm. For individuals with compromised immune systems, therefore, the mere possibility that organic foods may help protect and maintain their somewhat fragile health may present a choice worth making. If so, it's advisable for such individuals to guarantee the quality and reliability of these foods firsthand by researching the vendor who sells the product, the farmer who supplies the product and the production methods utilized in raising and growing the produce, and caring for the animals.

Drug Free/Complementary Medical Follow-Up Care

We already have discussed many non-drug approaches that are valuable tools in reducing and eliminating cancer-related pain. Several of these techniques, however, also have proven valuable tools in the post-cancer maintenance of general health. Therapeutic exercise, for example, can continue to increase one's joint flexibility and improve one's cardiovascular and respiratory functioning long after one's cancer pain and treatments have come to an end. Massage can continue to improve one's blood circulation and muscle tone while it continues to relieve tension and increase relaxation.

The suggestions induced during hypnosis may continue to help a survivor sleep more soundly, feel more relaxed and maintain a positive outlook in regard to health issues. Biofeedback can continue to help a survivor change physiological body functions such as blood pressure rates from involuntary to voluntary responses. Progressive muscle relaxation can continue to reduce one's anxiety and increase energy. Visualization and distraction can continue to provide relief from everyday stress and reduce the negative impact of any lingering side effects due to cancer treatment.

The disciplines of meditation or yoga can calm one's mind, relax one's body, reduce the risk of heart disease and stroke, maintain normal blood pressure and enhance the functioning of one's immune system. And chiropractic, acupuncture and acupressure also may continue to provide positive health benefits for many cancer survivors seeking to recover and maintain their pre-cancer quality of life and good health.

Maintaining Health

Maintaining one's health at any time can be a daunting task that requires an enormous amount of attention and diligence. For cancer survivors, however, this task becomes one of even greater magnitude. No cancer survivor, of course, wants to experience a recurrence of the same cancer or an occurrence of another. We've already discussed several of the medical procedures and techniques that can aid a survivor in preventing the disease from developing in the future. We also have discussed lifestyle changes that one may wish to incorporate into one's daily routine to improve their physical and mental well being.

Yet, we must remember that maintaining good general health is more difficult for a survivor than for one who has never experienced cancer. For although the disease itself may have been eliminated, the treatments responsible for its elimination may leave the body in a weakened condition. Surgery can alter the body in physical ways that impair movement, weaken muscles, distort balance and change one's ability to engage in certain activities. Chemotherapy and radiation can produce long-term effects that harm body organs and interfere with their proper functioning, alter one's red blood count resulting in anemia and fatigue, reduce one's white blood count resulting in an increased susceptibility to infection and compromise one's entire immune system that leaves one more vulnerable to any illness or disease. It's essential, therefore, for every survivor to take steps on a daily basis to protect one's overall health and avoid unnecessary discomfort or pain. While the following suggestions are simply an exercise in common sense that apply to all individuals, their practice is especially important for a cancer survivor who wishes to remain as healthy as possible.

Twelve Tips

Most important, perhaps, is the practice of washing one's hands thoroughly and frequently each and every day. Human hands may be the greatest source for harboring and spreading a variety of germs and bacteria. Our hands come into contact with hundreds, if not thousands, of surfaces throughout the day that have in turn come into contact with hundreds, if not thousands, of hands belonging to other people. These germs and bacteria can live for many hours on human skin and can proliferate and spread to everything we touch. Accordingly, regular hand washing must become a part of every survivor's daily personal hygiene.

1) When washing one's hands, one should use antibacterial hand soap under warm or hot water and lather for a minimum of fifteen seconds.[342]

There are obvious situations that require immediate hand washing, such as using a bathroom, touching and handling trash, picking up after pets and changing diapers on children. In these situations soap and water are usually nearby and available. Yet, one often finds oneself in situations where soap and water aren't available and where hand washing is not practical. Accordingly,

2) One should always carry a small bottle of waterless hand sanitizer in one's pocket or purse to use when regular soap and water are not available.

These products are quite effective in killing germs and sanitizing hands and can be used virtually anywhere at anytime. Indeed, many hospitals and other medical facilities encourage the use of these products among their staff and supply dispensers for the products in every examination room.[343] Moreover, waterless hand sanitizers prove extremely useful in situations where the need for hand washing is less obvious yet, just as necessary. For example,

3) One should always wash one's hands after putting on shoes that require the use of one's hands to tie or buckle.

If there's any doubt about this suggestion, one only need observe the path the next time she or he walks a city block, a country mile or a few parking spaces from a vehicle to a front door. Our shoes collect and dispense as many germs and bacteria as our hands, and even if we spend our time indoors where flooring is cleaned regularly, bacteria are constantly being tracked in on the shoes of others. During our days, most of us walk into public bathrooms, through hospitals, into libraries and schools, restaurants and from one office to another.

One's shoes become a magnet for dirt and germs, and in an effort to stay healthy it's advisable always to wash one's hands, with or without water, each time we touch our shoes. Furthermore, it's estimated that approximately eighty percent of the germs and bacteria in our own homes is brought in on the soles of our shoes. Accordingly, removing them before entering the home, a tradition commonly observed in many parts of the world, also is advised. In addition,

4)   One should always wash one's hands before eating.

Yes, this seems to be another obvious situation that most individuals recognize, and it's a simple suggestion to follow when one is dining in. When dining out, however, many individuals forget that by the time they pick up their first piece of bread, they have touched the knob of their front door, perhaps a steering wheel, a vehicle door handle, the public door of the restaurant, possibly the chair back and seat, the table, the glass and silverware and the menu, some of which may have been touched by hundreds of other individuals.

This is where a small bottle of waterless hand sanitizer truly comes in handy. Further, because it isn't possible to avoid contact with every surface that may contain bacteria, one should refrain from eating or touching food with one's hands if at all possible. At the very least, one should refrain from eating the portion of the food, be it a roll, a cracker or a carrot stick, that one holds with one's fingers.

5)   Avoid foods in public places that are communal.

Many establishments, including lounges, restaurants, bars and grocery stores, often offer bowls of nuts and chips or plates of free product samples. Unless these foods are replaced for every customer, there is no telling how many fingers have touched them or how many times they have been sneezed or coughed upon. For survivors trying to remain healthy, these offerings should be avoided.

6)   Make certain that the physician or medical attendant in charge washes her or his hands.

Cancer survivors will be on a tight schedule of follow-up medical appointments for at least the first five years following their initial treatment. Typically, all medical personnel wash their hands after examining one patient and before examining another. This practice, however, is conducted to protect the health of the personnel and not necessarily the health of the patient.[344] If one, therefore, encounters a situation in which the examining medical personnel fails to wash her or his hands, one should request that they do so.

Headline:

Antibacterial Soaps–
Should They Be Avoided?

There is a fair amount of confusion surrounding the use of antibacterial soaps in general, and the use of waterless hand sanitizers in particular. Let's try to clear this up. First, some sources suggest that the use of antibacterial soaps results in a phenomenon known as "bacterial resistance." This means that while the weakest bacteria are killed during a regular hand washing, the strongest are not. Further, these stronger bacteria continue to multiply and continue to gain in strength until they are immune to the chemical agents in the antibacterial soap.[345]

Such hand washing, therefore, may leave an individual more susceptible to coughs and colds, rather than less susceptible. The chemical agents also kill the "good" bacteria found on the skin, which may contribute to one's vulnerability to sickness and disease. In addition, the active ingredient in most antibacterial soaps is triclosan, a chemical some studies suggest kills normal healthy human cells as well as bacteria.[346] Several other studies from around the world, however, indicate that any risk associated with the use of antibacterial soaps has been overstated and that no link exists between triclosan and antibiotic resistance.[347] As such, the existing data on this issue remains inconclusive and controversial.

Moreover, it's important to understand that *all* soaps are essentially antibacterial. Those considered "regular" soaps kill approximately 99.4 percent of the bacteria on the skin, and those labeled "antibacterial" kill approximately 99.6 percent of the bacteria. This is a small increase, and for most individuals the additional protection afforded by this .02 percent may not warrant the use of antibacterial soaps and exposure to their possible risks.[348] Yet, for individuals with compromised immune systems and for the medical personnel who care for them, the extra protection afforded by antibacterial soaps may be warranted. This is a decision each individual must make for her or himself.

The use of waterless hand sanitizers, however, doesn't present the same issues. First, these instant sanitizers kill 99.99 percent of germs without water or towels, the latter of which can harbor a significant amount of bacteria in themselves. Second, these sanitizers use alcohol to destroy germs physically. They're antiseptics, not antibiotics, so bacterial resistance cannot develop. Indeed, in 2001 the Center for Disease Control in the United States issued new guidelines for hand hygiene in health care facilities.[349]

These guidelines called for a move away from regular hand washing, unless the hands are contaminated or visibly dirty, and a move toward the use of alcohol-based, waterless sanitizing gels. They recommended that all health care personnel carry individual containers and that waterless sanitizing gels be kept at all patient bedsides. Indeed, hand washing with sanitizing gels is even replacing the traditional "surgical scrub" in hospitals.[350]

Moreover, these gels have not only been found to be more effective than regular or antibacterial soap and water, they also are less drying and irritating for some skin types. For other skin types, some of these gels contain a moisturizer that helps combat dry skin. Of course, one can always apply a moisturizer after using a sanitizing gel. If one does so, however, one should wait a minute or so as the bacteria won't be killed until the gel has completely dried and the alcohol has evaporated.[351]

7) In other circumstances, make certain that individuals wear gloves to insure cleanliness.

The right to request an assurance of clean hands isn't limited to the medical profession. There are other situations in which one shouldn't expect or assume that the person in question has clean hands. The employee who spoons tuna salad in a delicatessen, prepares sandwiches at a fast food restaurant or selects cookies from a pastry counter should always use gloves as well as the proper utensils to do so.

Further, only those employees whose job it is to serve food should do so. The employee who handles the money and the cash register, for example, should never handle the food. The employee who throws the pizza dough shouldn't answer the telephone unless her or his hands are washed after every call. In certain countries and in certain professions this precaution is required by law, and in others it's practiced as a common courtesy. If one is confronted by a situation in which neither case appears to apply, however, the individual has the right to make this simple request.

8) When in public, one should touch as little as possible.

The less one touches, the cleaner one's hands will remain. Unless it's necessary to maintain balance and insure safety when no other means of support is available, one should avoid touching handrails on escalators, walkways and staircases. Instead of using fingers, one should try using an elbow to punch a button in an elevator. One can push swing doors open with a shoulder or pull them open with a scarf, jacket, shirttail or tissue covered hand. In these small ways, one can lessen one's exposure to the bacteria that proliferates in public places.

9)   One should take one's own reading material to public or medical waiting rooms.

Public waiting rooms typically are filled with magazines and books designed to occupy the client or patient as she or he waits. Indeed, some of this material remains in a waiting room for months and even years. Throughout that time, it may be used by hundreds of individuals and if the reading material is in a physician's office, medical clinic or hospital, many of those individuals most likely will have been sick. As a result, it's advisable to avoid touching these materials. If one expects a delay or enjoys reading while waiting, one should always take her or his own book or magazine to each appointment.

10) One should wait outside a medical waiting room if necessary.

Individuals in medical waiting rooms often are already ill. This may be obvious if those waiting are sneezing, coughing and blowing their noses. If this should be the case, or if one is uncomfortable for other reasons less obvious, one should wait in the hall, in the lobby or even outdoors if one wishes. Every individual has the right to protect her or himself from unnecessary harmful exposure to illness. If it appears that remaining in a waiting room may compromise one's health in any way, one should explain the situation to the receptionist or nurse, request an alternative place to wait and a time to return.

11) Try to avoid close contact with others who are sick.

It's not always possible to recognize when another individual is sick, and even when we do, it's not always possible to avoid contact with the individual. This is especially true for one who must spend a great deal of time in and around medical offices and hospitals. If another's illness is made apparent by coughing and sneezing, one should always try to leave the room or the area. The bacteria that spread from a simple cough or sneeze can travel several feet in a wide area. If this isn't possible, however, at the very least one should turn away from the source and cover one's mouth and nose.

12) Breathe through the nose.

When in public, or around others who are obviously sick, breathing through the nose can offer a great deal of protection from unavoidable air borne particles and bacteria. The small hairs in the nose act like a filter that prevents many harmful elements from entering the nasal passages, the throat and the lungs. Similarly, the filtering process of the nose can disarm many air borne elements that can cause problems when inhaled and absorbed by the tissues of the mouth.[352]

One must remember, however, that any filtering system must be cleaned regularly and maintained to insure maximum effectiveness. Accordingly, one should blow one's nose often. This simple act will remove much of the accumulated waste in the nasal passages and allow the nasal hairs to do their job properly. In addition, one must remember that any filtering system by definition will be filled with dirt, dust and airborne bacteria. As such, it's **always** important to use tissues or handkerchiefs to clean the nose and teach children from an early age **never** to play with or eat anything that comes out of the nose.

Paranoid? Not really. Practical? Absolutely. A bit extreme? Possibly. Yet, for one whose immune system has been compromised by cancer, chemotherapy, radiation, or for that matter, any other illness or condition, these precautionary measures will prove to be invaluable tools in maintaining the good general health that so many of us once took for granted.

Personal Note

While shopping in a bakery recently, I decided to purchase a dozen croissants. The employee was helpful and suggested she give me those that had just come out of the oven rather than those in the counter window. I agreed, of course, but noticed that as the employee walked to the baked goods by the oven, she pushed a trash can out of her way with her bare hands, then proceeded to pick up the croissants, again with her bare hands.

I didn't want to say anything to embarrass her or myself. Yet, I knew I wouldn't be able to eat the croissants after observing the way in which they had been handled. So, I stopped her and asked her to please use gloves or a utensil before picking up my croissants. She replied by saying the trash can wasn't really "dirty," but she would do as I asked. In spite of my initial reluctance, I realized my request was absolutely valid and I no longer hesitate to make such requests when necessary.

Chapter 9:
Survivorship: Emotional Concerns

Courage in danger is half the battle.
Titus Macci Plautus

One's life as a survivor will not only differ from one's pre-cancer life in physical ways, it will differ in emotional ways as well. Of course, it isn't really possible to separate completely the emotional concerns from the physical for these issues are intimately intertwined. Our physical state often dictates our emotional state and vice versa. It's only for the sake of organization that we attempt to make this separation within these pages.

To begin, each cancer survivor, similar to others who have faced life and death situations, has emerged victorious from a treacherous journey. For many, one's greatest fears have been realized and overcome. It's a time to recognize and embrace one's strength, one's courage and one's resilience. It also, however, is a time to recognize that some things will now be different.

In addition to the ways in which one's body may be different, one's expectations and goals may be different, one's ability to communicate with others may be different and one's image of oneself and the world in which one lives may be different. This isn't to say that these differences will be necessarily negative, for they may embody greater expectations and goals, an increased ability to communicate and an improved image of oneself and one's world. Yet, anyone who has survived a serious physical health threat may encounter a range of specific and difficult emotional repercussions as a direct result of that threat.

Good mental health and emotional stability are concepts extremely difficult to define. These concepts often have been determined by the way in which one acts and reacts to stress or difficult situations, and one's ability to move through those situations in a reasonable and thoughtful manner. Reactions to stress, however, and the appropriateness of those reactions differ from one culture to another. A variety of emotions expressed in one culture may be considered completely acceptable, while in another the same expressions may be considered quite odd.

Accordingly, a definition of these concepts depends, at least in part, upon an individual's cultural background and circumstances. With this in mind, a better definition of good mental health and emotional stability might be the simple ability to accept and cope with life and its changes, to overcome traumatic experiences and create and live a productive and useful life. Further, it's important to recognize that mental and emotional health don't result from the absence of conflict or the ability to repress conflict, but rather from the ability to accept and learn from conflict.

Every individual lives a unique life the responsibilities of which may include school, a career, caring for a family, friends and a variety of other issues. Regardless of one's culture or lifestyle, every well-adjusted individual strives to meet the demands of those personal responsibilities while maintaining some degree of harmony and balance with the demands of culture and society. In the most basic sense, therefore, we might say that good mental health and emotional well being equate to an individual's ability simply to function. And when physical illness and trauma enter the equation, this basic ability may be significantly compromised.

The relationship between physical illness and emotional well being isn't a difficult concept to understand. When our health is good, when we have sufficient energy, when we're sleeping well and getting adequate rest, when we're eating properly, receiving necessary nutrients and vitamins, and when our bodies are functioning according to design, getting through each day is a little easier. When we're in pain, when we experience fatigue, when we suffer from insomnia, when we cannot eat and when our bodies fail us in various ways, getting through each day becomes more difficult.

Meeting daily responsibilities becomes a significant chore, and as the control we thought we had over our lives begins to disintegrate, our confidence in our abilities and ourselves often begins to waver. Further, some illnesses have a direct impact upon the endocrine system, the central nervous system or other body systems that produce the chemicals and hormones necessary for proper mental and emotional functioning. Illness that's potentially fatal or results in disfigurement or disability also can trigger a number of emotional responses that greatly interfere with one's day-to-day activities.

In such difficult situations, the most common of these emotion responses may include **anger**, **anxiety**, **depression** and **grief**. Clearly, these types of responses may arise at anytime during a severe illness. Yet, there's a distinction between the time one spends being ill and the time one spends resuming life after the illness. Certainly in cancer cases, the individual may go through periods of anxiety or depression while undergoing treatment and recovery. During this time, however, the individual is fully engaged in a fight for survival, and one's focus remains upon the physical aspects of the disease.

Once treatment is completed and the individual is released from this intense medical care, she or he returns "home" to the life left behind. No longer a patient, a survivor may expect that life to be the same as it was before the disease interrupted it. A survivor may not be prepared for the many ways in which that life may be different. Relationships with family and friends may be altered, one's ability to work or attend school may be compromised and, of course, one may continue to be physically plagued by the long-term, chronic side effects of cancer treatments. With expectations dashed and the quality of life diminished on one side, and the pressure, need and desire to reclaim one's former life on the other, one's mental and emotional stability and well being may be significantly challenged.

In General

Anger

Simply defined, anger is an emotional reaction characterized by rage or displeasure, indignation or belligerence and hostility.[353] It's a response that often results from situations in which an individual encounters frustration or provocation. When one is unhappy or displeased with the circumstances in which one finds oneself, it's common to strike out at those circumstances, to take revenge on those circumstances and even find someone or something to blame for those circumstances.

Certainly, the circumstances in which a cancer survivor finds her or himself may be fraught with frustration and a variety of mental and physical obstacles. It may be difficult to regain one's strength and health, resume work and career and adjust to life at home with family and friends. There may be many days spent in physical pain, fatigue and mental confusion or hours chained to a toilet with nausea or diarrhea. While anger associated with these types of challenges is to be expected, some of it may be irrational.

One may ask, for example, "Why me? Why must I go through this pain? Why must I suffer?" This, however, is really the wrong question. The more appropriate question is, "Why not me?" After all, we know that if the statistics for cancer incidence continue to increase at their present rate over the next ten years, nearly one out of every two individuals will have or have had some form of cancer. Further, unless the question is asked with the intent of researching and tracing the cause of the cancer to one of the specific risk factors associated with the disease, it's not a particularly helpful question to ask. For cancer can strike anyone, of any race, of any age, in any part of the world, at any time.

So on the one hand, we have some emotional responses to having the disease and struggling through its recovery that are not driven by logic. On the other, the fact that one may be affected by pain, physical limitations or uncomfortable chronic side effects that interfere with one's ability to function and enjoy life after cancer are driven by logic and first hand experience. In either case, anger due to frustration under these circumstances is a completely natural and expected emotional response.

The key, of course, is to find ways of dealing with this anger that will help alleviate its intensity without further aggravating the situations causing the anger in the first place. To this end, most experts agree that anger shouldn't be repressed or ignored. It's a powerful emotion that shouldn't be allowed to fester, but rather, should be recognized and directly confronted. Recognizing one's anger, identifying the source of the anger, then talking about the anger has been a long-standing approach in managing anger. Doing so allows an individual to vent her or his frustration and possibly change or improve the situation or circumstance creating the frustration.[354]

One may choose to discuss one's anger privately and intimately with family, a friend or a physician. Or one may choose to join an anger management or cancer survivor support group and discuss the situation openly with others experiencing the same frustration and anger. In any case, every survivor must remember that they are not alone. Anger while one adjusts to her or his new post-cancer life is a common and natural phenomenon for which an enormous amount of help, both personal and professional, is available.

Anxiety

Defined as a vague, uneasy feeling the source of which may or may not be known, anxiety is characterized by numerous objective and subjective criteria.[355] Objectively, one may experience restlessness and insomnia, an increased heart rate, dilated pupils, trembling, a quivering voice or increased perspiration. Subjectively, one may experience tension, feelings of uncertainty and inadequacy, helplessness, fear and apprehension. Recovering from cancer is a critical time in one's life filled with new and stressful situations. It comes as no surprise that the threat of self image, the change in one's health status, pain or discomfort and the fear of being a burden to one's family and friends can result in anxiety.[356]

Like anger, anxiety is a powerful response that can significantly decrease one's ability to interact with others, think clearly or solve problems, retain self-confidence and face and overcome physical obstacles. Anxiety, however, is two fold in that the objective and observable physical characteristics of the response may be easy to detect while the thoughts and mental processes that give rise to these physical characteristics may not be. Pinpointing the true source of the anxiety, therefore, may require professional counseling with a psychologist or help from a social worker. It may require joining a support group or conversing with one's religious or spiritual community leader.[357]

In any event, talking about the problem is the first step in resolving the problem. It also may be helpful to increase activities one finds enjoyable and spend more time with close and trusted family members and friends. It's, of course, important to treat any physical condition created by the anxiety or any pain or discomfort that appears to be causing the anxiety. Finally, the practice of relaxation techniques, meditation, yoga and exercise should all be encouraged for their mental as well as their physical health benefits.

Grief

Also known as bereavement or mourning, grief is a universally recognized pattern of physical and emotional responses to extreme sorrow, separation or loss.[358] For cancer survivors, many different types of loss can trigger grief. It may be triggered by the loss of one's good health or the loss of a body part or tissue. It may result from the loss of one's self image or from the loss of one's quality of life. It may result from the loss of time spent in illness and recovery or from opportunities lost due to the disease. It may occur as one realizes that activities, life expectations, goals and relationships have changed and pleasures once enjoyed may not, in some cases, be resumed or recovered.

Regardless of the many possible origins of grief, however, the symptoms in each case remain typically the same. Physically, the symptoms of grief are similar to those produced by fear, rage and pain and occur when the sympathetic portion of the nervous system is stimulated. These symptoms can include an increase in heart rate and blood flow, tightness or pain in the throat and chest, bristling of the hair, dilation of the pupils and sweating. One may experience extreme restlessness, headaches, a shortness of breath or a lack of muscular power and lethargy.[359]

Grief also can produce emotional symptoms, such as feelings of guilt and anger, hostility, disorientation, as well as an inability to concentrate, initiate or maintain familiar patterns of daily activity. One may choose to withdraw from social and family responsibilities, one may become irritable and experience extreme mood swings, insomnia and crying spells.[360]

Grief, or the process of grieving, will vary from one individual to another. One may experience all of these classic symptoms or only a few. The symptoms may appear immediately after a crisis or their appearance may be delayed several weeks or months following the crisis. They may be extreme in nature or mild to the point they appear to be absent. Yet, enough similarities exist in the typical **grieving process** to allow it to be divided into five basic stages including 1) **denial or disbelief**, 2) **anger and blame**, 3) **bargaining**, 4) **depression,** and 5) **resolution and acceptance**.[361]

In denial, the first stage of grief, one may not be able to grasp the reality of the situation that has created the tremendous feelings of loss. One may refuse to accept the fact that life has changed in some significant way and may attempt to remove oneself emotionally from the new and painful situation. An individual may feel isolated and may have difficulty concentrating, relating to other people and performing everyday functions. Eventually, when the individual can no longer fight or ignore this new reality, she or he may be overcome with feelings of anger and a need to attach blame to someone or something for creating this new reality.

During this second stage of grief the individual may strike out at family and friends. The individual may hold one's physician, hospital or medical staff responsible for their pain. One may blame oneself for the crisis or doubt one's faith and belief system or target the world and the universe in general. Typically, such anger will dissipate, and when it does, this emotion may be replaced with apology and a search for comfort.

In this third stage of grief, the individual may begin to bargain with the world and make promises in exchange for comfort. One may, for example, vow never to smoke again if her or his lung cancer is cured. One may promise to live a more productive life if her or his health is restored or if the cancer-related pain is resolved. Such bargaining, however, won't produce immediate results and when the futility of one's good intentions and promises becomes apparent, one may enter the fourth stage of grief known as depression.

At this stage, one may feel like giving up. One may be overcome with feelings of hopelessness and defeat and the crisis creating these feelings may appear too powerful an enemy to fight effectively. Punctuated by extreme fatigue, sadness and mood swings, this fourth stage typically is the longest phase of the grieving process and can last for several months. Eventually, however, the individual will work through these various stages of grief and enter a final emotional state defined by feelings of resolution and acceptance of the crisis and the new reality it has created.[362]

One's mental and physical energy begins to return as will one's ability to think clearly and engage in daily activity. One's confidence increases and one's self image improves. Once insurmountable obstacles are now seen as challenges that can be faced and overcome. One's adjustment to a life that may differ in many ways from one's pre-cancer life begins to be seen in a new light that brims with promise and possibility.

Having stated this, the grieving process will nevertheless vary from one individual to the next. It isn't possible to determine how long a particular stage of grief will last or if the stages will occur in the typical sequence. One may stay in one stage for an extended period of time, skip another stage entirely or experience several stages simultaneously. Some may resolve their acute grief responses within a few weeks while others may not reach resolution for several months. Indeed, the residual effects of the milder symptoms associated with grief may continue for a year or longer. Further, one's cultural background will greatly influence the overall process of grieving and the ways in which one expresses that grief.[363]

In any case, grieving is a process that must be treated with respect. It's a necessary and healthy response to loss that needs to be exposed and experienced rather than repressed or prevented. Most individuals will move through the grieving process in their own time and in their own way without the need for formal intervention. Grief, however, is a response that also has the potential for developing into a number of pathological conditions and psychosomatic illnesses.

Grief or bereavement that is healthy, and that which is not, is sometimes distinguished by the terms **uncomplicated bereavement** and **complicated bereavement**.[364] While there is no specific standard for determining this difference, there are warning signs that may indicate a problem is developing. Avoidance and reluctance to face one's crisis may be one of those signs. A prolonged inability to function and conduct one's normal daily activity may be another. The development of new physical ailments in addition to those already present may be yet another.

If it appears one is experiencing complicated bereavement, it may be necessary to enlist the aid of a support group, social worker or mental health professional to help guide that individual through the process to resolution. For complicated bereavement can aggravate the healing process and lead to a number of physical and mental disorders, such as insomnia, bulimia and anorexia, asthma, ulcers and clinical depression.

Depression

Most individuals have experienced some form of depression to one degree or another at some time during their life, either through personal experience or through the experience of a family member or friend. It's, indeed, one of the most common of all psychological problems and is estimated to affect approximately seventeen million individuals each year in the United States alone. It's important, however, to distinguish normally occurring feelings of sadness and disappointment from true clinical depression.[365]

Every individual faces situations in life that create stress and at one time or another every individual feels sad, fatigued or discouraged. These emotional responses may result from serious problems in one's family life or work environment. They also may result from a personal loss or tragedy and, in most cases, these feelings are appropriate and in proportion to the event. They typically dissipate within a few days, weeks or months as we adjust to or eliminate the problem and learn to accept the loss. And, typically, these responses do not interfere with school, work or relationships on a long-term basis.

Clinical depression, on the other hand, can significantly alter the way one feels and thinks, and as a result, it can change one's inner sense of physical and mental well being as well as one's outer social behavior. It's defined as a mood disorder or an abnormal emotional state characterized by long lasting feelings of hopelessness, melancholy, despair and sadness that become exaggerated, inappropriate and out of proportion to reality.[366]

Further, clinical depression can have its origin in a number of sources other than personal loss or disappointment such as genetics, pharmacology and drug use, nutrition, infection, neurology or endocrinal imbalances. The symptoms of depression can be as numerous as its causes and may include oversleeping or insomnia, overeating or loss of appetite, fatigue and lack of energy, loss of enjoyment, difficulty concentrating and making decisions, excessive crying and even physical aches and pains that occur for no apparent reason.[367]

In extreme cases, of course, depression also may lead to alcohol and drug abuse as well as thoughts of self-harm and suicide. Regardless of the severity, however, or the cause or range of symptoms, depression can have a tremendous impact on one's ability to function and engage in normal daily activities. It can result in a loss of productivity, emotional pain and a disruption of life not only for the one who experiences the depression, but for those who care for and live with the depressed individual as well.[368]

Regrettably, the majority of individuals who suffer from depression fail to get proper treatment. All too often, the symptoms one may experience simply aren't recognized as clinical depression. Additionally, because depression can result in numerous changes that typically are associated with physical illness it often is misdiagnosed as being such. When this occurs, the symptom may be treated while the underlying cause remains untreated.

Further, some individuals experience symptoms so severe they lose their ability to recognize the problem and seek help, while those around the individual wrongly perceive the problem to be a matter of disinterest or laziness. Some individuals recognize they have a problem but are reluctant to seek help because of the unjust social stigma that sometimes attaches to one with the disorder or to one's association with professionals trained to treat the disorder.[369]

The entire process of facing cancer, undergoing treatment and enduring recovery is an exercise in overcoming one's fear, inhibitions, modesty and reluctance. It's a process that forces us to accept reality with all its unpleasantness and to take whatever action is necessary to restore and protect our health. Depression isn't a weakness and it isn't a condition about which one should feel embarrassed or inadequate. If one finds she or he is experiencing any of the symptoms we have discussed, and if their presence is interfering with one's ability to meet the demands of daily life, one should seek help immediately.

Once again, the first step in securing help is to consult with one's oncologist or quarterback doctor. Of course, it may be helpful to talk to any trusted person who cares for and understands the situation. This person, however, may be too emotionally involved in the situation to offer objective advice. And in most cases, this person also will lack the professional training required to diagnosis the condition and recommend the proper treatment.

One's oncologist or quarterback doctor, however, will have the experience necessary to evaluate the individual, ask the proper questions, enlist the aid of other specialists if required and decide upon a proper course of action. Typically, when depression is suspected, an individual will undergo a complete consultation with a psychologist. This consultation will determine if the individual actually is experiencing a depressive illness, and if so, how severe and what type of depression it is. This consultation also will include a complete medical history that becomes even more important when the individual is a cancer survivor and when the depression appears to be related in some way to the disease.[370]

A good psychologist will list every symptom the individual is experiencing and will inquire as to when they began and how severe they have become. A good psychologist will attempt to cross-reference each emotional symptom with a corresponding physical condition and vice versa. For those struggling through a post-cancer recovery, a good psychologist will rule out other less likely sources of the depression by inquiring about one's family history regarding depression, one's diet, additional illnesses and possible alcohol or drug abuse. Lastly, a **mental status examination** will assess an entire range of psychological symptoms and problems that will help identify any additional condition pertinent to the individual's emotional well being. In this way, a good psychologist can diagnosis and evaluate the type and severity of the depression and can determine the most appropriate treatment.[371]

While psychotherapy is the most common type of treatment for clinical depression, it's a therapy that can take many forms. **Supportive counseling**, for example, encourages the individual to recognize her or his emotional problems and to talk openly about them. Such counseling addresses the specific feelings the individual may be experiencing, such as hopelessness or helplessness, and strives to reduce the individual's emotional pain resulting from these feelings.

In contrast, **cognitive therapy** attempts to change the way the individual thinks and evaluates the world in which she or he lives. This therapy can help teach one to distinguish between problems that are important and critical to physical and emotional well being and those that are not. It can help an individual change unrealistic into realistic expectations, pessimistic into optimistic thoughts and overt self-criticism into balanced evaluations and acceptance.

Third, **problem-solving therapy** strives to teach an individual how to take action and change the areas of her or his life causing or contributing to the depression. If these problem areas require the individual to develop better coping skills to make these necessary changes, the treatment may include **behavioral therapy**. If these problem areas relate to one's personal relationships with family or friends, the proper treatment may include **interpersonal therapy**.[372]

When diagnosed with clinical depression, it's important for one to remember that there are two aspects to treating the disorder, initiating change on an internal level and initiating change on an external level.[373] Supportive counseling and having individuals around with whom one can talk, vent one's frustrations and compare notes feels beneficial and, indeed, is an important first step in overcoming depression. It can create internal changes that positively affect one's evaluation of self and others, one's expectations from a post-cancer life and one's ability to identify and focus on the problems that have become so overwhelming on a daily basis.

This type of help, however, is only skin deep. It's cosmetic therapy that addresses the various symptoms of depression and the way we think about them, but stops short of addressing the underlying external sources responsible for the depression. Change also may be required in the way we communicate with others, the way we manage relationships and the way we conduct the physical aspects of our life. This type of external change, for example, may require a cancer survivor to explain fully to family members the household chores she or he is capable of doing and those she or he is not.

The cancer survivor may need to curtail certain physical activities that have become too strenuous. The cancer survivor may need to rest more during the day, or reduce the hours one spends at work or equip one's home with special features to compensate for a resulting disability. By doing so, the cancer survivor can eliminate or improve many of the situations that create frustration and contribute to depression in the first place.

In cases of severe depression, however, chronic fatigue, insomnia and the inability to concentrate may be so debilitating that one is unable to make the necessary changes. One simply may not have the energy to mentally focus or physically act upon her or his behalf. Should this occur, the appropriate treatment for the depression may include medications in addition to psychotherapy. Known as **antidepressants**, these medications will be used only if it appears to be absolutely necessary and only after the individual has been completely informed about the pros and cons of their use.[374]

Once the individual has granted consent, one's oncologist or quarterback doctor, in conjunction with one's psychologist, will carefully monitor the medication of choice. In addition, the medication will be used only for a limited period of time and only after its compatibility with the individual's health history has been determined. In this way, a collaborative treatment approach between the individual, the primary physicians and the psychologist will insure one receives the care necessary for a full and complete recovery.

Recovery from clinical depression, however, won't be a quick and easy process. It's important for one undergoing psychotherapy for this condition to understand that positive and noticeable results may not be seen for several weeks or months. It takes time to recognize the aspects of our life that have helped create our depression. It takes time to change the ways in which we perceive our world and ourselves and to develop better communication skills. It takes time to make the necessary external changes in our daily activity, our home or workplace and our relationships. And, it takes time for medication to work and for one to fully recover from the physical and mental side effects that so often contribute to the cancer survivor's difficulties.[375]

Treatment itself may be a lengthy process. While most individuals may attend psychotherapy once a week, the sessions may continue for several months depending upon the severity of the depression and the number of life situations that must be addressed and altered. In any case, however, one suffering from clinical depression must acknowledge it's a condition that must be treated and a condition for which several treatment options and ample help are available.

Relationships

Let us state once again, surviving cancer is a process. It's a long-term commitment that requires great vigilance, awareness and persistence. It's a commitment in which one must accept and overcome a number of potential limitations, obstacles and challenges. Cancer is a disease the impact of which, in many cases, will continue to be felt by the survivor throughout her or his lifetime. It's a disease that alters one's perception of reality and creates a defining point in time by which other life events will be measured. Invariably, one will always compare life before cancer to life after cancer.

Yet, the demands of survival aren't limited to the survivor. For while one's health care team may slowly disengage from one's life, one's family and friends remain. And these individuals will face many of the same challenges that confront the survivor. The survivor, family and friends all will be required to explore and accept new ways of thinking about themselves and each other. All will be required to analyze their existing relationships with one another. All will be required to alter those relationships to accommodate a new reality. For survival demands that those who share in the victory of a loved one's battle with cancer also must share in the fight to overcome the emotional and physical challenges created by that victory.

Family

It's a simple fact that some people have an easier time accepting the realities of cancer than others. This is true for those directly affected by the disease as well as those indirectly affected. During the actual physical battle with cancer, the patient's loved ones as well as the patient are preoccupied with the disease itself. During this time, family relationships are focused upon helping the loved one survive. With survival and the completion of treatment, however, these relationships are forced to re-define their purpose and focus upon the future and the challenges that future presents. This, of course, can prove to be a daunting and difficult task.

To begin, family members may not understand that recovery isn't a fixed and static event. It isn't something that magically occurs when a tumor is removed or when chemotherapy and radiation are completed. It's a long-term process for which many family members may not be prepared. Just as the survivor often expects to pick up life exactly as it was left, one's family may share the same unreasonable expectation. Indeed, recovery from cancer treatment may take a much longer period of time than the treatment itself. One's post-cancer life will be different in many ways, a fact that must be acknowledged by the survivor's family as well as by the survivor.[376]

By definition, a survivor is someone who has overcome a life-threatening disease, condition or situation.[377] As such, a survivor is no longer considered to be "sick" and family members may feel the special efforts they have contributed to the survivor and the family during the long months of treatment are no longer necessary. Family members may expect the survivor to begin carrying her or his own weight and resume her or his prior responsibilities immediately. Family members may expect the survivor to reclaim her or his place in the family easily and without complication. Family members may be anxious to and insist upon a return to "normal" life and the relationships they all shared before cancer entered their lives.

Family members may not realize that the relationships within the family may never return to "normal."[378] They may be altered in permanent ways. In addition to the expectations family members may have for the survivor, they may have others for themselves. Loved ones may feel they aren't appreciated. They may feel their efforts aren't being recognized. They may feel that no one longer cares about their needs. They may feel unimportant compared to the overwhelming concerns now facing the family. All of these issues must be addressed if the family is to move forward together and build a future that provides comfort and support for each individual member.

Once again, the most important skill a cancer survivor can possess is that of clear and precise communication. No one can really understand cancer or cancer recovery and the ways it affects everyday life unless one has experienced cancer first-hand for oneself. Accordingly, it's the survivor's responsibility to explain the details of their physical condition and their emotional state to others. One needs to speak openly about one's feelings and the healing process. One needs to describe one's pain or discomfort and the ways in which it affects one's ability to function. One needs to define the responsibilities one is able to assume and those one is not. A survivor needs to assess one's needs to insure she or he will be able to meet the demands of those responsibilities.

If, for example, one needs a two-hour nap each afternoon before helping with dinner, say so. If one only feels well enough to run errands in the morning, let others know. If outdoor activities prove too exhausting, change the routine and work indoors instead. Let family members know what they can now expect of and from you, and what they cannot. For without this information, loved ones cannot properly assess the situation and replace old expectations that have become unrealistic. With it, new expectations can be adopted and an enormous amount of confusion, frustration and resentment can be avoided.

Clearly, this is easier said than done. There will be situations in which the best efforts and powers of communication will, nonetheless, prove inadequate. Successful cancer recovery isn't limited to the survivor, it's a process that involves an entire family. It must address the complexity of perhaps numerous and conflicting personalities, needs, expectations and limitations. It must employ creative and practical methods to balance these issues and resolve differences and misunderstandings. The survivor may not be up to the task. Family members may not be up to the task. Good communication skills may be lacking. Or, individuals simply may be too tired, too worried or too frightened to speak frankly to one another.

In these cases, it's highly advisable for the family to enlist some type of professional help. Once again, this help may come in the form of a support group, a clergy or spiritual leader, a licensed counselor, a social worker, a physician or a psychologist. Such help will provide an objective evaluation of the situation as well as suggestions and techniques for improving the situation. Further, recognizing the need and asking for help is in no way a sign of weakness or failure. Rather, it's a sign of perception and wisdom that illustrates one's desire to implement a successful recovery process that embraces the entire family.

Regrettably, not everyone or every family will be able to move through the cancer recovery process to a point of successful resolution. As we already stated, some people have a greater capacity for accepting and living with the reality of cancer than others. Regardless of the efforts of professional guidance, in some cases siblings, children, parents or spouses won't be able to rise to the challenge cancer and its recovery present, and they will leave.

Some may only distance themselves emotionally from the survivor. They may refuse to help around the house or decline to talk about the situation. They may choose to ignore the new reality of family life and pretend that nothing has changed. They may fail to acknowledge the fact that cancer affects them as well as the survivor. In some cases family members will abandon the survivor completely by moving out, by cutting all ties of communication or by divorce.

The reasons for these extreme and largely irrational reactions are enormously complex and can only be examined on a case-by-case basis. One would have to know the history and background of the individual in question as well as the history and background of the individual's relationship with the survivor. One would have to examine the individual's health and mental history, her or his expectations and goals for the future.

For some, such responses may be triggered by the survivor's new physical limitations. One may find that the survivor's inability to speak or walk without aid or to have children is unacceptable. One may be unable to face the reality of disfigurement, missing body parts or openings and tubes in tissue where once there were none. Many of these reactions, however, arise from the desire some individuals have simply to avoid illness and its aftermath.

Not surprisingly, such avoidance behaviors typically are triggered by fear.[379] Some individuals actually may suffer from clinical disorders such as pathophobia, the fear of disease, panthophobia, the fear of suffering and disease or carcinophobia, the fear of cancer.[380] And while no well-adjusted individual wants to be sick or suffer or get cancer, these phobias by definition are intense, abnormal and irrational fears that render an individual completely incapable of making intelligent choices or taking appropriate action.

Some individuals still may have the misguided belief that cancer is contagious. This, of course, is an erroneous belief that today is encountered rarely. For even cancers that result from contagious viruses such as HIV and AIDS, or the papillomavirus, are not contagious in and of themselves. It's more likely that avoidance and abandonment issues in family situations that involve cancer and cancer recovery are the result of misdirected attempts for self-preservation.[381]

This preservation, of course, may be directed to one's emotional and mental state as well as one's physical state. Essentially, contact with a person who has cancer or any other disease reminds some individuals of their own mortality and vulnerability. In removing themselves from the afflicted person, the disease and the unpleasant situation, these individuals hope to remove this constant reminder as well.

Clearly, if such avoidance behavior appears to be an issue, it's vital for a family to obtain some form of professional guidance. Identifying and addressing the attitudes and fears associated with avoidance behavior is demanding work that is best accomplished with the help of a trained and licensed counselor. Some individuals, however, won't respond to such help, and still others may refuse to even explore the option. Some individuals simply lack the mental and emotional maturity that realistic and practical problem solving requires. Once again, cancer recovery demands a great deal of sacrifice, compassion and courage from every member of the family.

If one member refuses to accept these demands or is unable to embrace this new reality, the other members may be forced to move forward without them. These situations aren't common and most families manage to work together through the recovery process. They find ways to face the situation together, set new goals together and work to insure a productive future together. For those engaged in the fight, professional support combined with personal commitment can lead family members to a resolution that is mutually rewarding for all.

Friends

Many of the same issues a survivor faces with family members also will surface with friends. The obvious difference, of course, is that unlike family, friends don't have to live in the same household with the survivor. They don't have to be with the survivor day in and day out, through bad days and good. Friends don't have to alter their lifestyle, change their personal habits or patterns or sacrifice their needs or comforts. Their lives aren't as intimately intertwined with the survivor as are the lives of family.

Friends don't have to sacrifice their daily routines or living accommodations. They don't have to share in a division of household labor and commit to additional chores and errands. They don't have to experience the emotional and psychological ups and downs sure to accompany one's recovery and survival. Friends, basically, can come and go as they please. As there may be less stress associated with friendly relationships than with family relationships, it may be easier for friendships to survive and maintain equilibrium in the aftermath of a cancer diagnosis.

On the other hand, intermittent contact with the survivor may leave friends in a quandary in which they don't really understand what's going on, aren't aware of how the individual is feeling and don't know what they can do to help. Friends may not know what the individual is thinking or what her or his physical limitations are. They may not know if it's acceptable to ask questions or talk about the situation. In any event, friends will depend even more upon guidance from the individual than family members.

Many will be unsure as to how to proceed, and it will be important for the individual to take the lead. Even if the survivor doesn't wish to share intimate details with friends, she or he can suggest ways in which they may be of help. For instance, it may be helpful to have a friend drive one's children to school. It may be helpful to have another vacuum the house or shovel snow from the driveway. Yet another may cook a meal, shop for groceries or mow the lawn. In these ways, friends also can take an active role in one's survival and remain a vital element of one's life.[382]

Similar to some family members, however, friends and acquaintances as well may prove disappointing and incapable of dealing with a survivor's post-cancer reality. Friends also may have difficulty adjusting to change. They may be uncomfortable around someone who is fighting cancer or they may believe any help they could offer would be inadequate. Consciously or subconsciously, they may harbor fear of the disease that prevents them from behaving or reacting in a rational manner. Some may lack the education required to understand the disease and, although rare, some may fall victim to the old misconception that cancer is contagious.[383]

Friends may be incapable of accepting the changes that have taken place in the survivor's life, abilities or appearance. Those with whom one has enjoyed physical activities in the past such as jogging, tennis or soccer may lose these friends if one loses the ability to participate in these activities. Some, of course, simply may choose not to engage in someone else's battle to survive.

Cancer awareness is much greater today than in decades past. These things do occur, and when they do, they create waves of emotional trauma for the survivor that can be extremely painful and disillusioning. Should this be the case, once again professional guidance in the form of individual therapy, emotional hot lines or support groups can be effective in helping one manage this additional and unfortunate loss due to cancer. Ultimately, one can only prepare for the possibility, accept it should it occur, then move forward with the steadfast who remain.

Sex

Sexual intercourse and intimacy after cancer will be a significant challenge for many survivors. This is an area in which it's particularly difficult to separate the physical issues of cancer survival from the emotional. First, the physical changes to the human body which directly impact one's sex life after cancer may be numerous. Stress, for example, is a common response to any emotional, physical, social or economic stimulus in which perceived or actual change may be required. When the body experiences stress, it reacts in a number of ways, one of which is to produce an elevated amount of stress related hormones.[384]

In turn, these bio-chemical agents produce a number of effects within the body, one of which typically results in a significant reduction and interference with libido.[385] Clearly, overcoming the enormous obstacles presented by illness requires a great deal of energy. As we've already discussed, to maintain its energy reserves, the human body may begin to shut down certain functions that it deems unnecessary or superfluous to the immediate process of recovery.

From the moment cancer is diagnosed, throughout its treatment and long into its recovery, one is under stress, and the last thing on the mind of many survivors is sex. In addition, not only may the desire for sex be lacking in one's life, but the actual physical ability to have sex may be lacking as well. Fatigue and anxiety that result from one's inability to eat or sleep properly or from pain and anemia due to cancer and its treatments may leave one too tired to engage in sex.[386]

Men who have survived cancers that directly affect the sex organs, such as prostate cancer, testicular cancer or cancer of the penis, may not be able to achieve an erection due to the disease or surgery, chemotherapy and radiation. Surgery for prostate cancer can result in rectal damage that can impose the need for a colostomy, radiation can damage the bladder resulting in incontinence and both can result in infertility. Other treatments can weaken a man's orgasm, produce dry orgasms and hot flashes and significantly decrease his sexual desire.[387]

Women who have experienced cancer of the reproductive organs, such as the cervix, the uterus and the ovaries, also may face considerable challenges in their post-cancer sex lives. These cancers and their treatments can induce menopause and the hot flashes, mood swings and vaginal dryness related to menopause. Sexual organs may be removed either through a partial or complete hysterectomy.

Regardless of the type of cancer, chemotherapy and radiation may result in infertility, and abdominal radiation may further damage the tissues of the vaginal and rectal areas, making sexual intercourse uncomfortable and painful. A colostomy may be required for some cancers in some cases and in others the individual may lose the ability to control her or his bladder or bowels. The emotional toll created by such physical conditions can be enormous.

In addition, many men and women psychologically will have to adjust to a new body image replete with missing parts and permanent scarring. In a world of less desire, fatigue and anxiety, limp penises, weak orgasms, menopause and hot flashes, dry vaginas, sterility, missing testicles and breasts, surgical scars, colostomies, incontinence, pain and emotional and psychological insecurity, having good sex can be a chore.

Having stated the obvious, however, there are numerous ways in which cancer survivors can overcome these problems to regain and enjoy sexual intimacy with their partners. To begin, men affected by post-cancer erectile dysfunction may find significant help in a variety of medications now available by prescription. In some cases, surgery can restore or increase one's ability to have an erection, and hormones may help increase libido. Penile rehabilitation programs teach men how to exercise their erectile tissues to reverse impotence.[388]

As discussed, women who experience severe symptoms of menopause may choose to undergo a low dose hormone replacement regimen for a limited period of time. Or, women can choose an estrogen substitute or a natural product that has been found to relieve these uncomfortable symptoms. Several products, such as lubricants and creams, can alleviate vaginal dryness, and dilators can improve tissue flexibility and reduce sexual discomfort or pain. By practicing control over the muscles that stop the flow of urine through Kegel exercises, women can improve the ability to control their bladders and increase their pelvic strength. Both men and women can explore new sexual positions to compensate for discomfort, pain, fatigue or shortness of breath.[389]

Both can explore new ways of sharing intimacy. If penis-in-vagina sex simply isn't satisfying, possible, or desired, there are many other forms of sexual contact that can provide pleasure and intimacy. Oral and manual stimulation, for instance, allow couples to give and receive sexual pleasure and achieve orgasm in ways that retain and promote physical closeness and intimacy. Intimacy itself can be achieved through simple sensual pleasures such as kissing, hugging and stroking. Indeed, by establishing sensual intimacy in this way before engaging in sexual intimacy, the insecurity, anxiety and fear that both partners may feel can be greatly alleviated.[390]

Coping with sexual dysfunction in the aftermath of cancer and its treatments, however, remains a difficult and daunting task. Once again, forthright communication among couples affected by the disease is an absolute necessity. Both individuals must discuss their fears, feelings and ideas regarding their sexual relationship openly and honestly. Insecurities about disfigured bodies, physical limitations and inabilities to perform or please must be aired.

This is a process the success of which often requires and depends upon professional guidance. Indeed, many cancer centers today include the services of a trained sex therapist as a part of their patients' overall treatment programs. Such a professional can be extremely valuable in helping couples identify their concerns, express themselves through effective communication and find ways to maximize their sexual pleasure and intimacy.

For the human body comes in all colors, shapes and sizes. Some are young, some old. Some have two breasts, some have none. Some are missing limbs. Some operate in one way, some in another. Each has strengths and weaknesses, abilities and limitations. And yes, cancer may accentuate or exaggerate, alter or create some of these characteristics. Yet, with all the variations, every human body is capable of giving and receiving pleasure and achieving intimacy both sexually and sensually. The key is to recognize one's new reality, effectively communicate one's feelings, make the necessary adjustments and move on, just as life itself moves on.

Headline:

Oral Sex Linked To Mouth Cancers

For some time, scientists have suspected that malignant tumors of the mouth may be linked with a sexually transmitted infection associated with cervical cancer. We know that the presence of the human papilloma virus has been linked not only to cervical cancer, but to cancers of the larynx, mouth and skin as well. Now studies have isolated two specific strains of the human papilloma virus, the dangerous HPV16 and HPV18, and the direct relationship each has to the development of oral and cervical cancer.[391]

These strains target the epithelial cells that are found in the oral cavity, as well as in the vagina. It appears that one form of HPV16 or HPV18 transmission may occur during oral sex when women infected with one of these viruses pass it to their partners. Once transferred from the mucous membranes of the vaginal area, the strain may proliferate in the mucous membranes of the mouth where it may lead to, or facilitate the development of, certain oral cancers.[392]

Indeed, additional research has found that individuals diagnosed with oral cancer containing the HPV16 strain were three times more likely to report having had oral sex than those without the viral strain. This risk, however, is small, especially when compared to the risk for oral cancers that results from tobacco use and alcohol abuse. Yet, it does reinforce the need for women to undergo regular gynecological exams and PAP smears, not only for their own protection, but for the protection of their partners as well.[393]

Career

Returning to work is another area of a survivor's life that may present significant challenges. Most individuals need to work. We need the income and the health benefits, we need to be productive, we need to be valued for our contributions, and we need to have a sense of routine in our lives. These needs for a cancer patient or survivor, however, must give way to the more immediate need of fighting and surviving the disease.

It's true that in some cases an individual may feel well enough to conduct personal business and continue working while undergoing cancer treatments such as chemotherapy and radiation. In other cases, an individual may need to make enormous adjustments in her or his work schedule or take a medical leave of absence from work until treatment is over. This will depend, of course, upon the form of cancer one is fighting, the strength and type of treatment one is receiving and one's stamina and physical ability to cope with the recovery process. Ultimately, the decision to work through treatment or return to work after treatment will be reached through a consensus of opinions, including those of the individual and her or his primary caregivers and physicians.

For those affected by cancer, however, feeling physically well enough to work is only half the story. Clearly, cancer recovery and survival demands one engage in a psychological battle as well as a physical battle, and the former may continue long after the latter has been resolved. We know the return of physical strength doesn't necessarily equate with the return of confidence, self-assuredness and emotional well being. While returning to work after any absence can be stressful and filled with trepidation, returning after a battle with cancer may be far more complicated.

One may feel nervous and apprehensive. One may question her or his ability to perform their job well. One may worry that lingering side effects such as incontinence or fatigue will interfere with productivity. One may dread being confronted by too many questions. One may be reluctant to share information with co-workers or discuss the details of one's recovery. One may fear that fellow employees or managers will treat them differently, view them with doubt or withdraw previous support. All of these are real concerns, yet there are several steps an individual can take to make the transition as easy as possible.

The first step is to speak with one's supervisor or manager before returning to the workplace. Through direct communication, one needs to explain the lingering physical side effects that may affect one's ability to assume previous responsibilities. For example, if fatigue is still present one may want to explore the possibility of working part-time immediately following one's return. In the alternative, one may be able to work flexible hours or work from home one or two days a week.[394]

If still undergoing treatment, one must discuss the need to create a new schedule that accommodates both one's work and medical appointments. One may need to work a four-day week, for instance, undergoing treatments on Fridays to rest over the weekend. One needs to describe pain or discomfort that may temporarily interfere or limit one's ability to perform her or his previous job. Men who have survived prostate cancer may not be able to lift heavy objects or operate heavy equipment. Women who have survived breast cancer and mastectomies may lack the arm strength or manual dexterity to work on a computer.

One also should share the emotional concerns one has about returning to work. One needs to discuss one's feelings about confidentiality. The supervisor must understand the perimeters of one's comfort zone. For example, is it all right for co-workers to know about the cancer? If so, is it all right for co-workers to ask questions about the situation, and if so, how much should they be told? Should co-workers feel free to approach the survivor and discuss the issue? What will be comfortable for the survivor and what will not? Will the individual prefer to inform co-workers her or himself or should the supervisor be the one to do so?[395] By addressing these concerns with one's supervisor before actually entering the workplace, the emotional trauma that so often accompanies one's return can be greatly reduced.

Once in the workplace, however, the second step in the transition process begins. One still has to face and work with fellow employees on a daily basis, and many will have concerns and questions. Typically, one's involvement with colleagues upon returning to work will depend upon the relationship one shared prior to the cancer. Co-workers with whom one has worked closely in the past may be particularly anxious to understand the situation and, indeed, may need to understand the situation to plan projects, create timetables or schedule completion dates effectively.

No one wants to say the wrong thing, no one wants to appear nosey and no one wants to violate the survivor's privacy. And while one's supervisor may have initially paved the way to help insure the survivor's comfort on returning, it's important for the survivor to take additional steps to help insure the comfort of fellow employees. In fact, most colleagues want to be supportive and are simply waiting for the survivor to set the tone and issue the guidelines.

Accordingly, one should let others know what information can be shared comfortably and what cannot. Let them know if it's all right to approach with questions. Explain any physical condition that may temporarily affect one's ability to participate in group projects. If fatigue is a problem, let them know if mornings or afternoons are better for tackling new assignments. Inform co-workers of any change in personal work schedules so that they can plan accordingly.[396]

Once the ground rules are laid out clearly, one needs to reassess the entire situation on a regular basis. One should engage in weekly progress reports with one's supervisor. Compare notes regarding the needs and expectations of both the survivor and her or his co-workers. Discuss the health issues that continue to affect work or productivity. Together, determine if more personal accommodations are required or if the return is progressing as smoothly as possible. In these ways, the emotional stress associated with a return to work can be decreased and the level of comfort can be increased for all concerned, including the survivor, one's supervisor and one's fellow employees.

Once again, however, problems regarding the understanding and acceptance of cancer and its aftermath can arise in the workplace as easily as in the circles of family and friends. Some colleagues may choose to ignore the returning individual. Some may resent the survivor's return or fear contact with the survivor. Others may request transfers or new work assignments to avoid the individual. And, these misguided reactions may not be limited to one's co-workers.

One may face a situation in which one's manager or supervisor is similarly influenced. A supervisor may be reluctant to grant the necessary medical leave or to schedule work around treatment days. A supervisor may refuse to make reasonable accommodations upon one's return to work. One may find her or his prior job gone and the resulting reassignment unsatisfactory or find one's wishes regarding personal privacy have not been honored.

Some employers may be concerned about the emotional and psychological effect a survivor's cancer history will have on other employees. Some employers may incorporate needless or, perhaps, illegal barriers to a survivor's employment opportunities. Some may refuse or simply neglect to revise their policies to comply with new personnel laws and guidelines regarding a survivor's rights. Some employers may fear a loss of productivity and be reluctant to incur increased costs related to additional health benefits and insurance.[397] Ignorance and misinformation aren't limited to family and friends, and business decisions aren't made on the basis of charitable considerations. When these factors impact negatively upon one's livelihood, the results can be financially as well as emotionally devastating.

Apparently, the most frequent workplace problems reported by cancer survivors include the failure to hire, dismissal and demotion, undesirable transfers, the denial of promotions and benefits and hostility in the workplace. One of the first of its kind, a 1992 survey conducted among two hundred supervisors working in the United States revealed that sixty-six percent were concerned that employees with cancer would no longer be able to perform their jobs adequately. Further, fifty percent of these supervisors stated that a current cancer diagnosis would affect their decision to hire an otherwise qualified applicant.[398]

This survey also interviewed five hundred employees of whom thirteen percent believed that a co-worker with cancer wouldn't be able to perform her or his job. One in four of these employees feared they would have to work harder to pick up the slack. Another survey randomly conducted by telephone in 1996 in the United States interviewed five hundred survivors who were employed during their cancer treatment. Of this sample group the percent of individuals fired or laid off was five times greater than that of other workers in the United States.[399]

Further, a 1997 follow up survey also conducted randomly by telephone in the United States questioned 662 employed adult Americans who had never been diagnosed with cancer. Of these, however, over forty percent said they would fear losing their job if they ever were diagnosed with cancer and nearly twenty percent reported their fear of discrimination following a diagnosis would be so great they wouldn't disclose the fact to anyone within their workplace.[400]

Clearly, the fear of discrimination in the workplace is not without a substantial base in reality. The fact also remains that the physical and emotional demands of cancer treatment and survival often make it difficult for a survivor to maintain an identical or uninterrupted work schedule or career path. Every cancer survivor, therefore, must know how to protect her or his rights within the workplace. To do this and reduce or avoid the emotional and financial trauma associated with cancer-related job discrimination, it's necessary for every survivor to be familiar with the laws that address these sensitive issues.

Rights in the Workplace

As we've discussed, the legal support regarding cancer patients and survivors varies depending upon the state or country in which the individual resides. In the United States, there are three primary pieces of legislation with which a cancer survivor returning to work must be familiar.

The first is called the **Family and Medical Leave Act of 1993,** or **FMLA**. This Act is triggered when the employer is a public agency on the local, state or federal level, when the employer is a school or when the employer employs fifty or more employees within the private sector. In addition, the employee in question must be one who has been employed for a minimum of twelve months and has worked a minimum of 1250 hours during those twelve months. The employee also must be employed at a worksite where fifty or more fellow employees work within a seventy-five mile radius.[401]

When these conditions are met, however, this Act provides numerous workplace protections enforced by the United States Department of Labor. Among these, FMLA states that the above covered employers must provide eligible employees with up to twelve weeks of unpaid leave during any twelve-month period of time for any of the following reasons. First, the Act may be triggered by the birth of the employee's child and for care of the child. Second, the placement of a child with the employee for adoption or foster care will qualify for leave under the Act. Third, the employee may take leave to care for a spouse, child or parent who has a serious health condition. And fourth, the Act may be triggered when the employee is experiencing a serious health condition that renders the employee incapable of performing the essential functions of her or his job.[402]

While an employee may not accrue benefits while on leave under FMLA, the employee is entitled to retain coverage under the company's health care program. This holds true even if the employee is unable to pay her or his share of the premiums while on leave. Indeed, the employee has the choice to pay the premiums in regular intervals during the leave or to pay upon returning to work. The employee also has the right to substitute paid annual or sick leave for an unpaid leave under FMLA or may take such accrued paid leaves in addition to any leave taken under FMLA.[403]

Protection under the Act also extends to the employee's return from leave. For example, the employee must be returned to the same position she or he held prior to the leave or to an "equivalent position with equivalent benefits, pay, status, and other terms and conditions of employment." Finally, the employee is entitled to be fully informed of all the above provisions in a clear and concise manner by the employer.[404]

In addition to the responsibilities the employer has to the employee, however, FLMA also outlines the responsibilities the employee has to the employer. Among these, the employee must notify the employer of the intent to take a family and medical leave at least thirty days before the leave is to begin. If this isn't possible due to an emergency situation, the employee is required to give notice as soon as is "practicable." Under no circumstances may an employee invoke entitlement to FMLA leave retroactively *after* the employee has already been absent from work.[405]

If FMLA is invoked as the result of a family medical situation in which the employee's spouse, child or parent has a serious health condition, the employee may need to provide her or his employer with a medical certification from a doctor or other health care provider. Similarly, when the leave is concluded and the employee wishes to return to work, FMLA requires that the employee provide an additional "return to work" medical certification.[406]

It's important to clarify some of the terms found within The Family and Medical Leave Act. When the Act refers to a "health care provider," it refers to those recognized by the Federal Employees Health Benefits Program, those certified under federal or state law, those who practice in countries other than the United States and those recognized as Native American "traditional healing practitioner(s)" within the United States.[407]

The term "serious health condition" has been revised significantly since 1993 and now includes conditions that require multiple treatments such as chemotherapy or radiation for cancer and kidney dialysis, as well as chronic conditions such as diabetes and asthma. The third term that requires clarification to understand and properly invoke a leave of absence under FMLA is "spouse." In defining this term under the Act, the United States Office of Personnel Management relied upon the definition put forth by the **Defense of Marriage Act** in 1996.[408]

In this public law, "spouse" refers to an individual who is a husband or wife in a marriage that's a legal union between one man and one woman. This includes a common law marriage between one man and one woman in states in which common law marriage is recognized.[409] Although the requirements vary from one state to another, common law marriage typically is defined as one in which one man and one woman have co-habitated for a significant period of time, have held themselves out to the world as husband and wife and have intended to be married.[410]

Clearly, this definition as stated by the Marriage Act and adopted by the Family and Medical Leave Act doesn't consider either partner in a homosexual relationship a "spouse" regardless of any commitment ceremony that may have taken place between the partners or the duration of their relationship. Unless or until the appropriate legislative bodies change this terminology, one homosexual partner may not invoke FMLA to care for the other who may be affected by a serious health condition. In these domestic partner situations, one may need to apply accrued vacation and sick days to acquire a leave or, if possible, make special arrangements with one's employer to accommodate the necessary absence.

The second important law that protects one's rights within the workplace is known as the **Americans with Disabilities Act**. It also is known as the **ADA,** although this Act shouldn't be confused in the United States with the American Diabetes Association, which also is referred to as the ADA. The Americans with Disabilities Act offers protections to disabled individuals similar to those provided to other individuals on the basis of sex, race, age, color or national origin and religion. It guarantees equal opportunity and requires "reasonable accommodations" for the disabled in the areas of public accommodations and transportation as well as, of course, employment.[411]

In particular, employment discrimination is prohibited under the ADA and applies to all private employees with fifteen or more employees, state and local governments, the legislative branch of the federal government, employment agencies and labor unions against "qualified individuals with disabilities." This phrase means that the individual, apart from the disability, is fully qualified to perform the "essential functions" of the job that she or he is applying for or that she or he currently holds.[412]

The term "disability" is a little more complicated and applies to three separate scenarios. The first is when an individual has a **current physical or mental impairment that substantially limits one or more major life activities**. The second is when an individual has a **record of such impairment,** and the third is when an individual is **regarded as having such impairment**.[413]

The first part of the definition clearly applies to those whose impairments obviously limit a major life activity such as seeing, walking, breathing, learning or working. An individual, therefore, who's affected by blindness, paralysis, lung disease or mental retardation is an individual with a "disability" to whom the provisions of the ADA apply. In contrast, the provisions typically won't cover an individual with a nonchronic condition of short duration such as the flu or a broken limb.

The second part of the definition applies to those who may be healthy at the present time, but whose past health history includes a recovery from a chronic physical or mental illness such as those mentioned above. The third part of the definition applies to those who may not have an impairment that substantially limits a major life activity, or may not have a past record of such impairment, but are *perceived* by others to have such impairment.[414] For example, this part of the ADA would protect an individual with a severe and obvious physical disfigurement from being denied employment simply because the employer feared or wished to avoid the "negative reactions" of colleagues or customers.

For cancer patients and survivors, the question of whether the protections of the ADA will apply in a particular circumstance typically will be decided on a case-by-case basis. This decision will be based in part upon whether or not the individual currently has cancer, is undergoing treatment for cancer or has recovered or is in remission from cancer. In the first case, the Act considers most individuals with cancer to be "disabled." These cases fall into the first part of the definition of disability as a current cancer is widely recognized as a health condition that can significantly limit one or more of an individual's major life activities.[415]

One's physical ability to walk or speak may be impaired, one's ability to breathe may be impaired and one's basic ability to work or conduct everyday activities such as driving or caring for oneself may be impaired. In addition, cancers that are ongoing such as many of the leukemias and lymphomas also would generally fall into the first part of the definition of disability as a current impairment.

In the second case, individuals who are receiving treatment for cancer typically can rely on the first and second part of the definition. In these instances, the individual may no longer have cancer. The known tumor or tumors may have been surgically removed, leaving the individual technically free from cancer. Yet, cancer treatments including chemotherapy and radiation can create physical and mental conditions that, in and of themselves, substantially may limit the individual's major life activities.[416]

In the many ways we've already discussed, cancer treatment greatly can impair one's ability to conduct her or his personal or professional life in a normal and productive manner. Thus, the first part of the definition generally will apply to one undergoing treatment for cancer. The second part of the definition, however, also may apply as an individual who technically is cancer free during treatment nevertheless has a record of cancer, an impairment we already have established as a disability under the Act. Accordingly, the ADA most likely will apply to individuals who may not have a current cancer, but are receiving treatment for cancer.

In the third case, individuals who have survived cancer and are cured or are in remission still may be covered by the ADA based upon the second part of the definition. One who has experienced cancer will always have a record of that disability in one's health history. This fact alone may be enough to trigger the protections afforded by the Americans with Disabilities Act.

Further, cancer patients or survivors who may be left with a physical disfigurement due to the disease or to surgery related to the disease may qualify for ADA protection based upon the third part of the definition of disability. This disfigurement, however, would most likely have to be obvious such as a bone cancer that results in the loss of a limb or, perhaps, a tobacco-related oral cancer that requires extensive surgery.[417]

Individuals with cancer related to HIV or AIDS also are covered by the ADA not only because of the cancer, but because these infections themselves, like some cancers, have a continuous and detrimental effect upon an individual's lymphatic and hematologic systems that may significantly limit life's major activities. Finally, cancer patients and survivors who have become infertile as a result of a particular cancer or its treatments are significantly limited in the major life activity of reproduction, and as such may be afforded the continuous protections of the ADA on this basis alone.[418]

Once the Americans with Disabilities Act has been determined to apply to an individual whose life has been touched by cancer, it's important to understand the protections that may be available. First, the ADA requires an employer to provide "reasonable accommodation" to an employee covered by the Act. Such accommodation typically involves flexibility in the workplace, and for cancer survivors it may include time off for treatments and medical appointments, a change in job duties due to a temporary physical limitation, a shorter workweek, job sharing or telecommuting.[419]

Such changes are considered "reasonable" and are in contrast to changes that would be disruptive, excessively expensive or would fundamentally alter the nature or operation of the business creating "undue hardship" for the employer. The ADA prevents an employer from denying employment or from firing a survivor based solely upon an actual or perceived disability. This doesn't mean, however, that an employer must hire one with a disability or that an employer may never fire one with a disability.

It does mean that if an individual is qualified for a position to which she or he applies, an employer cannot reject the individual based upon her or his disability due to a cancer history. The employer can only reject the individual if the individual isn't fully qualified to perform the essential functions of the job. This also means that an employer retains the right to fire an individual who would have been fired anyway, regardless of her or his disability due to a cancer history.[420]

For example, if an individual is unable to perform the essential functions of her or his job because of a lack of education or skill and not because of a disability, the employee may be legally fired. Simply put, the ADA requires that all employers must treat all employees similarly whether a disability exists or not. Let's suppose two individuals possess exactly the same qualifications for a specific job. The only difference between the two candidates is that one has a disability and the other doesn't. If the one without a disability is considered qualified for the job, then the one with a disability must similarly be considered qualified for the job and cannot be denied the job solely because of the disability.

Likewise, consider two individuals who hold the same or comparable positions within the same company. Both employees, one disabled, the other not, are exactly alike in that they both perform their jobs poorly. If the employee without a disability can be fired for incompetence on the job, then the employee with a disability similarly can be fired for incompetence as long as the dismissal isn't based solely upon the disability.

Unlike most employment discrimination laws, the Americans with Disabilities Act is broader in that its protections extend not only to a survivor, but to a survivor's family as well. This is extremely important as there may be many times throughout one's battle with cancer when the care of the individual will fall to family members. Under the ADA, an employer may not discriminate against an employee based upon the employee's relationship or association with an individual considered disabled under the Act.[421]

Accordingly, an employer may not deny employment or fire an individual because the individual is caring for a disabled person. The employer may not assume that the individual's job performance would suffer or be negatively affected by the need to care for a family member with cancer. In addition to matters of hiring and firing, the ADA prohibits discrimination in most job-related activities, including benefit packages and health insurance.[422]

In fact, in most instances an employer may not even ask a prospective employee if she or he has ever had cancer. Within the context of a job interview, the employer only has the right to know if the applicant is able to perform the essential functions of the job for which the individual is applying. If employment is contingent upon the individual taking and passing a medical examination, the exam must be applied similarly to all prospective employees *and* an employer has the right to question one's health history only after making a job offer.[423]

A great deal of leeway exists in the courts, and while some have fairly assessed the impact of cancer upon an individual's life and have awarded damages for violated rights, others have not. If one is to be protected from workplace discrimination under the ADA, one must be found to be "qualified" to do the job yet "substantially limited" by the disability.[424]

Some courts have found that if a cancer survivor cannot perform the essential functions of the job she or he isn't qualified, *and* if a cancer survivor is capable of working she or he isn't substantially limited. This forces a survivor into a box and creates a no-win situation in which the provisions of the ADA won't be triggered either because the survivor is too ill to work or too healthy to be considered disabled. By and large, this "catch 22" interpretation of a disability under the Act is now being replaced by judicial opinions that recognize the long-term effects and limitations of cancer and its treatments upon an individual's ability and right to work.[425]

Moreover, many survivors find themselves in a position in which they begin work for the first time or change jobs following a cancer recovery. In these situations, there are several steps one can take to protect her or his personal privacy and perhaps prevent workplace discrimination from occurring in the first place.

To begin, one isn't required to volunteer information about her or his cancer at a job interview or on any employment application. Indeed, one should keep her or his cancer history private unless it impacts directly upon the position for which one is applying.[426]

If, for example, one has difficulty lifting heavy objects after undergoing surgery for prostate cancer, one need not divulge this fact unless one is applying for work in a warehouse or on a loading dock. Second, one should only discuss one's ability to perform the essential functions of the job in question. In this case, if a technician's computer skills aren't impaired, the individual need not share the fact that she or he may not be able to participate in company retreats requiring physical stamina.

Third, one shouldn't inquire about an employer's benefits or insurance packages until one has received a firm job offer. Once the offer has been accepted, one may ask questions about these matters to determine if her or his personal coverage is fair and adequate. Finally, one must always stay apprised of one's legal rights as they pertain to employment in case one believes she or he is being treated differently by an employer due to one's cancer history.[427]

The third important piece of legislation that directly affects the rights of workers with disabilities is the **Federal Rehabilitation Act,** or the **FRA**. Under the FRA, disability is defined as "a physical or mental impairment that constitutes or results in a substantial impediment to employment" or "a physical or mental impairment that substantially limits one or more major life activities."[428] Clearly, the second part of this definition will apply to the same individuals to whom the ADA applies, including many survivors of cancer.

In addition, this Act offers protection from workplace discrimination for the disabled and pertains specifically to organizations both private and public that receive more than $2500 annually in federal funding. This is especially important as the FRA extends protection to individuals who cannot benefit from the ADA because their employers do not meet the requirements of the ADA. For instance, the FRA will apply to employers who receive federal contracts in excess of $10,000 and have fewer than fifteen employees.[429]

It also applies to employers who have fewer than fifteen employees and operate federally funded services and programs. Accordingly, the Federal Rehabilitation Act will cover all individuals working for these employers, as well as all employees who work for the executive branch of the federal government. In this way, the FRA helps to fill the gaps that exist the ADA and offers protection from job discrimination to disabled individuals who otherwise would have none.[430] Privacy in the workplace regarding an individual's health history can be a tricky issue. We already have discussed the **Health Insurance Portability and Accountability Act**, which addresses these issues concerning the maintenance and protection of health-related information. The HIPAA, however, only applies to "covered entities" such as health insurance plans, health care providers, hospitals and clinics. It doesn't apply to other types of employers such as universities, law firms, utility companies or department stores.

Certain principles of the HIPAA, however, may be used to encourage and set an example for employers not directly impacted by its provisions. It would be reasonable, for instance, for any employer to keep all employee medical records locked in file cabinets or offices. It also would be reasonable for any employer to limit access to this confidential information to only those employees in personnel who work directly with the company benefits and insurance programs.

Further, a failure to comply with such reasonable requests or expectations may result in discrimination that occurs when such private information becomes public knowledge. Should this be the case, such discrimination, if based upon a disability, may become actionable under the provisions of other previously discussed workplace legislation including the Americans with Disabilities Act or the Federal Rehabilitation Act.

In addition to the above federal statutes, **state laws** prohibiting discrimination against the disabled exist in each of the United States. These laws typically cover both private and public employers and many apply to employers who employ fewer than fifteen individuals. In this way, state laws also help fill in the gaps that exist in federal legislation. Employers who may not be covered by the ADA or the FRA because they employ too few employees and don't receive federal funds may nevertheless be covered by applicable state laws. When a particular law applies to an employer, the employees are entitled to the legal protections of that law.[431]

Many state laws offer workplace protection from discrimination for individuals who have a real or perceived disability. Some states expressly prohibit discrimination based upon a cancer history even if the individual isn't considered disabled under federal or state guidelines. Moreover, several states have medical leave laws the provisions of which are often more generous than those provided by the federal provisions of the FMLA.[432] It's important, therefore, to be aware of all the applicable federal and state regulations regarding employment, disability and the ways in which each regulation may impact one's personal situation.

Having discussed the positive aspects of invoking protection under the above federal and state laws, however, it also is necessary to discuss the negative aspects. Filing any lawsuit can be a complicated and time-consuming process. It can be a process that dominates an individual's life for several months or years. It can be costly, and there's no guarantee that the lawsuit will result in the fair or equitable solution for which the individual is hoping. For cancer survivors who need to concentrate on restoring and maintaining their health, the attention and energy a lawsuit requires may prove detrimental and exhausting.

For these reasons, lawsuits filed under federal and state laws regarding workplace discrimination are typically not the best way to enforce one's rights. They should be used *only* as a last resort and *only* after all other means of resolution have been exhausted. Fortunately, most employers in the industrialized countries of the world have a grievance process clearly outlined for the benefit and use of their employees. These informal solutions should be investigated thoroughly by any survivor who believes she or he is being treated differently on the job because of a cancer history.

In the event these procedures fail to produce a satisfactory result, one then can proceed to the higher federal and state laws for protection. In fact, if these procedures fail, it's important for one to preserve one's right to seek a legal remedy by keeping a carefully written record of the discriminatory acts in question and by knowing the filing deadlines for the laws one wishes to invoke.

Lastly, one's health care provider or a branch of the local government may provide information regarding the appropriate legal regulations governing employment discrimination and disability related to cancer. Pertinent information also may be obtained by contacting the World Health Organization, the specialized health agency of the United Nations, which operates in 192 nations around the world. One also may contact the American Cancer Society and the National Cancer Institute, both of which can help refer individuals to the proper legal sources and local authorities regardless of their place of residence.

Chapter 10:
Survivorship: Financial Concerns

Want of attention to these matters has impeded the progress of science and of genius itself.
William Cobbett

Health Care: An Overview

Unfortunately, there's no escaping the fact that cancer creates an enormous economic burden not only upon society, but also upon each patient and each patient's family. Cancer treatment is an expensive process, the impact of which will affect both society and patient differently depending upon a number of various factors.

First, the cost of cancer treatment itself will vary with the type of treatment required. Clearly, if chemotherapy and/or radiation therapy are recommended in addition to surgery, the cost of treatment will escalate. The kind of drug and the dose or strength of drug that may be used will affect the overall cost of treatment. The length of time the treatment lasts and the frequency with which it's administered will affect the cost. Also, the location in which the treatment is administered, be it a clinic, an office or a hospital, will affect the cost.

Second, the financial impact upon society and the patient, and the delegation of the cost between the two, will depend in large part upon the country in which the patient resides or has citizenship. In this respect, it will be helpful if we divide the countries of the world into two groups, those considered to be less or undeveloped and those considered to be developed.

The former, often referred to as "third world" countries, are those in which the importance of health care is often eclipsed by the simple survival priorities of securing adequate shelter, nourishing food and clean water. These countries typically share high national debts, low per capita gross national profits and a scarcity of natural resources that can result in crippling poverty. In addition, they can be characterized by political unrest and civil war.[433]

Under these circumstances, proper health care may be non-existent, rare or available to only a chosen few. The common people are too poor to visit a physician or purchase necessary medications as such necessities often cost more than an individual's monthly, or in some cases, yearly income.[434] Adequate health care as well as hospital services and beds are reserved for the rich who can afford to pay in advance. Accordingly, many diseases including cancer remain undiagnosed within the general population.

It's often not until the disease reaches epidemic proportions, or until the individual becomes terminal that the disease is discovered. It's this scenario, for example, that accounts for the high mortality rate of cervical cancer among the world's female population. For although we know cervical cancer typically is highly treatable and rarely life threatening for women who have access to adequate medical care and are diagnosed early, women living in the undeveloped countries of the world don't share in this luxury. Nor do the thousands of other individuals living in these countries who are diagnosed with other forms of advanced cancer each year.

In these parts of the world, individual wealth and health insurance policies are far from common, and the cost of cancer care primarily falls to the regional or national governments. Unfortunately, the effectiveness of these governments often is undermined by inexperience and instability such that their health care systems, if existent, remain poorly organized and inadequately funded. As a result, the bulk of financial responsibility for cancer care in the less developed countries of the world often falls to the numerous privately and publicly supported organizations, foundations and charitable institutions springing from the world's more developed countries.[435]

This brings us to our second group, the developed or industrialized countries of the world. In most of these countries, the cost of cancer care is borne by their respective governments through national health care plans that extend to each individual who is a citizen of or resides in the country. In France, for example, the health care system is a state subsidized plan in which doctors and dentists are allowed to establish private practices and the patient is allowed to visit their physician of choice. Coverage extends to all residents of the country who are reimbursed by the state for up to eighty-five percent of the incurred medical costs.[436]

Japan's health care system is characterized by universal coverage in which all residents of the country benefit regardless of existing medical conditions or one's risk of developing a serious medical condition. It relies upon a system of employment-based financing in which an individual's premiums are based upon income and the ability to pay. Similar to Australia, Canada and most other European nations, the government-sponsored health care systems in these countries are compulsory.[437]

Granted, these systems may not operate perfectly in all situations. Some lack the necessary governmental management and attention required to insure the smooth running of a reliable and efficient operation. The number of hospital facilities may be inadequate or prone to overcrowding, physicians may be concentrated in urban areas rather than rural, and "state of the art" equipment may not always be available in all facilities.

Yet, these systems offer a medical safety net for all citizens regardless of income level or ability to pay. They guarantee medical coverage for those who otherwise would be without, while allowing those with personal wealth to either use the existing system or purchase private health care elsewhere. Overall, these systems generally have proven to be cost effective, and in offering affordable and subsidized health care to all members of the population, the economic impact of cancer upon both society and the individual is more evenly distributed, and neither is hopelessly overwhelmed.

In the United States, however, things are not so simple. With the exception of two states now taking action to implement state-sponsored universal coverage plans, the United States is the only industrialized country in the world that doesn't have in place some type of national health care system that offers coverage for all its citizens. As a result, paying for cancer care can be a complicated and financially devastating under-taking for cancer patients and their families. Indeed, a new health care bill recently was passed in the United States in 2010. Accordingly, we'll first discuss insurance issues within the present health care system. We'll then discuss insurance changes the new bill may present once the bill has been enacted.

Basically, issues of individual health care for those living in the United States fall into two categories, those who have health insurance and those who don't. Of those who have health insurance, the coverage is provided either through **government insurance** of which the major programs include 1) Medicare, 2) Medicaid, 3) military health care programs, 4) the Indian Health Service, and 5) a variety of state funded plans, or **private insurance** which includes 1) employment based plans, and 2) direct purchase plans.[438]

In whatever form insurance may come, however, be it governmental or private, state or federal, employment, poverty or military-based, having it doesn't guarantee freedom from financial stress. Dealing with and making sense of health benefits can be an extremely frustrating and confusing undertaking. Medical plans and insurance poli-cies vary significantly in their coverage and terms of payment. What one may pay for, another will not.

Financial pitfalls abound, and it's essential for one to thoroughly understand the scope and limitations of her or his policy and the contractual obligations set forth by that policy. For regardless of the type of policy one might have, its effectiveness will be limited unless it's applied in a way that *insures* payment for allowed medical care will be forthcoming. Obviously, no cancer patient can afford to have unnecessary and unwanted money problems competing with the attention and energy one needs to focus upon physical and emotional recovery.

To begin, each individual must obtain a copy of any and all insurance policies under which coverage may be claimed. One also must take the time necessary to learn about the specific benefits that may apply to the current situation. This clearly isn't an easy task, and it's highly advisable for each individual to contact her or his insurance broker or representative, or any other appropriate personnel, social or governmental office to aid in this task.

First, one must make sure she or he understands the basic provisions of the policy in question as it applies to any medical situation. For example, does the policy, or policies, require the covered individual to make a co-payment at the time of every medical visit and if so, what is the amount of that co-payment? Does the policy set forth an annual deductible that must be paid by the individual before medical expenses are paid under the policy? Does the policy have an annual or lifetime limit beyond which medical expenses won't be covered under the policy, but rather become the financial responsibility of the individual? Does the policy offer coverage for check-ups, testing and procedures on an ongoing basis or only when the individual is ill? If more than one policy is in question, which is considered the primary coverage and which is supplemental?[439]

More specifically, cancer patients and survivors must determine which cancer treatments and procedures are covered by their insurance and which are not. Patients and survivors also need to determine if those covered treatments must be administered in a particular manner or in a particular location. For instance, does the insurance cover treatment administered in cancer centers, hospitals, physician offices, hospices or at home? Can chemotherapy be administered in the privacy of one's home and still be covered by insurance? Must radiation therapy be performed only in specific hospital settings?

Can medical supplies needed at home or prescriptions be purchased anywhere or will coverage only apply if such items are purchased from a specific pharmacy? Does the individual have a choice as to the manner and location of required treatment? Does the coverage extend to out-patient services as well as in-patient services? Does lab work such as blood tests, pap smears or urinalysis need to be sent to a specific laboratory or facility before its cost is covered by the insurance? One must determine if the policy requires one to see specific physicians and specialists to qualify for reimbursement for any of these services or medical treatments, and to what extent that reimbursement may apply.[440]

Federal and State Sponsored Insurance Plans

We'll begin with the government-funded insurance programs that in 2007, when combined, offered health coverage to approximately twenty-seven and a half percent of United States citizens.[441] Of the federal government insurance plans, **Medicare** is the most common, affording approximately thirteen and a half percent of American citizens medical coverage. Medicare provides this coverage for individuals who are sixty-five years of age, have been legal residents for five years and qualify for social security.[442]

In addition, it provides coverage for younger individuals who have been determined by Social Security to be "disabled" for a period of twenty-four months as well as individuals with end stage renal disease requiring dialysis or a kidney transplant and those diagnosed with Lou Gehrig's disease or amyotrophic lateral sclerosis. Medicare covers hospice care, in-patient hospitalization and skilled nursing services. The individual, however, is responsible for paying certain premiums, deductibles and co-payments. Individuals receiving out-patient care also are responsible for a $155 deductible and twenty percent of the expense with Medicare paying eighty percent of the covered services.[443]

Further, Medicare will only cover out-patient prescription drugs if they're administered in an out-patient facility or in a physician's office. As drugs can be extremely expensive, it may be advisable for an individual to purchase private health insurance supplements or enroll in a Medicare HMO to reduce the impact of this expense, although Medicare now offers a new Part D prescription drug benefit that began in 2006.

This benefit was established under the **Medicare Modernization Act** or **MMA**.[444] In addition to a $310 deductible, an individual must pay twenty-five percent of the cost of covered prescription drugs up to a cap of $2,830. Once this coverage limit is reached an individual must pay the full amount of her or his prescription drugs until their out-of-pocket expenses reach a total of $4,550. At this point, the benefit kicks in again. The individual now becomes responsible for paying $2.50 for a generic drug and $5.30 for a brand-name drug, or for a five percent co-payment on both, whichever is greater.[445] This coverage gap is commonly referred to as the "Donut Hole." It's a highly debated issue that will be impacted by the new health care reform bills.

In addition, under the Act low income individuals are eligible to receive a subsidy that helps cover the cost of the drug co-payments, deductible and premiums. Premiums for Medicare once again are paid on a monthly basis, which in the case of those receiving social security benefits is deducted from the benefits check.[446]

Medicaid is the largest public health insurance program offering health insurance for Americans who don't qualify or cannot afford private insurance or other types of government insurance. It's a joint federal and state program based upon a set of general federal guidelines, yet allows the states wide discretion in determining individual eligibility. Accordingly, eligibility requirements will vary from state to state, but typically one may qualify if one has high medical bills and if one meets certain income, resource and age or disability standards.[447]

In general, Medicaid is designed to provide medical coverage for most low-income seniors, children from low-income families and individuals with disabilities, coverage that applies to approximately eleven and one half percent of the American population. Under this plan, the states pay a portion of the cost while the federal government matches every dollar of state expenditure with $1.00 to $3.22 of federal funds.[448]

The third type of government insurance includes programs that cover personnel of the military and armed forces. Depending upon an individual's status, the **Civilian Health and Medical Program of the Uniformed Services,** or **CHAMPUS,** is a federal program that provides coverage for active duty and retired military members as well as those of the Guard or Reserves, family members and certain veterans. It offers free or government-subsidized medical and dental care to qualifying individuals most of which falls under an overall program known today as **TRICARE**.[449]

The **Civilian Health and Medical Program of the Department of Veterans Affairs,** or **CHAMPVA,** is another federal program that is administered by the Department of Veterans Affairs. It's a fee for service program that provides reimbursement of most medical expenses incurred by eligible veterans, veteran's dependents and survivors of veterans. Similarly, the federally funded **Department of Veterans Affairs** offers assistance to certain eligible members of the Armed Forces, and when combined with the other military health programs, covers approximately three and one half percent of Americans.[450]

In addition to these programs, the Department of Health and Human Services of the federal government provides medical assistance to eligible Native American Indians through the **Indian Health Service,** or **IHS**. This program helps pay the cost of medical care at government-sponsored IHS facilities as well as selected medical services provided by non-IHS facilities.[451]

Finally, many states have their own health insurance programs that offer assistance to low income individuals who may not qualify for any of the other private or governmental programs. Of these, one of the most common is the **Children's Health Insurance Program (CHIP)**, a program administered at the state level to provide medical care for low income children whose parents don't qualify for Medicaid.[452] Each of these government insurance plans, however, may be known by a different name depending upon the state in which the programs are administered.

The states also sponsor public benefit programs that supplement the federal Medicare program. Once again, the name of each program will vary from state to state, but usually are identified in part by the name of the state. In California, for example, the program is known as **Medi-Cal**. This program may apply to those who wish to supplement their Medicare, but cannot afford to buy private health insurance. To qualify, however, an individual must meet the same disability standard as Social Security recipients and must possess a certain financial profile.[453]

Another form of Medicare supplemental insurance is **Medigap**. Medigap insurance is regulated by both state and federal law and provides reimbursement for many expenses that are not covered by Medicare. To date, there are ten standard Medigap policies and each offers a different package of benefits. Clearly, one must first be eligible for Medicare before one becomes eligible for Medigap. Once eligible, however, individuals applying for Medigap cannot be denied coverage due to a prior health condition and all Medigap policies are guaranteed renewable. In addition, one enrolled in Medicare may purchase a Medigap policy at any time and, for one who leaves or is terminated from a Medicare HMO or managed care plan, the right to open enrollment in a Medigap insurance plan is assured.[454]

State Health Insurance Assistance Program (SHIP)

Matters of insurance can be extremely confusing and difficult to understand. One is inundated with issues of eligibility, rules concerning claims and reimbursement, covered expenses, deductibles, co-payments and one's rights and obligations under the various plans. Among these plans, Medicare may be one of the most difficult to fathom. Fortunately, an organization known as the **State Health Insurance Assistance Program** is available to provide guidance and information to those individuals who subscribe to or are interested in Medicare.[455]

As a state organization, the name once again will change, depending upon the state of origin. For example, in California the organization is known as the **Health Insurance Counseling and Advocacy Program,** or **HICAP**, in New York it's known as the **Health Insurance Information, Counseling and Assistance Program** or **HIICAP**, in Washington it's known as the **Statewide Health Insurance Benefits Advisors,** or **SHIBA,** and so on.

While the names may differ, the goals and functions of this organization nevertheless remain the same. It specifically trains personnel to help individuals understand all aspects of Medicare and the Medicare managed health plans. It will research and compare the available private supplemental health plans when one's coverage under Medicare proves inadequate. It also will develop personalized systems to organize one's medical bills and to file claims under both Medicare and private insurance plans. In the event either Medicare or one's private insurance carrier denies one's claims, the relevant SHIP office will prepare and file the appropriate appeal or legal challenge.[456]

SHIP offices also are extremely useful in helping individuals explore long-term care options and learn about the available government assistance programs. The organization offers local and community educational presentations and all its services are provided free of charge. Fortunately, information on the SHIP organization in each state can easily be accessed by contacting the State Department of Insurance or, because SHIP handles matters related to Medicare, the State Division of Senior Services.[457]

Private Insurance Plans

The most complicated of the insurance programs, however, typically are found in the private sector of the business. Accordingly, the bulk of our discussion will pertain to these plans, the most common of which are offered through one's own employment or that of a spouse or family member. Employment-based plans also may be sponsored by an employer or a union and according to the United States Census Bureau approximately fifty-nine percent of all individuals in the United States in 2007 were covered by such plans.[458]

In these plans, the employee typically contributes a minimum amount each month from her or his paycheck and in return receives benefits based upon a group policy that represents all the company's employees. Direct purchase plans differ in that an individual contacts a private insurance carrier personally and pays premiums directly to that company. Much less common, these plans account for approximately nine percent of the country's medically covered individuals.[459]

In the United States, there are five basic categories of private insurance plans that include 1) **Self-Funded/Self Insured Plans**, 2) **Indemnity Plans**, 3) **Health Maintenance Organization Plans** or **HMO**s, 4) **Preferred Provider Organization Plans** or **PPO**s, and 5) **Point of Service Plans** or **POS**s. The first, Self-Funded Plans, are those in which money is set aside by a company or union in order to pay the health claims of employees or members as the claims are filed. This type of insurance coverage isn't strongly regulated, and the specifics of each policy may vary greatly.[460]

Self-Funded Plans are similar, however, in that most severely limit benefits during the first year of enrollment for pre-existing conditions. It's essential, therefore, for each covered individual to review her or his policy thoroughly before making any decisions about and moving forward with specific medical care and treatment.

The second type of coverage, known as an Indemnity Plan, has the advantage of allowing covered individuals to seek medical care from the hospital or physician of one's choice. These plans usually have a deductible that must be paid by the individual before the plan will cover any medical expenses. Once the deductible has been met, the plan will begin to cover approximately seventy to eighty percent of one's expenses in a payment known as co-insurance. The remaining thirty to twenty percent is still considered the patient's liability and must be paid by the individual.[461]

These plans, however, typically set an "out of pocket" maximum for each covered individual. This means that if one's policy has an out of pocket maximum of $3,000, the plan will pay one hundred percent of the medical expenses once the individual has paid this amount. Similar to Self-Funded Plans, the provisions of Indemnity Plans vary significantly and must be carefully reviewed by the individual prior to making any important health care decision.[462]

Unlike an Indemnity Plan, an HMO typically doesn't allow a covered individual to choose and receive medical care from any hospital or physician. Although there are some exceptions to this rule, an HMO usually contracts with a pre-approved panel or list of doctors from which a covered member must choose.

Further, members of an HMO plan have one physician who is deemed the "primary" physician and is ultimately responsible for the member's medical care. If the member chooses to receive care from another physician or specialist, the member first must obtain permission from the primary care physician before doing so. If these additional physicians or specialists also are within the HMOs network of providers, the patient will only make a small co-payment per visit and the plan will cover most of the remaining charges.

The advantage of an HMO is that there are no deductibles for the patient to pay and no claim forms to fill out as long as physicians within the plan provide one's care. The disadvantage is that if one chooses to see someone other than one's primary physician, whether that physician is within the HMO network or not, the procedure can be complicated and time-consuming. Accordingly, this requirement of gaining permission by "referral, "pre-certification" or "authorization" to see additional physicians will be discussed separately.[463]

A PPO insurance plan incorporates some elements of both an Indemnity Plan and an HMO. First, PPOs are similar to Indemnity Plans in that they have a deductible that must be paid by the individual. Second, PPOs are similar to HMOs in that they contract with a pre-approved panel or list of specific physicians and medical providers. If one has paid the deductible and sees a physician within the network, a PPO typically covers eighty to one hundred percent of the remaining expenses. The covered individual also is required to pay a deductible if she or he chooses to visit a physician outside the network.

In these situations, once the deductible is met, the plan will cover part of the bill at a lower percentage leaving the individual responsible for the remaining cost in a co-insurance payment. Once again, similar to an Indemnity Plan, a PPO typically sets an out of pocket maximum for this co-insurance responsibility. Therefore, if one's maximum is limited to $3,000, the PPO will pay one hundred percent of the bill once this amount has been reached.[464]

Finally, we have the Point of Service Plans. These are the most versatile of the major insurance plans in that they provide three types of coverage. These three different levels of coverage are referred to as **tiers,** with the first operating like an HMO, the second operating like a PPO and the third operating like an Indemnity Plan. Under the first tier, an individual receives care through a primary physician within the designated network of medical providers. This primary physician can refer the individual to other medical providers within the network, and as there is no annual deductible, the individual is only responsible for a small co-payment at the time of each visit.[465]

Under the second tier, a member can visit any medical provider within the PPO network with the plan covering a set percentage of the charge. The member remains responsible for paying the annual deductible as well as covering the remainder of the medical charges through a co-payment. Under the third tier, members can visit their physician of choice. A certain percentage of the charge will be paid by the plan, although this percentage will be lower than that covered under the second tier. This means that the member will be responsible for a higher co-payment in addition to paying the annual deductible.

Once the member has reached the annual out of pocket maximum outlined in the policy, the plan will cover one hundred percent of her or his medical costs. Further, members of a POS have the option of using any one of these tiers at any time and can even switch back and forth between them, depending upon the form of medical care one wishes to receive or the physician one wishes to see.[466]

Special Insurance Concerns
Permission Requirements

Referral

To insure payment or reimbursement by one's insurance company for medical expenses is managed in a timely and efficient manner, the covered member must follow the terms of her or his policy precisely. If some form of permission is required from the insurance company before the member can receive certain medical care, the member must follow the appropriate steps dictated by that policy to the letter.

To begin, we know that some insurance plans, including HMOs, PPOs and certain tiers of PSOs, contract with a pre-approved list of physicians and medical care providers. Under these plans, a covered member typically can only visit a physician not on the pre-approved list of providers by obtaining a **referral**, or permission, from one's primary physician. A referral also is required if one needs to visit a specialist, usually defined as any medical practitioner who is not a "general" practitioner or pediatrician, or not in family practice or internal medicine. In addition, because most surgeries and diagnostic procedures such as MRIs, CT scans, colonoscopies and some x-rays are conducted in a hospital or an out-patient facility rather than in a primary physician's office, a referral is often required in these cases as well.[467]

The process of obtaining a referral can vary according to the specifics of the insurance policy in question. It can be a time-consuming process, however, and as such each individual must understand the demands of her or his policy before an emergency arises. Some primary physicians, for example, require the patient to make an appointment with them before they will refer the patient to another physician or specialist. Clearly, if a visit to one's primary physician must precede a visit to an out-of-network physician the process of obtaining a referral may take approximately seven days. On the other hand, some primary physicians will forego this required office visit if the patient has seen the primary at least once in the last six months for the same condition or complaint. Either way, once the primary physician agrees to refer the patient to another physician for any reason, the matter becomes an issue for the primary physician's **referral**

specialist to address. A referral specialist is an individual specifically trained to interact with and transmit information to the multitude of companies with whom patients may be insured. Some physicians, however, don't employ a specialist, and when this is the case, the liaison between a patient and her or his insurance company is a job that often falls to a physician's office manager, medical assistant or nurse.[468]

In any event, it's up to this individual to contact the insurance company with all the necessary medical information required to obtain the referral. As this information is processed by codes, the information easily is transmitted by the physician's office and automatically recorded by the insurance company either through touchtone telephone signals or typed computer entries. For instance, every physician has a special identification number that she or he uses when conducting business with any insurance company.

Similarly, every patient has an identification number on her or his insurance card. Each facility and each procedure has its own code number. And, each diagnosis and body part as well possesses its own numerical code. Accordingly, when this information is transmitted, it will include code numbers for the primary referring physician and the referred physician, the patient, the facility to which the patient has been referred, the procedure to be conducted, the problem suspected and the part of the body affected.

The referral specialist also will be required to enter the number of visits the primary physician believes will be necessary to treat the problem or condition. Once transmitted, a staff of nurses or physicians employed by the insurance company may review this information. And, once all the information has been entered and processed, the system will notify the referral specialist whether the referral has been denied or granted.

A denial generally will be the result of misinformation or a lack of required information generated during the transmittal process, a situation easily remedied by the referral specialist.

By law, it's illegal for an insurance company to deny an individual necessary medical treatment. The determination as to what treatment is necessary, however, and who is best qualified to deliver that treatment often becomes a matter of opinion.

In most cases if the information has been properly transmitted and the insurance company review staff has determined that the out of network specialist is the physician best qualified to treat the patient, the referral will be granted. Once this occurs, a referral number, the number of allowed visits and the dates when the visits can take place will be faxed or otherwise transmitted on a special form back to the referral specialist. This form also may be transmitted to the referred physician or facility as well as to the patient.[469]

In a perfect world, the referring and the referred physician both will file this information independently and retrieve it when needed. This isn't a perfect world, however, and as a result, copies of important information can be lost, mislaid and misfiled.

Accordingly, it's highly advisable for each patient to continue the practice of personal responsibility by obtaining copies of all pertinent documents and keeping them in her or his private files.

Notification

In the past, many PPO insurance plans didn't require a referral before a covered member visited an out-of-network physician or underwent a specialized medical procedure. Typically, members of a PPO choosing to go out-of-network for medical care could do so simply by paying the deductible and assuming responsibility for each visit's co-payment. While technically this remains true today, some PPO plans require members to obtain a form of permission known as **notification** before visiting any out-of-network physician or facility.[470]

Some office referral specialists will call a patient's insurance company to see if notification is required. Others, however, often assume that a referral and a notification are the same thing, and if the former isn't required, then neither is the latter. This is an often incorrect assumption that can create numerous financial headaches for the member and interfere with prompt reimbursement from the insurance company.

To be safe and avoid confusion, therefore, each member should request the referring physician's specialist to contact the insurance company and inquire about the need for notification or, the member should contact the customer service department of her or his insurance company directly and make a personal inquiry. When contacting customer service directly, however, members should be careful, as the turnover in these departments is great.

It's possible to receive incorrect information from a departing employee who no longer has the member's best interests at heart or a new employee whose genuine desire to help may be impeded by a lack of knowledge and experience. As such, an additional call by the member to a different customer service representative to verify previously given information is always advisable.

Pre-Certification

Another form of permission often required by insurance companies before a member undergoes certain medical procedures is known as **pre-certification**. In most cases, the need for a pre-certification won't arise until one has seen her or his primary physician and has received a referral or notification to see a specialist for a diagnosis. If this diagnosis indicates that an MRI, CT scan, colonoscopy or other procedure is required to validate or refute the diagnosis or suspected medical condition, a pre-certification may be necessary.[471]

If this is the case, the process for obtaining this permission typically will be initiated in the physician specialist's office by an individual known as the pre-certification specialist. It's the job of this individual to contact the patient's insurance company and inquire if the particular insurance plan and the recommended medical procedure require pre-certification. If so, the pre-cert specialist will fill out the proper forms, make copies of the physician specialist's notes as well as copies of any biopsy, pathology or lab work reports and fax all this material, along with a copy of the original referral, to the insurance company.

Once the insurance company receives this information, a staff of company nurses will review the information and decide if the patient qualifies for the recommended procedure. The company will then fax its decision back to the pre-cert specialist. As with a referral, if the request is denied, the denial generally is due to the transmittal of incomplete or inaccurate information from the pre-cert specialist.

It's particularly important that all diagnostic test results that help substantiate the seriousness of the patient's condition are included in the information packet and, if this is overlooked initially, the pre-cert specialist must begin the process again. When this is finalized, the pre-cert specialist will complete the paperwork and retain one copy in the office to insure that two copies of the records, one by the insurance company and one by the physician specialist, will be retained.

Once all the pertinent information and documents have been transmitted, the request for the medical procedure is approved and the required pre-certification is obtained, an "approval form" will be faxed to the pre-cert specialist. This form will include a number by which the pre-certification is identified and an effective date upon which the procedure may take place.

The allowable time frame for undergoing a procedure varies from company to company. While some will provide a two-month window in which the covered member may have the proposed procedure, others give only one day to undergo the procedure. In the latter case, if it isn't possible for the member to have the procedure on the designated date, the pre-cert specialist must contact the company again and request a new date. Fortunately, this doesn't take long and a new date typically will be provided with little delay.[472]

Legal and Other Protections

In Case of Emergency

Medical conditions and problems don't always occur gradually or give an individual ample time to react and prepare. In case of an emergency in which the covered member needs to see a specialist or undergo a procedure immediately, she or he should contact the primary physician and clearly explain the situation. Typically, the primary will try to expedite the process by immediately contacting the specialist or facility, as well as the patient's insurance company, and relaying the appropriate information.

In such circumstances, a referral, notification or pre-certification can be obtained within a matter of hours or, at the very most, within one or two days. In case of an emergency in which the covered member needs to go directly to an emergency room, the member still must contact her or his primary physician to inform the primary of the situation. The primary must then call the insurance company to let it know that the member has been admitted as a patient into the hospital. This is important as the time line for informing one's insurance company about one's receipt of any medical care is strict.

If the member is unconscious or incapacitated in any way, the insurance company must still be contacted if the insurance company is to pay its share of the expense. If the company isn't notified in a timely manner according to policy guidelines, and the steps for obtaining the proper permissions haven't been taken, the member's claim for payment or reimbursement may be rightfully denied. In emergencies, therefore, a family member or friend may conduct this vital communication. It also may be conducted by a nurse or hospital representative, as having the proper permission in place will insure the hospital gets paid as well.

Emergency situations, however, can be surrounded by chaos and confusion. Many problems and omissions can occur and if the proper steps for receiving medical care aren't taken, an individual with valid insurance coverage could be billed for the entire expense. The cost could easily reach tens of thousands of dollars, and once such a mistake occurs, it can take enormous amounts of time, energy and paperwork over several years to correct.

Furthermore, the sequence of obtaining insurance company permission must be followed exactly as dictated by policy. For instance, if the necessary referral or notification isn't properly obtained, a subsequent pre-certification that may be properly obtained will nevertheless be considered invalid. Each step of permission is only as valid as the steps preceding it.

To fully understand the importance of proper sequencing, with or without an emergency situation, and the relationship of each step of permission to the other, let's look at an example. Let's suppose an individual with valid insurance is admitted to the emergency room to set a broken bone. A hospital representative contacts the insurance company, explains the situation and obtains a referral. This allows the patient to receive treatment and assures both the patient and the hospital that the insurance will pay its share of the expense.

During this procedure, however, the attending physician notices an anomaly of the surrounding skin and summons a visiting specialist in dermatology. This specialist is concerned about the anomaly and orders a biopsy, which is performed while the patient is in the hospital. The patient is released from the hospital and a few days later the results of the biopsy indicate the existence of a melanoma. The specialist notifies the patient of the malignancy and informs the patient that surgery will be required to remove the cancerous tissue.

The specialist then contacts a second specialist, a well-known surgeon in the area who specializes in the removal of advanced skin cancers. This new surgical specialist makes an appointment for the patient to come in the following day and after an examination recommends a Moh's surgery to remove the melanoma. As Moh's surgery is an aggressive and expensive procedure, and the surgeon is outside the patient's network of physicians, the surgeon's office contacts the patient's insurance company to see if a pre-certification order is needed before the procedure can take place.

After learning a pre-cert is indeed required, the office faxes the necessary paperwork and the pre-certification for the Moh's surgery is approved. The surgery is performed within the week in an out-patient facility and the patient is sent home. This is followed by a few medications and follow-up visits, all prescribed and conducted by the surgery specialist. During this time, the patient made the required co-payment for each visit and procedure as required by the insurance company.

The patient, however, began to receive bills for the entire amounts from the hospital for the first specialist and the biopsy, by the second specialist for the Moh's surgery and follow-up visits, and by the pharmacy for the prescribed medications. The bills totaled thousands of dollars and the patient's insurance company rightfully denied any financial responsibility.

Although it appears confusing at first glance, we can see how and why such a scenario develops if we retrace the steps of the treatment process. The initial visit to the emergency room and the treatment received for the broken bone was covered by insurance because the hospital representative called the insurance company and obtained a proper referral. It was an emergency situation, so it was only necessary for the hospital to contact the insurance company, it wasn't necessary to contact the primary physician. Further, even if the hospital and the attending physician weren't within the patient's network of approved physicians, the referral made the emergency visit subject to insurance coverage.

The first problem occurs when the emergency room physician consults the visiting dermatology specialist. This specialist wasn't within the approved network of physicians and the consultation received from this specialist wasn't a part of the emergency situation. Accordingly, any examination conducted by or treatment received from this specialist wouldn't be covered by insurance unless the primary physician had been contacted and a proper referral had been obtained.

The second problem occurs when the first specialist contacts and sends the patient to the second specialist for surgery. This surgeon, like the first specialist, was outside the patient's network of physicians. To see this surgeon, therefore, the patient's primary physician once again should have been contacted and a proper referral should have been obtained. It's true that the surgeon's office took the appropriate step to obtain a pre-certification before performing the surgery. This pre-cert, however, would be invalid because there was no valid referral preceding it. Consequently, none of the treatment, including the surgery, the examinations or the medications prescribed by the surgeon, would be covered by the patient's insurance.

Unfortunately, these situations are all too common, and while there are steps one can take to correct the problem, the process of correction can be extremely complicated and time-consuming. Should this occur, the first step the covered member must take is to contact her or his primary physician and explain the entire situation. The primary physician must then contact the other physicians who, in this case, include the emergency room physician, the dermatology specialist and the surgical specialist. All four must work together and combine the information each one has collected on the patient in question.

This information may include the original referral, all physician notes, evaluations, test results, pictures, additional attempts to obtain proper permission and any other material that pertains to the patient's treatment. Once collected, this information must be transmitted to the insurance company where the company's Medical Director most likely will review it. The Medical Director is always a physician, and although she or he may confer with others within the company, the Director has the final word as to whether the company will change its position and assume financial responsibility for the patient's treatment or not.

It also may be possible for one's primary physician and the relevant specialists to contact the patient's insurance company and request a "back date" for the referral, notification or pre-certification that wasn't properly obtained. If this is an acceptable method of review, the insurance company again will analyze the pertinent information and if it approves, will issue the appropriate form with a date that reflects the past date of service or treatment.

Clearly, an attempt to obtain proper permission for medical treatment after the fact is a difficult and risky proposition that requires significant documentation. There is no guarantee that such a request will be approved, and even if it is, the final approval may be months or years away. In the meantime, one is left to deal with not only the medical bills but also the bill collectors and credit problems that also may arise from the situation. This, of course, is something that should be avoided at all costs.

Meet Your New Best Friend

Obviously, the importance of an experienced and thorough referral or pre-certification specialist cannot be overrated. A good one will never take anything for granted or assume that the necessary requirements for proper insurance coverage have been addressed by another and are in place. A good one will start at the beginning of the process by making sure that the patient's insurance is valid. Insurance validity means that the premiums have been paid regularly, the payments are up to date and the policy hasn't expired. This is very basic and important, and it's surprising how often those who should know better omit this obvious step of research.

Once certain that the patient's insurance is valid, a good specialist will then contact the insurance company and inquire if any type of permission is needed before the patient receives treatment from the out of network physician or before the patient undergoes a particular medical procedure. A good specialist also will contact the patient's primary physician to make sure the initial required referral has been secured and is in place, then will contact every other physician the patient has visited for the current condition. This allows the specialist to retrace each step of referral, notification and pre-certification to insure that the prior physician offices properly performed each.

This is essential as there are many ways for mistakes to occur, and a good specialist will never assume that others have performed their jobs properly. For instance, individuals in the insurance company referral department typically are deluged by telephone calls from hospitals, physician offices, medical facilities and covered members. These individuals spend hours on the phone each day performing this detailed work, and it's not uncommon for the codes designating the physicians in question, the facility, the procedures, the body parts or the diagnosis to be incorrectly entered into the records.

Similarly, pre-certifications may be rendered invalid if the patient is unable to receive treatment on the date set forth by the insurance company. If this date is changed, the pre-certification also may need to be changed to reflect the new date of treatment. Accordingly, in conducting this business a good specialist will document each conversation with the date, time and name of the insurance company employee so that any mistake that might occur can be more easily identified. A good specialist also will keep a logbook that details the history of the patient's condition, the attending physicians, as well as the tests and procedures conducted in order to protect the records from loss.

Even if the insurance plan in question is one that typically doesn't require company permission for visits to certain physicians or undergoing certain procedures, a good specialist will still contact the company by calling the member or customer services number. And, once the specialist has double-checked every prior step of obtaining such permission, she or he will carefully gather and transmit all the necessary documentation and paperwork concerning the patient's immediate need to insure the company can make an intelligently informed decision.

No matter how experienced and thorough the specialist or designated insurance company liaison may be, however, the patient must still take charge of her or his own care. The patient must work closely with the specialist and be aware of every step of communication conducted on the patient's behalf. The patient should understand the full process and, if unsure, should ask the specialist for a list of the pertinent insurance benefits, approved physicians and procedures and the relevant telephone numbers of customer and member services.

Similarly, the patient should request copies of every document and record that passes from the physician's office to the insurance company and vice versa. Keeping a separate personal file of all information in this way will help insure the process is conducted properly and moves forward in a timely fashion. In the event an omission or mistake has been made, the problem can be detected early in the process, the documentation can be retrieved and the problem can be solved before significant financial turmoil results.

It should be noted that even in emergency cases where the member isn't admitted to the hospital, but is sent home, the primary must be notified of the emergency room visit after which she or he must inform the member's insurance company. Remember, this procedure of contacting the insurance company isn't conducted to obtain a referral or notification. Indeed, by law no individual faced with a true emergency needs insurance company permission in any form before visiting an emergency room. This procedure does, however, assure an individual, as well as the hospital, that the cost of the visit will be properly paid.

Typically, the member will be responsible for the co-payment, which generally runs approximately $50 for an emergency room visit, and the hospital will be responsible for the remainder. This amount may vary according to one's insurance plan, yet the required co-payment for emergency room visits should be printed on the member's insurance card. Moreover, if for any reason one is turned away from an emergency room **without** treatment the individual must still call 1) her or his primary physician as well as, 2) the insurance customer service department whose number also appears on one's insurance card. This is a necessary step that will apprise both one's physician and insurer of the situation and will provide the member with the proper instructions as to how she or he should proceed.

How to Insure Reimbursement

As we've already discussed, the most important step in assuring proper and timely reimbursement from an insurance company is for the member to fully understand and comply with the policy guidelines. To do this, it's essential for each member to obtain a copy of the relevant policy and read it thoroughly. Yes, these documents can be lengthy and confusing yet, this problem can be solved in the following ways.

In cases in which the member is affected by cancer, the member must have a basic understanding of the type of treatment to be required for her or his form of cancer. Open communication with one's physician or oncologist will yield this information and allow the member to limit the focus of future inquiry. Once a list of specific questions has been compiled, the member may call the customer or member services department of the insurance company in question. Once again, these numbers should be clearly printed on the member's insurance card, and once contact with the appropriate department is made, the member can present her or his questions one at a time.

One needs to remember, however, that not all company employees will have the same level of experience or knowledge. The member, therefore, must be patient in obtaining the correct responses and must ask to speak to another representative or a supervisor if the responses are unsatisfactory or ambiguous in any way. The member also may speak to a representative of the hospital or facility in which the treatment is to take place.

These individuals are familiar with a variety of insurance companies and plans and can be extremely helpful in dissecting the particulars of a policy. Further, they have a vested interest in making sure the policy guidelines are followed, that the plan covers the intended treatment and that reimbursement will be forthcoming. Similarly, a hospital social worker often can put one in touch with services and individuals who can explain the details of an insurance policy and help the insured make the correct choices and take the appropriate action.

Personal Note

Insurance policies include guidelines that detail specific medical procedures and the recommended standard frequency with which those procedures should be conducted. It's standard, for example, for one to have one's teeth cleaned once every six months. In line with this recommendation, most insurance policies that include a dental plan will pay for teeth cleaning twice a year. Similarly, the frequency with which cancer screening procedures are conducted also is based upon a medically recommended standard.

For instance, it's recommended that the average individual over the age of fifty undergo a colonoscopy every five years. As this is the accepted standard, colonoscopies conducted according to this time frame will be covered by most insurance policies. When an individual, however, is at high risk for a particular type of cancer, screening must be conducted more frequently than the standard.

My mother, for example, has never had colon cancer but she has three first-degree relatives who have, two brothers and a daughter. Further, she's now over eighty years of age and has a history of colon polyps. These factors combine to create a high risk for my mother for developing the disease. Accordingly, she must undergo a colonoscopy once every two or three years, depending upon her physician's advice.

In such circumstances, based upon a show of medical necessity, insurance companies generally will follow the advice of the treating physician and cover the cost of the procedure even though it may be conducted far more frequently than the typical standard. Indeed, in such cases a simple cost/benefit analysis clearly illustrates that paying for a few more colonoscopies is much more cost effective than paying for extensive cancer treatment after the fact.

Understanding the requirements and limitations of an insurance policy, however, is only one step in insuring a prompt response from one's insurance company. As we already have made abundantly clear, the second step is to keep accurate and complete records of each phase of medical treatment received. One must maintain a medical diary and record and file the dates of each visit to a physician's office or hospital. The names of these individuals and facilities also must be recorded and filed as well as a detailed description of the services provided.

Again, one should never assume that another individual is keeping track of this important information. Each member must continue to assume personal responsibility for their treatment and the records pertaining to that treatment. Similarly, each member should make copies of all her or his medical bills and after carefully reviewing all correspondence received from the insurer, should make copies of these documents as well.

In addition to maintaining careful records of all one's claims and covered expenses, it's absolutely essential for one to file these claims in a timely fashion. There's a limit as to how much time an individual has to submit a legitimate claim after the treatment has taken place. For if a claim is not filed within this designated period of time, the insurance company has the legal right to deny financial responsibility for treatment that otherwise would be covered.[473]

In addition to filing claims within the specified time frame, the claims must be filed according to a specified format. For instance, if a preprinted form is required to substantiate a claim, that form must be used. If a claim needs to be submitted in triplicate, then three copies of that claim must be presented to the insurance company. If certain telephone numbers, health history details, family member names and other personal information such as birth dates and social security numbers are required to process the claim properly, this information must be submitted to validate the claim. If any part of the claim is prepared incorrectly or if required information is missing, the claim for payment or reimbursement may be denied. Even if the claim is re-submitted in a proper form and eventually approved, the time delay may prove problematic for the claimant.

Accordingly, it's helpful for each member filing a claim to enlist the aid of others. It's always helpful to have an extra pair of eyes review the requirements for filing. Friends or family members may be available to help. If not, the hospital social worker may be able to personally help file the claim or at the very least, refer the member to another source who can help. Finally, there are private companies, community groups and organizations as well as free legal aid services that offer help in filing insurance claims.

How to Appeal Rejections

Rejection from an insurance company regarding health coverage typically may occur in one of two ways. First, the company may refuse to grant authorization or permission for a member to see a particular specialist or to undergo a specific procedure. If either request is denied, the member should insist that the primary physician or the medical facility repeat the request immediately. Before transmitting this second request, however, it should carefully be reviewed for accuracy and any additional information that may help document the need for the specialist or procedure should be added to the request.

When this "new and improved" request is transmitted, it once again will become an issue for the insurance company's referral and pre-certification department. Any information missing or inaccurate will be corrected, and just as important, this new request probably will be reviewed by a different employee. These departments employ hundreds of individuals who quite often analyze information differently and arrive at different conclusions. It's always possible, therefore, for a request for any type of insurance authorization or permission to be denied on the first submission and approved on the second or third.

The insurance company also may exercise its right to deny coverage for a specific claim after one has received medical care. In the case of cancer patients, many experience problems in collecting benefits for certain forms of cancer treatment. It's not uncommon for insurance companies to label many types of accepted treatment as "experimental" and, therefore, outside coverage under the policy. Claims for new chemotherapies and bone marrow transplants are often rejected as covered treatments under a policy. When this occurs it becomes the member's burden to "prove" that the treatment she or he received was medically accepted and necessary.[474]

The first step in fighting the denial of any claim is for the member to contact the company customer service department directly and inquire about the decision. One needs to ask for a list of reasons the company used to support its decision. One also needs to have the treating physicians in question contact the company and explain why the medical care the member received meets the requirements for coverage under the policy. Physicians have a great deal of experience dealing with insurance companies, they understand the language and they are familiar with the ways in which such business is conducted. One's physician also can write a letter of "medical necessity" that explains the nature of and need for one's treatment or medication. One also needs to review the guidelines for submitting a claim to make sure the submission was properly prepared and conducted.[475]

Once these steps have been taken, the member should file the claim again, and again if necessary, and include complete medical documentation that supports a favorable decision on behalf of the member. If, however, in spite of these efforts one's request for company permission or claim coverage is denied, one should inquire as to whether the company has an appeals process. It's often worthwhile to appeal a decision as the process typically involves a panel of individuals who review the material with the final decision being made by the Medical Director of the company or someone of similar education and training. In addition, one appealing the rejection of either an authorization or claim can request an oncologist rather than a nonmedical employee within the insurance company review the issue.[476]

If the appeals process itself fails and the member still believes she or he is being treated unfairly, the member may want to enlist the help of an attorney. One who specializes in medical issues and insurance company benefits may be found through the hospital social worker or legal department, a legal aid office, the BAR Association or any number of internet searches that list and rank the attorneys in one's area. This is only recommended as a last resort, however, and it doesn't mean that the case will end up in litigation. Indeed, the mere knowledge that one has engaged an attorney often prompts a surprisingly quick reversal of a company denial without the respective parties ever stepping inside a courtroom.

Extending Group Health Insurance

Having insurance coverage, however, is a different and separate issue from that of keeping it. Most medical benefits in the United States are made possible by and related to one's employment, and if or when that employment comes to an end, one's insurance often comes to an end as well. For one who has been diagnosed with cancer and requires long-term medical care and evaluation as a result, it's vital to understand the ways in which personal insurance coverage can be extended.

There are three major laws that address this issue, including two federal laws known as the **Consolidated Omnibus Budget Reconciliation Act,** or **COBRA,** and the related **Omnibus Budget Reconciliation Act,** or **OBRA**, and a state law derived from COBRA. The first, COBRA, is a law that applies to companies that have employed twenty or more employees for fifty percent of their regular business days in the prior year. It applies to plans sponsored by state and local governments as well as plans in the private sector. It doesn't, however, apply to plans sponsored by certain religious organizations or the federal government.[477]

Under the law, the employer is required to offer any terminated employee the option of continuing coverage with the same group plan she or he enjoyed as an employee. Moreover, with the exception of gross misconduct, the law applies to any reason for termination, including retirement, layoff, reduction in hours, illness or a voluntary decision. Typically, the extension of coverage under COBRA will last up to eighteen months for the employee as well as the employee's spouses and dependents. This coverage, however, may continue for twenty-nine months if the employee is determined to be disabled during the first sixty days of COBRA coverage.[478]

COBRA coverage may extend for thirty-six months for spouses and dependents faced with losing their health insurance as a result of the covered employee's death or a legal separation or divorce from the covered employee. Group coverage under COBRA is more expensive for a terminated individual than for an employed individual, yet it's usually less expensive than individual health coverage. Until recently, an individual was required to pay the entire insurance premium plus two percent and to reimburse any portion of the premium previously paid by the individual's employer.[479] Beginning in 2009, however, the **American Recovery and Reinvestment Act** provided for premium reductions and additional election opportunities for benefits under COBRA. Under ARRA, eligible individuals pay only thirty-five percent of their COBRA premiums while the remaining sixty-five percent is reimbursed to the coverage provider in the form of a tax credit.[480]

COBRA is an important law for cancer patients and survivors as well as any individual who has experienced recent health problems, ongoing health problems or is taking expensive medications. It's important for those who have a history of any medical condition, those who already have been declined for private insurance and those who find themselves in a new job where group health insurance isn't available. It's an important safety net for those who need continued health insurance, and one that guarantees coverage for basic medical care including physician care, in-patient or out-patient hospital care, surgery, prescription drugs and often dental and vision care.

Before the protections under COBRA can be triggered, however, there are two mandatory items that must be processed. The first is called the "initial notice," a communication that must be given by the employer or administrator of the group health plan to the employee at the time the employee becomes eligible for coverage. This notice describes the benefits and obligations of COBRA and informs the employee of her or his rights under the plan.[481]

The second item is called the "qualifying notice." When an event occurs that qualifies one for coverage under COBRA such as a termination, an employee death or divorce the employee has sixty days to notify the plan administrator. The administrator must then send this second notice to each employee and beneficiary affected by the event. Typically, this notice will include 1) a cover letter that again explains one's obligations and rights under COBRA, 2) the payment, election and notice deadlines, 3) a premium schedule, 4) an election form, and 5) an ACH notice. The employee then has sixty days from the date her or his coverage is terminated, or if later, sixty days from the date of the qualifying notice from the administrator, to elect coverage under COBRA.[482]

As rules and regulations often change over time, however, each individual must be certain she or he understands the current rules related to COBRA coverage, for COBRA is a law. It isn't an endorsed insurance plan or company. As a result, any deviation in the requirements of the law or any mishandling of the mandatory notices may create significant liability for the company health plan and prove a lengthy source of litigation.

OBRA is a federal law that allows an individual to extend her or his COBRA coverage for an additional eleven months. Like COBRA, OBRA isn't health coverage in itself. Rather, it's health coverage protection that allows an employer-sponsored group health plan to continue uninterrupted after an employee termination or other "qualifying" event. This law is restricted, however, and only applies to individuals whose COBRA coverage was chosen due to a Social Security approved disability. Remember, individuals determined to have certain disabilities, have been disabled for twenty-nine months and are approved for Social Security are eligible for Medicare.[483]

For these individuals, OBRA can take over when COBRA expires and provides extended health coverage during this period of disability. If the individual is still considered disabled at the time OBRA expires, the individual will be eligible for Medicare. While providing another safety net for these individuals who otherwise would lose their group coverage, OBRA is not cheap. Qualifying individuals are required to pay one hundred and fifty percent of the total insurance premium, including any portion that may have been previously paid by one's employer.

In addition, eligible individuals must 1) obtain an "award letter" from Social Security that certifies their disability began within the sixty day period of the COBRA qualifying event and, 2) provide a copy of the award letter to the COBRA administrator within sixty days of its receipt. Further, once one becomes eligible for Medicare, one will lose one's group health extension protection under OBRA.[484]

The states also have group health extension protection laws that work much like the protections offered through COBRA. As we know, the name of state laws vary from state to state, but typically will begin with the name or abbreviation of the state followed by COBRA as **Cal-COBRA**, a California state law enacted in 1997. This law helps protect employees who work for companies that employ less than twenty individuals. Cal-COBRA, for instance, requires companies that employ less than twenty employees, yet more than two, to offer employees the right to continue group health benefits for eighteen months following a termination.[485]

Once again, with the exception of gross misconduct, this protection extends to all forms of termination including retirement, layoff, reduction in hours, illness or a voluntary decision. Under these state laws, the employee is required to pay one hundred and ten percent of the total insurance premium for the first eighteen months. After this time, if coverage is then extended due to a Social Security approved disability, the employee is required to pay up to, but not exceeding, one hundred and fifty percent of the premium for the remaining eleven months. This brings us to twenty-nine months, which means that if the individual is still disabled at this time, she or he will be eligible for Medicare. The guidelines for applying for Cal-COBRA or any other state form of health extension protection may vary according to the state. As a result, those employed by smaller companies must consult with their employer or health plan administrator to insure their options and rights are clearly understood.[486]

Disability Income Benefit Programs

As we've discussed, recovering from cancer and its treatments can be a debilitating and lengthy process. In many cases, this recovery legally qualifies as a disability under various guidelines, and as such, disability insurance is often available to the survivor. The federal

Social Security Administration oversees two programs that offer disability income benefits to legal residents of the United States, including **Social Security Disability Insurance,** or **SSDI,** and **Supplemental Security Income,** or **SSI.**

The first, SSDI, provides benefits based upon one's work history of Federal Insurance Contributions Act, or FICA deductions. Eligibility for SSDI depends upon one's age. For example, an individual less than twenty-four years old must have paid into Social Security a minimum of one and a half years in the three years before the disability began. An individual thirty-one years of age or older must have paid into Social Security a minimum of five years in the ten years before the disability began.[487]

This program isn't need-based, and there's no limit placed upon one's net worth or assets for one to become eligible. Rather, it's based completely upon one's medical eligibility and one's FICA contributions throughout one's years of employment. There is, however, a five-month waiting period for SSDI during which no payment is made to the individual. Eligibility doesn't become final until the sixth month after application, and the first payment isn't made until the seventh month.[488]

The second program, SSI, provides benefits for individuals who have limited resources. SSI is need-based. One's assets cannot total more than $2000 for an individual or child and no more than $3000 for a couple. One's home, however, won't impact one's eligibility as long as the individual lives in the home. One vehicle is allowed, regardless of value, if it is used for transportation for the individual or someone in the individual's household. Finally, SSI is only available if one already has applied for other available disability programs, such as SSDI or the appropriate state benefit programs.[489]

State benefits typically are administered under a program known simply as **State Disability Insurance,** or **SDI.** Although the program may vary from state to state, the premium for state disability insurance generally is paid through one's employer. The benefits usually last for fifty-two weeks with the payments issued every two weeks. While this program isn't need-based, the disabled individual will only qualify for the full benefit of fifty-two weeks if she or he has contributed to SDI through their employer for a minimum of twelve months.[490]

There are, of course, private insurance companies that provide both short-term and long-term insurance for one determined to be disabled. Private disability insurance may be offered to company employees on a voluntary basis or the employer may automatically provide it. **Short-Term Disability Insurance,** or **STD,** insures one will receive a short continuance of one's salary if one can't work due to the disability. Although the benefit under STD can be a flat dollar amount, the benefit usually is based upon one's gross salary prior to the disability. This means that any income received after the disability, such as that derived from sick leave or other disability programs will not be considered. After one's gross salary is calculated, STD can provide a benefit of forty to one hundred percent of the amount and typically lasts for up to one year.[491]

Unlike STD, **Long-Term Disability Insurance,** or **LTD,** can provide benefits for several years or until one reaches the age of retirement. Once again, the amount of the benefit under LTD can be a flat dollar amount, and it usually will be based upon one's gross salary prior to the disability. Once calculated, LTD can provide a gross benefit of forty to seventy percent of that amount. It's possible to obtain both STD and LTD insurance through an individual policy, but this is difficult if the individual has had what is considered a "pre-existing condition" anytime during the prior ten years. For one who has been diagnosed with cancer, therefore, private disability insurance should be obtained through one's employer if at all possible.[492]

What Is A Pre-Existing Condition?

A pre-existing condition is an insurance term that describes any illness or disability for which an individual has been advised or treated within a certain period of time prior to applying for an insurance policy.[493] First, the illness or disability may be anything from a broken toe to a diagnosis of cancer. In the former case, the injury may not sound substantial. Setting the bone or immobilizing the fracture until it's properly healed easily can treat a broken toe. If this fracture occurs within a designated time frame prior to purchasing a new policy, the fracture is considered a "pre-existing condition."

Now, if the bone heals properly, no problems should arise. There's always a chance, however, that an injury won't heal properly. If this particular fracture fails to heal properly, the individual may experience discomfort and pain at some future time. Walking may become difficult and medications may be required. In some instances, surgery may even be recommended to correct the problem. Unfortunately, because the initial condition, the broken toe, was a "pre-existing condition," no medical care or treatment associated with that pre-existing condition would be covered under the new insurance policy.

In the latter case, a diagnosis of cancer is an obviously significant medical condition. Problems related to the disease may continue for several months or years, as may the necessary medical care and medications. Once again, however, if the initial diagnosis took place within a designated time frame prior to obtaining the new insurance policy, the cancer will be considered a pre-existing condition.[494]

Even with this new insurance in place, therefore, any medical care related to this initial diagnosis of cancer, be it x-rays or CT scans, MRIs, office visits, medications or subsequent surgery, radiation or chemotherapy resulting from the initial diagnosis or a recurrence of the same cancer, won't be covered by the new policy. Clearly, the financial burden an individual may face as a result of such a pre-existing condition could be devastating.

It's important to understand, however, that significant problems relating to a pre-existing condition can occur even if a definite diagnosis of cancer is not a part of one's health history. For instance, many women discover lumps in their breast that turn out to be benign and completely harmless. Many insurance companies will use this information to substantiate a pre-existing condition of the breast. The company reasons that the existence of a lump in the breast tissue, whether it's malignant or not, indicates an abnormality of the tissue.

Further, lumps in the breast tissue and benign conditions such as fibrosis may be indicative of a higher risk for developing breast cancer. As such, any disease of the breast, including cancer, that develops after the insurance has been obtained, may be considered a condition related to the pre-existing abnormality and, as a result, won't be covered under the policy.

This same logic may be used in a number of situations regarding a number of different medical conditions. Let's suppose, before obtaining new insurance, one undergoes a colonoscopy during which a benign and harmless polyp is detected and removed. Now, let's suppose that five years into the new policy, this same individual develops colon cancer. An insurance company may deny coverage for any medical care pertaining to the cancer by using the same logic. Once again, the reasoning is that a polyp, even if it's benign, may indicate the existence of abnormal tissue within the colon.

Further, a history of such polyps may be related to the development of colon cancer and other diseases of this large intestine. As a result, colon cancer or another intestinal disease that occurs even while one's insurance is valid may be determined to be related to the pre-existing abnormal condition of the colon and, therefore, not covered under one's current policy.

Moreover, it isn't necessary for one to actually have received medical care for a condition before it can be considered pre-existing. A simple consultation with a physician or a specialist about a particular condition before insurance is obtained is enough to trigger the pre-existing clause in the policy. This means that should the covered individual eventually develop a medical problem that relates to the subject of the past consultation, the treatment for the problem may not be covered under the policy. This applies as well to any prescription medications one may have taken within the designated time frame. If the individual develops a medical condition related to these drugs after the insurance has been obtained, the condition similarly can be considered pre-existing and coverage can be denied.[495]

Finally, one must consider the time periods associated with a pre-existing condition. There are two such periods of which one needs to be aware that we'll refer to as the **occurrence period** and the **exclusion period**. The first relates to the period of time before which an insurance policy becomes valid. In some cases, any condition that occurred in the three months prior to the policy's activation may be considered pre-existing. In others, any condition that has occurred within eighteen months prior to obtaining the policy will be considered pre-existing.[496] This means that any diagnosis, consultation or medical prescription that took place during this stipulated period of time may be considered pre-existing *and* any condition resulting from any of these events may be excluded from coverage under the policy.

The second or exclusion period refers to the length of time after a policy has been activated in which a pre-existing condition won't be covered under the policy. This period of time also will vary depending upon the type of plan in which one is enrolled. Typically, the shorter time frames for both occurrence and exclusion periods are found within group health policies. The longer time frames are more commonly found with individual health policies.[497]

Fortunately, many employment based group health plans offer an "open enrollment" plan which means there is no pre-existing condition clause. Accordingly, one will be covered fully for any condition even if one has a history of cancer prior to obtaining the new insurance. One must remember, however, that if the policy does have a pre-existing clause and the individual fails to reveal such a condition, the insurance company may cancel the entire policy upon discovery of the omission.

Health Insurance and Survivor Rights

The rights of a cancer survivor regarding her or his insurance coverage are closely related to the employment rights we already have discussed. This, of course, is because most adults in the United States who have insurance receive their coverage through an employer's group health plan. Clearly, those with a history of cancer are entitled to the same rights under their policy as those without. Simply having rights doesn't mean they automatically will be enforced. One sometimes has to fight for those rights, especially when an insurer fails to pay for medical treatment in accordance with one's policy or discriminates by denying coverage for one with a cancer history. Just as the issues are similar, the steps for protecting one's insurance rights mirror those regarding employment rights.

The laws governing health insurance and one's attempts to secure and maintain adequate coverage changed significantly in the United States during the last decade. There are now four federal laws that provide limited protection for those striving to keep health coverage obtained through employment. We already have discussed some of these including the **Americans with Disabilities Act,** or the **ADA**. To review, this Act prohibits employers from treating employees who are cancer survivors differently from other similarly situated employees. Regarding insurance matters, therefore, the ADA prohibits employers from denying health coverage to cancer survivors if other employees with similar jobs receive coverage.[498]

We also have discussed the second applicable law, the **Health Insurance Portability and Accountability Act,** or **HIPPA**. In addition to addressing medical health privacy issues, this Act allows individuals, even those with a history of cancer, to change jobs without losing coverage if the individual has been insured for a minimum of twelve months. This provision alleviates "job lock" and eliminates the need for a survivor to remain in an unfulfilling job simply to retain the health benefits.

Further, for individuals previously insured, the HIPPA limits the time frames that group plans can impose for pre-existing conditions. Specifically, coverage for a pre-existing condition can only be denied for a maximum of twelve months after the policy is enacted, and only conditions for which advice, treatment or drugs have been received in the six months prior to obtaining the insurance can be considered pre-existing.

The Act also disallows group plans from denying health coverage based upon current and past health or genetic information. These plans, however, may place lifetime limitations on benefits and may exclude certain conditions from coverage, but only if these policies are uniformly enacted for all covered individuals and not one specific group such as cancer survivors.[499]

The third law is the **Employer Retirement and Income Security Act,** or **ERISA**, which regulates self-insured and employment-based health plans. This Act prohibits employers from discriminating against employees and preventing them from collecting benefits under the employer's group health plan. On the other hand, however, ERISA prohibits state legislatures and courts from holding self-insured HMOs liable for medical malpractice. This is very important to understand, as the majority of health plans today are self-insured.

Accordingly, if a cancer survivor's health plan comes under the jurisdiction of ERISA, she or he will be limited exclusively to those rights and benefits defined by the terms of the HMO. This means that even if a survivor has a legitimate claim against an insurer for failing to pay rightful benefits or for harm that results from negligence or from the limited choice of providers or treatment as defined by the HMO, the survivor may not be able to pursue legal satisfaction in the courts.[500]

We already have discussed the fourth law, which is the **Comprehensive Omnibus Budget Reconciliation Act,** or **COBRA**. This law, as well as the related OBRA law, enables individuals to extend their group health benefits for themselves and their dependents. In addition to these federal laws, the states also have laws that further define the rights of individuals. Each state, for example, highly regulates all insurance policies sold within the state. Some states have incorporated laws that specifically protect cancer survivors. Some require insurance companies to pay for a minimum hospital stay following cancer surgery, for off-label or "experimental" chemotherapy and for other types of newly recognized cancer treatments not expressly covered under the policy.[501]

State laws don't apply to self-insured policies, and individuals must contact the state's department of insurance on a regular basis to remain up to date on these constantly changing rights. Ultimately, the comprehensive umbrella of federal legislation must be combined with the applicable state laws to offer the maximum protection and guarantee that coverage for cancer patients and survivors will be determined on a medical rather than financial basis.

Getting Insurance

As we know, most individuals in the United States obtain their health insurance through the group plans of their own employment or that of their spouse or parent. As a result, many problems regarding insurance coverage arise from employment discrimination or a loss of employment. If coverage through a group health plan isn't available, individuals with a pre-existing condition and those who have survived cancer suffer the brunt of this loss.

Several studies conducted upon this very subject indicate that cancer survivors experience more barriers to obtaining adequate health insurance than those who have no history of the disease. It's been found, for instance, that survivors experience more new application refusals, policy cancellations, problems changing from a group to an individual plan and higher premiums than other individuals. An early survey conducted by the Mayo Clinic Rehabilitation Program in the 1980s reported that approximately twenty-five percent of a sample group of 940 cancer patients experienced "discrimination" of some type in obtaining health insurance.[502]

Another study concluded that approximately one half of individuals who survived leukemia or Hodgkin's disease experienced health insurance problems related to their cancer history. It appears that breast cancer survivors with inadequate health insurance receive lower quality hospital care and treatment, fewer medical services and fewer major procedures. Regional studies report that approximately thirty percent of employable cancer survivors in the state of California experienced problems in obtaining insurance, and that the denial of insurance in North Carolina is more common for young adult survivors of childhood cancers than for their siblings.[503]

Many survivors find they cannot choose their treatment and treatment provider based upon their medical and personal needs. Rather, they find they are forced to make these decisions based solely upon whether or not their insurance plan provides coverage. The impact of this reality compromises one's emotional, physical and financial being resulting in poorer health and higher mortality risks. For the truth remains that individuals who have higher incomes and can afford private insurance experience better access to medical facilities, physicians, cancer screening and treatment and, therefore, have a greater chance for overall well being and survival.

For the majority of survivors, obtaining adequate insurance with a pre-existing condition remains a complicated and difficult process. There are ways, however, to reduce the frustration associated with this process and insure that one will obtain the best possible health plan under the circumstances. To begin, when seeking proper insurance, one should always work with an insurance broker or agent recognized and licensed by one's state insurance department. A call to this department or an Internet search will provide several names of reputable agents who work in one's area and specialize in insurance matters for cancer survivors.

In turn, the agent will provide the individual with a list of insurance companies and a number of different insurance plans. The agent will help one compare all the options, determine the overall cost of each, outline the provisions of each and make recommendations based upon one's personal circumstances and needs. Once this is accomplished, however, the individual must read the policy her or himself and become familiar with all its terms and provisions. And, if questions remain, one shouldn't hesitate to contact the agent and request the necessary explanations.

While it's the job of an insurance agent to research and present a variety of insurance plans and advise and consult with an individual regarding each plan's benefits, upon reaching a decision one should make payment only to a company or agency and not to an individual agent. Further, in supplying personal information to that company or agency, one must be certain that the information is accurate as false information, or an omission of required information, may result in a sudden cancellation of the policy or a denial of benefits. One should never, of course, cancel an existing health plan until a new one becomes effective. Finally, one with a history of cancer or another pre-existing condition should, if possible, always choose a policy that has a guaranteed renewable clause.[504]

If possible, one with a pre-existing condition also should obtain health insurance through a group health plan rather than an individual plan. Typically, the benefits of a group plan are greater, the cost is lower and the restrictions on pre-existing conditions are more lenient. Fortunately, there are many groups and associations to which one may already belong or be able to join. For instance, attorneys may be able to obtain group coverage through their state Bar Association. Medical personnel may be able to obtain group coverage through the American Medical Association. Group policies may be offered through membership organizations and unions such as the American Automobile Association, the American Association of Retired Persons, the American Federation of Teachers, the Aircraft Mechanics Fraternal Association or the Metal Workers Association.[505]

Many possibilities exist and, indeed, many individuals may qualify for membership in one or more of these organizations and may simply be unaware of their eligibility. It's true that once one qualifies for membership in and obtains group coverage through such an organization, payment of the premiums becomes the financial responsibility of the individual. Yet, the cost will remain lower than the premiums associated with an individual plan. Further, obtaining group coverage through an organization such as those above may offer an individual a choice of health care plans.

If this is the case, it's important to balance the cost of the premiums with the type of benefits provided. For example, the cost of an indemnity plan or a PPO may be lower than other plans. Both, however, may decline coverage for pre-existing conditions for an exclu-sionary period of six months if the individual lacked prior medical coverage. On the other hand, the cost of an HMO plan may be higher, but this type of plan is required by law to cover a pre-existing condition immediately without imposing an exclusionary period.[506]

Another option for obtaining group health coverage may be explored through the applicable state Department of Insurance. Many states offer health insurance plans for individuals who work for small businesses or for those who have their own small busi-ness. These plans group together large numbers of workers who don't otherwise qualify for group insurance plans or have access to group insurance plans. By combining these uninsured individuals, a new group is formed through which many health care options previously offered only to large businesses become available.

Typically, these options include a choice of several different POS and HMO plans and a variety of costs and benefits. Similarly, many states have implemented a medi-cal insurance program for individuals who cannot obtain health insurance in the open market. In California, for example, this is known as the **Major Risk Medical Insurance Program,** or **MRMIP**. For those who have a pre-existing condition, have been denied health insurance coverage through private companies and don't qualify for benefits under Medicare coverage through a major risk program may be available.[507]

If this is the case, one may have a choice of numerous medical plans and providers as well as coverage for prescription drugs. These plans, however, are similar in that each typically has a lifetime maximum coverage and an annual limit, which in many states such as California are $750,000 and $75,000 respectively. Most also will have an annual deduct-ible, a co-payment for each medical visit and an annual out of pocket maximum. For those who may find themselves in need of a state major risk insurance program, it's important to know that a waiting period of up to a year may exist before an eligible individual may enroll. Furthermore, many states have programs that will help individuals pay the premi-ums for their private insurance plans when the individual cannot do so her or himself.[508]

Once again using California as an example, this program is known as the **Medi-Cal Health Insurance Premium Payment Program,** or **Medi-Cal/HIPP**. To be eligible for this program one must have coverage under a private health plan that has no exclu-sions for one's pre-existing condition or other serious medical condition. One also must be enrolled in Medi-Cal, but may not be enrolled in any of the HMOs under Medi-Cal or MRMIP. These programs won't make any retroactive payments on an individual's behalf, but they will help cover the cost of one's private health insurance and allow one to keep this insurance while on Medi-Cal.[509]

And Now, For Those With No Insurance

The financial burden imposed by any illness, including cancer, upon an individual or family without health insurance is painfully obvious. Just as important, but perhaps less obvious, is the financial burden the lack of personal health insurance places upon society. In 2004, for example, seven hospital closures in southern California alone were attributed in large part to the high and non-reimbursable cost of treating individuals without health insurance.[510] In the United States, nearly 14 million low income adults do not qualify for public health insurance programs. Indeed, even though two out of three of these individuals work, they still lack health insurance because their employers don't offer medical plans or because the employee cannot afford the premiums.[511]

Moreover, the irony in the United States is that those employers who do offer adequate health benefits for their employees are increasingly finding themselves unable to absorb the skyrocketing costs associated with their health care plans. As a result, employers are being forced to fire or lay off thousands of employees in an effort to cut costs. Further, this problem is shared not only by small companies, but by major corporations such as General Motors, which in 2005 sliced 25,000 employees from its payroll due in large part to escalating and unmanageable health care costs.[512]

Such action results in more unemployed individuals who possess inadequate or no health insurance at all. Non-workers, of course, retain the option of purchasing individual health insurance policies directly, however, the premiums for these types of policies often are more expensive than those for employment based group policies, and as non-workers are by definition unemployed, the cost of such policies may be prohibitive.

According to the United States Census Bureau, the share of the American population without health insurance rose in 2007 for a fifth consecutive annual increase. Indeed, this increase rose to over fifteen percent, which means that nearly forty-six million Americans were without health insurance in the year 2007.[513] This figure also contributes to the fact that the United States places 25th among the world's developed countries in its average life expectancy of 77.6 years.[514]

Moreover, while Medicaid is the largest public health insurance program, the federal government's broad definition of eligible individuals can be significantly limited at the discretion of the states. It's the responsibility of the states to determine the income levels that trigger eligibility for Medicaid, and most states have set these levels quite low. Typically, people with disabilities and most low-income seniors can receive coverage under public insurance plans. In addition, most children from low-income families will qualify for health coverage from public programs. Nevertheless, the number of children without insurance in the United States in 2007 was over eight million.[515] Further, parents employed in low wage jobs have even fewer options when it comes to health insurance programs than do their children.[516]

To explain, a poverty level income in the United States for a parent in a family of three was determined to be less than $17,600 in the year 2008. Such parents who work full-time jobs at minimum wage to earn an annual salary of approximately $15,000 would, therefore, be considered poverty level income earners.[517] Even so, this income would be considered too high in twenty-four states to qualify the parent for public health insurance. For this same parent, an annual salary at or just above the poverty level would similarly disqualify her or him from Medicaid and other public programs in thirty-one states. As a result, nearly seven out of ten low-income parents remain uninsured and ineligible for Medicaid.[518]

Unfortunately, the news doesn't improve for low wage adults who are childless. Indeed, this segment of the population experiences the greatest limitation in health insurance options in the country. Medicaid only covers childless adults if they're severely disabled. Some states have federal approval to use CHIP funds to offer coverage to childless adults, but otherwise each state must decide independently if it will make its own public funds available to these adults or not.[519]

At present, only twenty-three states and the District of Columbia provide health insurance programs for low income childless adults. Of these, ten states finance their programs completely through the use of state dollars, while the remaining states finance their programs through Medicaid. Regardless of the way in which the program is funded, eligibility remains strict. In one third of the providing states, enrollment is limited to childless adults whose incomes are at, or below, the single person federal poverty limit of $10,400. Furthermore, as of 2008, most of these programs have either capped their enrollment or capped their funding due to constraints on state and federal budgets. Accordingly, many of these programs have long waiting lists.[520]

As a result of these limitations, low income childless adults are the population group most likely to be uninsured in the United States. As of 2006, approximately nine out of every ten of the country's low income childless adults had no access to public health coverage under Medicaid or other similar programs. Indeed, this group accounts for approximately thirty-four percent of the total number of Americans who live without health insurance which, in 2007, rose to a staggering forty-seven million individuals.[521]

Fortunately, for these tens of millions of American citizens who lack insurance and remain ineligible for federal and state public funding, financial assistance still may be available through a variety of resources. The first step, of course, in finding ways to solve a financial problem is to recognize that a problem exists. It's important for one to be realistic when assessing one's ability or inability to pay for medical care. It also is important for one to take those responsible for one's medical care into one's confidence regarding these concerns.

One should discuss the situation with one's oncologist, one's primary physician or the business or social assistance office of the facility providing the treatment. If, for example, one has some insurance, but cannot afford to make the co-payments, the oncologist or facility may arrange an individual payment program. In some cases, the physician or facility may accept the insurance as payment in full, thus relieving the individual from additional responsibility. If no insurance exists, but one has some income, it may be possible for the facility to set up a payment schedule that allows the individual to make small payments over a longer period of time. Finally, if one has no insurance and no income, there are organizations and programs that may still offer help.

The **American Cancer Society** and the **National Cancer Institute** are two wonderful resources that can provide information and advice on a number of different issues. Both have trained personnel who can discuss the emotional, physical and financial aspects of cancer and can refer an individual to other sources for additional specialized help. The **Patient Advocate Foundation,** or **PAF,** is a non-profit organization that offers educational programs and legal counseling to individuals with cancer. The Foundation also provides referrals and information regarding insurance matters, employment or job discrimination and, of course, financial and debt management issues.

Another program that specifically addresses financial concerns is the **Hill-Burton Program**. Hill-Burton refers to construction funds provided by the federal government. If a hospital or other medical facility was built in part by using these funds, the facility is required by law to provide some medical services to those individuals who cannot afford to pay. There also are other programs that provide aid to specific segments of the population.

The **Candlelighters Childhood Cancer Foundation,** or the **CCCF,** is a non-profit organization that provides information on available financial aid programs to eligible children and their families. This foundation also provides peer support to children and their families and maintains a referral network of additional local support groups in one's area. Similarly, the **Leukemia and Lymphoma Society,** or the **LLS**, offers financial aid and medical information to individuals who have leukemia, Hodgkin's and non-Hodgkin's lymphoma as well as multiple myeloma.

Women can find help through the *AVONCares* **Program for Medically Underserved Women**. As its name implies, this program provides financial assistance to under insured, uninsured and low-income women who have been diagnosed with breast or cervical cancer. It also provides a number of other supportive services to these women including childcare, home medical care and transportation as needed.

In addition to these foundations and programs, there are numerous community and service organizations that may be able to help cancer patients and their families. Some of these include the Lions Club, the Rotary Club, the Elks, the YMCA and YWCA or the Salvation Army. Different religious organizations such as the Catholic Charities, the Lutheran Social Services or the Jewish Social Services as well as individual churches, mosques, temples and synagogues may be able to provide needed services or financial aid to cancer patients and their families. Another method of securing essential financial aid may be through fund raising in which community members and businesses are asked, via flyers or the media, to contribute funds to help specific cancer families in need.

The cost of certain treatments and medications may be paid for, at least in part, by **Patient Assistance Programs** in which pharmaceutical manufacturers help cover the cost of specific drugs produced by specific companies. This is especially important in that sixty to seventy percent of American citizens, even those who have some form of medical insurance, have no insurance that pays for prescription drugs. Moreover, the cost of prescription drugs in the United States ranges from twice as much to ten times more than the cost of the same prescription drugs in the world's other industrialized countries.

In this particular matter, one's physician, medical social worker or facility manager can help one determine the drugs to which such programs may apply and can help navigate the sometimes complicated terrain. For one having difficulty paying medical bills, these individuals can help in a number of other practical ways as well. It may be possible to find a company sponsor willing to pay for the required cancer treatment for low income and unemployed cancer patients. It may be possible to find volunteers willing to clean or cook for low income and unemployed cancer patients.

Grocery and department stores may have programs in which the cost of food and household necessities is reduced for such cancer patients. Programs whereby utility companies solicit donations from customers to help cover the electric and gas bills for the less fortunate may be available. Other organizations such as **Locks of Love** provide haircuts to volunteers whose shorn tresses are then used to create and provide wigs or hairpieces free of charge for child cancer patients.

Additional programs may help provide low or no cost housing for patients who must travel to nearby cities for overnight treatment that may take several days or weeks. Ground transportation services often can be arranged for patients traveling to and from treatment, and for those who have engaged family and friends to drive, one's local American Cancer Society or Department of Social Services may reimburse the cost of mileage.

Similarly, nonprofit organizations such as the **AirLifeLine** service or the **Corporate Angel Network** arrange free air transportation for cancer patients who must travel for critical treatment. The first engages private pilots who own or rent aircraft to volunteer that aircraft and their time to fly needy cancer patients, family members and caregivers to medical treatment centers from their homes. Financial need, however, isn't always a requirement for a patient to utilize such services. The second organization, for example, arranges for cancer patients traveling to treatment centers to use the empty seats on corporate aircraft that are already flying the same route as a part of normal business. In this way, an essential service is provided for cancer patients at no additional cost to the patient or the provider.

United States Health Care Reform

As promised, this section briefly will try to explain the impact the new health care bills in the United States may have on the issues we've discussed. Specifically, these bills include the Patient Protection and Affordable Care Act and the Reconciliation Act of 2010, both of which were passed in March, 2010.[522]

To begin, we need to remember that health care in the United States is a business. In fact, it's really a combination of two businesses. On one side we have the business of providing health care. This includes our hospitals, medical centers, clinics, rehabilitation centers, pharmacies and all the physicians, nurses and technical professionals who work in them. On the other side we have the business of providing payment for the health care providers. This, of course, refers primarily to our insurance carriers.[523]

For many years, we found ourselves in the middle of the two. When we were sick we worked directly with our physicians on the one side. We received a diagnosis and then we received treatment. Once this was accomplished, we presented our bill to our insurance carrier on the other side who paid our physicians for their work. Over the last several years, however, insurance has jumped in between us and our physicians. Insurance now commonly dictates who can treat us, where we can be treated, what kind of treatment we can receive and how much it can cost.

Now these two businesses, that of providing care and that of providing payment, both depend entirely upon us to keep them in business. We are the only source of money for both. And as providers continue to prescribe and treat us to keep their money flowing in, the insurers continue to charge more (for premiums) and allow less (in services) to keep their money flowing in. In the process, we and/or our employers get financially squeezed as our costs keep going up.

In response to this increasing financial burden facing individuals and employers the government passed the two above mentioned bills. It's important to understand, however, that most of the changes required by these bills affect the business of providing payment, not the business of providing care. In essence then, what we can expect for now is not so much health care reform, but rather, insurance reform.[524]

Now, some of the changes we can expect to see immediately. Others, however, will be implemented over the next several years. So, let's begin by listing several bullet points that directly pertain to the insurance issues we've already discussed.

- Insurance companies can no longer deny children coverage based upon a pre-existing condition. This provision takes place in 2010.
- Adults with pre-existing conditions will be afforded the same protection by 2014 through an "exchange." An exchange will allow these adults to purchase insurance through private, non-profit co-operatives at a lower cost. Until then, these adults can join a temporary "pool" where many adults with pre-existing conditions come together as a group and purchase group policies at a lower cost.
- Children may remain as an insured on their parent's policies until the age of twenty-seven. This becomes effective in 2010.

- Known as a "recission," insurance companies can no longer drop an individual's coverage when she or he gets sick. Again, this takes place in 2010.
- A cap on the amount of insurance an individual can have over a lifetime will be banned in 2010. Annual policy caps must be reasonable. They too will be limited over time and banned by 2014.
- New insurance plans must cover check-ups and preventive care. This provision will take place gradually over the next eight years. All plans must conform by 2018.
- As of 2010, new plans will be prohibited from charging co-payments or deductibles for preventive care.
- New plans also must include an appeals process to address coverage denials that are challenged by the insured.
- Seniors who have Medicare Part D coverage for drugs will receive a rebate to offset the coverage gap known as the "Donut Hole." This gap will be eliminated by 2020.
- Medicare will be extended to small, rural hospitals and health care facilities.
- Small businesses with fewer than fifty employees will receive tax credits to cover up to fifty percent of the cost of employee health care premiums.
- Businesses that provide costly early retirement health benefits will receive temporary financial aid until the appropriate exchange or co-op is established.
- New screening procedures will help control health insurance fraud and waste while insuring transparency.
- Insurers must reveal the amount of money spent on overhead including administrative and executive expenditures.
- Non-profit Blue Cross organizations (those that qualify as an exchange or co-op) must maintain a medical-loss ratio before they can receive IRS tax benefits. For small business and individual policies, the insurer must spend eighty percent of incoming money on procedures. For other policies, the insurer must spend eighty-five percent of incoming money on procedures.
- A credit program will be established for private investment in disease prevention and treatment.
- A web site to help small businesses and individuals find affordable health care will be established by the Secretary of Health and Human Services.[525]

Clearly, many additional provisions will be enacted over the next several years as a result of this reform. While tax credits will be offered to some businesses, others such as indoor tanning facilities will have to pay new taxes. Many of the state and federal programs such as CHIPS, TRICARE and CHAMPUS will be impacted in a variety of ways. To clearly understand this impact, therefore, it's important for every individual who relies upon or is involved with any of these programs to consult with an expert.

Even with all of the changes, however, under the new reform individuals with private insurance may keep their existing coverage as well as their existing providers. And, of course, of the forty-seven million individuals nationwide who had no insurance as of 2010, many now will have access to this precious and necessary commodity.

Clinical Trials

The only limit to our realization of tomorrow
will be our doubts of today.
Franklin Delano Roosevelt

Another approach one may take to reduce the financial burden of cancer care involves enrollment in a specific clinical trial. First, a clinical trial is a research study that utilizes human participants in evaluating specific medical treatments. The data generated from such research may aid in the development of new treatments, establish the effectiveness of current treatments or illuminate the need to shelve outdated treatments.[526]

When a clinical trial focuses on cancer, the data may provide essential information concerning new drugs and chemotherapies, improved combinations of drugs and the methods in which they are administered, new approaches to radiation therapy or advanced and improved surgical techniques. In addition to treatment, cancer trials also may provide vital information on early cancer detection and prevention, short and long-term side effects resulting from cancer treatment and even new insights into patient quality of life issues and behavior modification.[527]

Clinical trials are sponsored by numerous national and international governmental agencies and private industries throughout the world, as well as community hospitals, teaching or academic medical centers and physician practices. Each clinical trial, however, is carefully scrutinized before becoming active by a number of groups and committees, including an **Institutional Review Board,** or **IRB**. Such boards, composed of researchers, scientists and physicians as well as individuals outside the field of medicine, determine the reasonableness of the study and whether it's properly designed and safe for patient participants.[528]

There are three different types of clinical trials categorized as a **Phase I trial**, a **Phase II** or a **Phase III**. The first focuses upon the effect a new drug has upon the human body, its safety and its proper dosage and method of delivery. Generally, the risk associated with Phase I trials may be the greatest because the drugs being studied are experimental and haven't been used before to treat human beings.

As such, these studies generally are limited in size with no fewer than twenty and no more than eighty participants. Moreover, these studies generally are limited to patients who have advanced forms of cancer, or another disease, that have become resistant to standard treatments. In this respect, they offer new hope to patients for whom other treatments have failed and provide another chance for a successful recovery.[529]

Phase II cancer trials attempt to measure the response of a malignancy to a specific drug or treatment that has survived the previous trial. As the drug or treatment in question has already been determined to be safe during Phase I, the goal of a Phase II trial is to determine how well the new treatment or drug works. The effectiveness or efficacy of new combinations of drugs also may be tested during this phase, which typically includes between one hundred and three hundred patients.

Phase III trials are those that compare the new drugs and treatments that have survived the first two phases of clinical trials to standard approaches that already are in use. Participants in this third phase may number from one to three thousand and each is randomly chosen to receive either the new treatment or the standard treatment. The resulting data will provide information that pinpoints the advantages or disadvantages of the new treatment and help assess its overall usefulness in a standard medical setting.[530]

The research and medical communities of the world are continually trying to identify and isolate more efficient and effective ways to treat cancer. Clinical trials are an essential part of this quest and, indeed, today's cancer treatments owe their existence to yesterday's clinical trials. They're crucial to the development of a progressive health care system and the generation of vital health care statistics. They're available for almost every type of cancer, offer patients the opportunity to benefit from treatments that are not yet available to the general public and provide close personal medical surveillance and follow up.

The benefit of clinical trials to both participants and future cancer patients is great, and the risk is minimal, yet participation in these studies remains extremely low especially among American adults. Indeed, of all adults in the United States who are treated for cancer, only three to five percent typically participate in a clinical trial. The rate of participation among American adults is so low, in fact, that the issue itself has spawned several studies. Overall, it appears the major reason these patients are reluctant to volunteer for clinical trials is their fear that their insurer won't cover the cost of the trial.[531]

In contrast, approximately ninety percent of American children with cancer and one third of European adults are treated through a clinical trial.[532] This, of course, makes sense as children in the United States have more private and public funds available to pay for their health care, and Europeans don't have to rely upon private insurance companies to pay their costs. Further, this fear common to so many American adults isn't without foundation, as many private health insurance companies have a policy of categorically denying coverage for treatment considered "experimental." We have to dig a little deeper, however, to understand the whole story.

Financially, there are two separate areas of fiscal responsibility in every clinical trial. The first includes the costs associated specifically with the trial, such as the cost of the new drug or treatment itself, the testing procedures and the gathering and analyzing of the data produced by those testing procedures. The governmental or industry sponsor of the trial typically covers these costs.

The second area of fiscal responsibility includes the costs associated with the remaining "routine care" involved in the trial. These costs generally are defined as those that a patient would receive anyway were she or he being treated in a non-trial setting. They might include physician office visits, in-patient hospital care, diagnostic procedures or intravenous infusions, and it's these costs for which insurance coverage is sometimes denied.[533] Of course, the resulting argument is that these "routine" costs are by definition not "experimental," and that the costs of the "experimental" portion of the trial have already been or will be covered by the sponsor.

While this fear, however, is fueled by reality, to a certain extent it also is fueled by a certain amount of rumor and misinformation. For example, the **Summit Series on Clinical Trials**, **Harris Interactive** and the **American Society of Clinical Oncology** were enlisted to conduct surveys designed to investigate this very issue. Independently each found that American insurers ultimately paid approximately seventy-five to eighty percent of the claims submitted for treatment received in a clinical trial setting. This would seem to indicate that about one fifth of clinical trial claims are denied.[534]

Yet, this figure may not be accurate because the data only indicates that approximately twenty percent of trial costs aren't paid by insurers but by patients and institutions. We don't know if this twenty percent is the result of claims that have actually been denied or the result of costs never submitted for payment in the first place. Furthermore, a study conducted by the **University of California Davis Cancer Center** among individuals who chose not to participate in cancer clinical trials found that the fear of insurance denial was only a factor for three of the 276 individuals.[535]

The more common reasons for nonparticipation appeared to be the lack of an appropriate trial for the individual's specific type of cancer, the treatment offered in the trial wasn't what the individual desired, the physician or oncologist in charge didn't consider the individual for participation or the trial was being conducted too far from the individual's home. In addition, the demands many insurance policies enforce such as authorization, notification or pre-certification before certain procedures may be required, and delays in reimbursement also may negatively influence one's choice to participate in a clinical trial.[536]

The fear of non-reimbursement and the denial of claims, however, remains a real concern for many individuals when considering participation in a clinical trial. Fortunately, many states, private insurers and third party payees are working to minimize this particular obstacle. Some states, for instance, have enacted laws that require insurers to cover all or some of the routine care costs generated by clinical trials. Some states have joined forces with insurers to develop voluntary agreements by which routine care costs will be paid. And, some insurers have elected to cover these costs independent of any related state law or mandate.[537]

Some public insurance programs such as Medicare began covering the cost of clinical trial routine care in 2000 and the Department of Veterans Affairs and Tricare/CHAMPUS have since followed suit. For those without insurance the same programs, organizations and foundations that offer help for regular medical care also may offer help in covering the routine care costs of clinical trials. For those with insurance, the same rules of assuming personal responsibility and researching one's coverage regarding regular medical care apply to clinical trials as well.[538]

Quite often, the availability and amount of coverage offered for clinical trial routine care by insurers, be it state mandated or voluntary, is a matter of public record. This information is commonly available from one's state Department of Insurance, the Coalition of National Cancer Cooperative Groups, local social or medical welfare offices and numerous cancer or insurance-related web sites. Many insurers, however, have policies regarding clinical trials, but choose not to make the information available to the public.

In either case, it's essential for one to confirm or deny this information directly, although this can be a somewhat tricky proposition. Unfortunately, some patients report that by contacting their insurer personally they raised a "red flag" which, in the patient's opinion, hurt their chances of securing proper trial coverage. Accordingly, a better way to handle this situation may be to enlist the help of the oncologist's office staff, an attorney or a medical social worker to make the contact for the patient. These individuals may extract specific information about insurance company policy without providing the name of the patient or client in question.[539]

Regardless of who makes this contact, however, the questions that need to be asked remain the same. First, one must assess the "goodwill" the insurer may or may not exhibit toward clinical trials in general. Does the state in which one resides have any laws that require and/or regulate insurance coverage for clinical trials? Does the insurer have a positive history of involvement in clinical trials devoted to the treatment of cancer? If so, was this involvement the result of state law or mandates, voluntary decisions or a combination of both? What percentage of clinical trial costs was denied by the insurer in the prior one or two years? Does the insurer treat all clinical trials equally in determining coverage or does coverage only apply to certain types of trials or trials with certain sponsors?[540]

Second, one must inquire about the practical aspects of an insurer's policies regarding clinical trial coverage. For example, one must determine if there are any restrictions upon the location of the trial or the type of facility in which it's conducted. Are there restrictions upon the number of patients participating in the trial? Does the insurer require the same steps of authorization or pre-certification in a clinical trial setting as it may for medical procedures outside a trial setting? Who reviews the claims submitted for payment from the trial? Is it a board of business executives? Medical staff members? A physician or oncologist? What paperwork is required from the trial specialists and sponsors before the insurer can consider coverage? Are there special forms to fill out and submit at the beginning of the trial, during the trial and when the trial is completed? Is trial coverage provided in a standard policy and does the coverage extend to the "routine care" costs of the trial?[541]

What does the insurer consider routine care costs? Is there a coverage exception for "experimental care," and what procedures does the insurer define as experimental? If trial coverage is provided, to what extent is it provided? Does the insurer pay seventy percent, ninety percent or one hundred percent of the cost? Is the patient responsible for co-payments during trial treatment, does the treatment cost apply to one's lifetime maximum of insurance coverage, and does the insurer cover the entire cost of care above a certain amount?[542]

Third, one must consult directly with one's physician or oncologist when considering participation in a clinical trial. This is the individual who can provide information on many of the other participants in the trial. Without compromising patient/physician confidentiality, she or he may be able to discuss the general medical history of the other participants and the reasons why each has decided to participate. She or he may be able to determine how many patients in this or similar trials have received satisfactory payment from their insurers. She or he may be able to provide a list of insurers that have paid claims consistently as well as a list of those who have not.

It's highly likely one's physician will have information regarding the sponsor of the trial, the potential success of the new treatment being tested and any risk that a patient may face while participating in the trial. One's physician and her or his staff also may be able to pinpoint any consistent problem pertaining to coverage and the reasons for that problem. One's physician also should be familiar with the paperwork the patient's insurer requires. This is particularly important as decisions granting or denying coverage often depend upon the way in which one's physician describes a trial and its treatment.

Further, many insurance companies are reluctant to set forth blanket policies that govern each clinical trial and claim submission in exactly the same way. Some prefer to handle these situations on a "case by case" basis and make decisions regarding payment according to the facts of each case. Under these circumstances, it's the physician's skill and experience with clinical trial protocol that may determine whether a patient's claim is paid or not. And should a claim be denied, one must inquire as to the reasons, then proceed through the same appeal process as outlined for medical claim denials outside a trial setting.[543]

As with all aspects of cancer treatment, patients must remain informed and pro-active when choosing to participate in a clinical trial. Indeed, each participant typically will be asked to sign an informed consent agreement before she or he is accepted as a participant. It's through such diligence that most cancer patients can take advantage of the "cutting edge" treatments and techniques found in a clinical trial while keeping the cost of such innovations to a minimum.

Having so stated, clinical trials unfortunately may not be the answer for all cancer patients. Clinical trials are carefully designed to insure they do more good than harm. And patient participation in a trial is dependant upon that patient satisfying a number of pre-determined requirements. Accordingly, many cancer patients over the age of sixty-five are often denied participation in clinical trials because they're too ill or have too many health issues in addition to the cancer.[544]

Known as **comorbidities**, forty percent of older cancer patients in the United States were found recently by the National Cancer Institute to have more than five comorbidi-ties, with hypertension and heart disease being the most common. The problem is that most patients with such comorbidities are required to take a variety of drugs for these various conditions. And, of course, these drugs may interfere with the drugs and treat-ments being tested in the trial. As a result, the data and findings from the trial may be rendered inaccurate and unreliable.[545]

As a rule, therefore, most clinical trials will only accept patients without serious comor-bidities, or without specific comorbidities that may compromise the integrity of the par-ticular trial in question. Clearly, this means that much of the research resulting from clini-cal trials is based upon cancer patients of a younger age who, other than the cancer, are in relatively good health. This also means that the findings will in all probability only be applicable to cancer patients with a similar health background and medical profile.

This is indeed a dilemma, because the majority of cancer patients are older indi-viduals. The findings derived from most clinical trials, however, are the result of research conducted with younger cancer patients and, therefore, will primarily pertain and be of importance to only other young cancer patients. Recognizing this dilemma, researchers have energized their efforts to expand the role of the clinical trial to include all popula-tion groups, including the elderly and the infirm. Only in this way will all cancer patients be assured of partaking in the important research opportunities provided by clinical trials and in benefiting from that research.[546]

Further Financial Matters

We already have discussed the importance of maintaining complete and accurate records throughout one's cancer treatment. Accurate medical records are important in tracking one's treatment and in communicating the history of this treatment to new physicians and specialists who may become essential to one's overall medical care. Accurate medical records also will prove a valuable source of information in the future should one experience complications from the cancer treatments or a recurrence or occurrence of the same or another cancer.

Financially, the maintenance of complete medical records will help insure that proper and timely reimbursement from one's insurance, should it exist, will be forthcoming. In addition, accurate records will be necessary if one has insurance and an income and hopes to receive tax deductions for medical expenses not covered by the insurer. Such expenses may include the purchase of recommended medical equipment, prescription drugs, meals during medical visits, the cost of taxicabs, trains or buses required to travel to and from appointments, or mileage if one uses one's own automobile. A tax consultant or certified public accountant can help determine which expenses meet the criteria of a legitimate medical expense deduction, and those that do will be deducted from one's income before taxes.

Maintaining accurate medical records, however, also is important in protecting oneself from a multitude of hospital and medical facility billing errors. In fact, hospital billing errors in the United States have become so common that companies specializing in auditing hospital bills for patients are today a rapidly growing business.[547]

Hospital Billing Errors

After credit card debt, medical debt is the second leading cause of personal bankruptcy in the United States.[548] Further, this significant development isn't simply the result of the forty-seven million men, women and children in the United States who live without health insurance. Indeed, according to one study approximately eighty percent of those families who had declared bankruptcy as of 2004 due wholly or in part to medical bills had health insurance.[549]

Rather, this development is due to a complicated maze of economic and social policies, and the fact that the average American wage increases about two to three percent annually while health costs are increasing at a rate of ten to fourteen percent annually.[550] In addition, many medical conditions, including cancer, can be very expensive to treat. It's not uncommon, for example, for a week of intensive in-patient radiation treatments to total fifty or sixty thousand dollars. An oncologist's bill may exceed thirty or forty thousand dollars, a two-hour surgery can reach approximately twenty-five thousand dollars and a CT scan can weigh in at about twenty-five hundred dollars. While there is little one can do to decrease the amount charged by hospitals for such services, there's a lot one can do to insure she or he is not overcharged and that the amounts one is billed are correct.[551]

To do this, one must invest a significant amount of time and energy, and if one is unable to commit to this endeavor due to the illness at hand, one must appoint a family member, friend or even one's physician or quarterback doctor to assume the responsibility. The first step in this undertaking once again depends upon the patient's medical diary with the complete list of all treatments, tests, equipment, medications and procedures that the patient has received, including the most basic services such as urine analyses, x-rays and the number of times one's blood was drawn.

If one hasn't been keeping a medical diary, one can request a copy of the patient's medical records from the primary physician or specialist. Yet, this may not be as dependable as one's own notes. A medical record, for example, will reflect everything that one's physician has ordered for the patient. It may not, however, reflect subsequent changes made to those orders. There will always be instances in which an order has been changed, one test has replaced another, an ineffective medication has been discontinued or the patient wasn't available for, or refused, the test.

If, for example, one's physician orders a chest x-ray and later decides an abdominal x-ray is preferable, a new order will be submitted for the new x-ray, but an order canceling the original x-ray may not be submitted. If the physician initially orders a CT scan and later deems it unnecessary, an order reflecting the cancellation may not be submitted. If the physician orders eight days of one antibiotic, then changes to another antibiotic after three days, an order reflecting the new antibiotic will be placed, but an order canceling five days of the first antibiotic may not be. Additionally, if a patient refuses a service or is out of the room when a technician arrives to perform a service, the physician may not even be aware the service was never performed.

The patient must remember that orders are designed to document services to be performed, they aren't designed to document services that are not performed. The problem with this system is that when an order is placed, the patient is automatically charged for the ordered service, and this charge will remain in place unless a subsequent order removes it. This is why errors found in hospital billing typically will reflect an error in favor of the hospital rather than the patient.[552]

Personal Note

Different medical facilities possess a variety of different strengths and weaknesses. Some facilities simply lack the proper management and organization to insure accurate patient billing. Over the course of my recovery and survival I've come to know numerous health care practitioners many of whom refuse to have their own personal medical tests performed in the facility in which they're employed because the billing departments are so inadequate. From my own experience I know that once a billing mistake is made, it can take two or three years before it's corrected.

It's interesting, to say the least, to hear similar stories from those who are themselves in the field of medicine and employed by such facilities. Clearly, billing inaccuracies are more prevalent in some facilities than others, and if this is the case, it's probably common knowledge among those employed by the facility. To protect oneself, therefore, from such mistakes and the unnecessary stress they create, one should simply ask one's health care practitioners for their opinions. Most will be happy to accommodate the request.

Ideally, a combination of both the patient's medical diary and the physician's medical record will provide the most complete information as to the services actually performed or that the patient actually received. For without such information, determining correct hospital charges from incorrect charges simply won't be possible. Once this information has been obtained, one must then request a copy of an **itemized bill** from the hospital in question. An itemized bill differs from other bills in that it lists each service, including medications, procedures or equipment, separately and typically contains data on each including an item description, a reference number, a medical code, a quantity, the date of service and the cost.[553]

With these documents in hand, the patient's records and the hospital's itemized bill, one can compare the two and isolate any charge on the latter not substantiated by an entry in the former. For any itemized charge that appears on the bill and is not substantiated by the medical records is likely to be an error. Further, such a charge should be considered an error by the patient unless and until the hospital proves otherwise.

The second step in this process is to have a clear understanding of how hospital billing errors occur and which billing errors occur the most frequently. The most obvious billing error and perhaps the easiest to detect pertains to the **number of days one was hospitalized**. The dates of one's admission **and** discharge must be checked carefully on the bill as most hospitals charge for the day the patient was admitted yet don't charge for the day the patient was discharged. If the bill, therefore, reflects a charge for the day of the patient's release it should be brought to the attention of the hospital billing department immediately to discern if the charge is in line with hospital policy or not.[554]

The second easiest billing error to detect pertains to the **type of room** in which one was hospitalized. Miscalculations in this area, for example, may include extra charges for a private room when the patient, in fact, stayed in a semi-private room. In some cases, the patient may have requested a semi-private room, but was given a private room because there was no semi-private room available. If so, the patient should only be charged for the less expensive room, not the more expensive.[555]

Similarly, patients may be charged for more days in a specialized unit such as cardiac or intensive care than they actually spent. Moreover, certain services performed by technicians and nurses such as equipment monitoring should be included in the cost of the room and shouldn't reflect additional charges.

If surgery was involved in one's treatment, the next most obvious error may involve the **operating room** charges. This charge typically is determined on an hourly basis, and one's physician or specialist can verify the time one spent in surgery. The anesthesiologist's records also can verify the correct amount of time spent in surgery and in the operating room. Both sources can be used to confirm or deny the charges itemized on the hospital's bill.[556]

Continuing, another common error in billing occurs with **work or services that have been canceled** by one's physician **or refused** by the patient her or himself. If, for instance, the patient has been scheduled for an expensive procedure ultimately deemed unnec-essary and canceled, the patient must make sure she or he wasn't charged for it. If the patient was scheduled for three CT scans to be performed at the same time and only two were actually performed, the patient needs to make sure the charges only reflect two. If an order is placed for additional blood work or x-rays by one's physician and the patient refuses to comply for some reason, the patient must make sure the hospital billing depart-ment, as well as one's physician, is aware of the refusal.[557]

Similarly, patients must check their bill for **phantom** charges. These are charges that relate to the standard fees some hospitals charge for procedures often performed auto-matically when another procedure or service is performed. For instance, when a patient is admitted to a hospital, a predetermined battery of tests typically will be conducted. If the patient, however, doesn't need some or any of these tests or simply refuses to have them performed, the patient must make sure she or he isn't charged for them.[558]

One must review one's bill for a multitude of **small services or supplies** that she or he **never received** as well. This area is somewhat difficult in that it requires more attention and a little digging to determine charges that are correct from those that are incorrect. For example, was the patient charged for items or tests never ordered by the patient's physician? Was the patient charged for medications never ordered by the phy-sician or received by the patient? Was the patient charged for a full bottle of aspirin when she or he only consumed three? Or was the patient charged for two weeks of penicillin, as ordered by one's physician, when the patient only used the antibiotic for one week?[559]

Was the patient charged for a service never canceled? For example, had a blood test been ordered for Tuesday when the patient left the facility on Monday? Was the patient charged for services associated with equipment monitoring when the equipment was, in fact, never in use? Was the patient charged for the use of routine equipment such as thermometers or heating pads? Similarly, was the patient charged for the use of rou-tine supplies commonly used by hospital personnel, including surgical masks, gloves or lab coats? Was the patient charged for other routine supplies, such as ice bags, linens including pillows or towels, gauze or intravenous tubing, bedpans or urinals?[560]

Hospitals often provide each patient with a toiletry kit of personal supplies when admitted. If a patient only uses the comb and not the hairbrush, or the toothbrush and not the toothpaste, she or he shouldn't be charged for the entire kit. Was the patient charged for an item taken from the patient's room by hospital staff to supply another patient's room? Was the patient charged for long distance telephone calls the patient never made? One must check for erroneous charges for personal items or services that are dated before the patient was admitted to the hospital or after the patient was released. Although this list is extensive, by knowing what to look for and by comparing the charges to one's medical record, many of these small errors and overcharges can be discovered and corrected.[561]

Another common billing error pertains to **duplicate charges** in which, for whatever reason, one is billed twice, or more, for the same item or procedure. The key here, of course, is to review the reference number, item description and date of service on the itemized bill. If any duplicate entries appear, the information easily can be compared to one's medical diary or personal record of services. This may be a little more complicated if one has several bills for both in-patient and out-patient services.[562]

In these cases, one must review each bill separately to make sure the same charge doesn't appear on more than one bill. For example, was the patient billed for more than one "initial" visit or consultation? One also must be aware of procedures or services that had to be performed more than once due to hospital error. If, for example, an MRI was performed twice because of equipment failure or because the initial test results were mislaid or lost, the patient is only responsible for the cost of one test, not two.

In addition, one must guard against errors that are the result of **incorrect data entries**. And, although this type of error may be one of the most common, it isn't always one of the most obvious. If a member of the hospital staff or a computer operator makes an error while entering an item description, it may be easy to spot. After all, a man charged for a tubal ligation or a hysterectomy, or a woman charged for prostate cancer surgery will be obvious. If, however, the error relates to the quantity or cost of the item or service, the mistake may be more difficult to see. Did the patient receive two shots of antibiotic or three? Is the cost of a box of Kleenex three dollars or four? If an extra zero were accidentally entered, would the patient know the charge for an electrocardiogram should only be $500 and not $5000?[563]

Similarly, do the reference and code numbers match the item description on the bill or reflect the proper service? Coding, which refers to the way in which medical procedures performed by health care providers are described, is particularly troublesome. Instigated by the **Health Care Financing Administration,** or **HCFA,** these codes were developed to help identify and assign the appropriate amount of reimbursement to Medicare providers. In other words, each procedure code triggered a specific dollar amount for which Medicare providers could expect to be reimbursed.[564]

Today, in addition to Medicare, many other providers in managed health care and insurance companies have followed suit. Since the 1970s the HCFA has encouraged the American Medical Association to actively work with physicians of every medical specialty to adopt this system of uniform procedural definitions and reimbursement. Most large hospitals, however, cater to in-patient services and CPT coding isn't required for in-patient services. As a result, these hospitals are allowed to use their own unique coding systems that don't lend themselves well to patient auditing. These situations, of course, raise questions for which the patient may not have answers, and for which a consultation with one's physician may be necessary.

Other common billing errors that are perhaps the most difficult to catch involve hospital practices known as **upcoding, unbundling** and **nickel and dime** billing. Up coding refers to the practice of substituting the code for a lower cost medication or service with the code of another medication or service that costs more. This may occur when one has been prescribed a generic drug, but ultimately was billed for a more expensive brand name drug. This also may occur when one received treatment from a technician, but was billed for the services of a physician.[565]

Unbundling, or nickel and dime billing, are basically the same thing and refer to a creative accounting practice in which hospitals separate each step of a procedure and charge a separate fee for each. An example of this type of billing might take place when a patient has undergone a CT scan with contrast. Using this type of billing practice a hospital might separate the procedure in the following way: 1) the lab work required prior to the procedure, such as blood tests, 2) the procedure room, 3) the specialist conducting the procedure, 4) the attending technician or nurse, 5) the iodine or other contrasting material, 6) the syringe used to administer the contrast material, 7) the intravenous equipment, 8) bandages, tape or gauze, 9) any sedative that might have been requested by the patient, 10) earplugs, 11) the scan or scans performed, 12) the review of the scan or scans and even 13) the slippers, drape or blanket that covered the patient's body during the procedure.[566]

The hospital then lists each item separately, assigns a separate code to each and, of course, bills the patient a separate charge for each. It's difficult to determine the cost of a standard procedure when this type of billing is used, and it's difficult to decipher and audit one's bill. In addition, when these separate charges are added up they typically will exceed the amount insurers consider to be standard or reasonable.

If inflated charges are denied payment by an insurance company, it becomes the patient's responsibility to cover the unpaid excess. Clearly, one shouldn't see separate charges on one's bill for tests that generally comprise a panel and for which there should be a single charge. Nor should one see separate charges for any item or service that should be automatically included in the overall charge of another item or service.

Research suggests that approximately sixty-five percent of all hospital bills contain at least one error, usually in the hospital's favor.[567] It also has been reported that ten percent of the average hospital bill of $10,000 or more is composed of inaccurate and inflated charges. Many hospitals have inefficient billing systems to begin with, and hospital billing is designed to protect the hospital, not the patient.[568]

The enormous number of public and private insurance providers and the differing policies with which each hospital must work further complicates this fact. Not only is proper billing difficult, but uniform and appropriate reimbursement is difficult to determine as well. Overall, the system works with hospitals granting volume discounts to private insurers. The insurers, in return, include the hospital on their preferred list of medical providers. This, of course, funnels millions of patients who have coverage through the insurer to the hospital.[569]

As these private insurers continue to bargain for discounts, the hospitals continue to raise their prices in an effort to recoup the monetary shortfalls created by the discounts. In addition, these increasing hospital costs also reflect an attempt by the facilities to balance the deficit created by unpaid and delinquent bills as well as the free medical care provided to the indigent and the uninsured. Some insurers, in fact, are reluctant to bring attention to inaccurate hospital billing or improper billing practices because they're satisfied with the volume discounts they're receiving. By bringing attention to problems that may exist in a hospital's billing, the insurers fear they may risk damaging their business relationships with the hospital.[570]

Obviously, the most vulnerable patients to such practices remain those who are uninsured. These individuals often will be responsible for the entire amount of the bill, accurate or otherwise, and many have few alternative resources available to them. Yet, even for those fortunate enough to have insurance, the cost of hospital billing errors can add up in a very personal way. For even when the insurer is willing to pay a share of an inaccurate or inflated bill, the patient is still victimized.

First, while the insurer may pick up the tab for the bulk of the error, the patient remains responsible for the portion of each bill that insurer won't cover. Moreover, the amount of one's co-payment increases dramatically as the total amount of the bill increases. Second, most insurers have policies that set a lifetime maximum or "cap" for the insured, and when that limit is reached, the policy becomes inactive and the insurer is no longer responsible for any of the insured's medical expenses.

Clearly, billing errors, especially gross billing errors, that result in excessive costs will reduce one's lifetime resources under the policy much more quickly than costs reflected by accurate billing. Similarly, one must carefully review bills from one's physician as well, as many are prepared not by the physician, but by an assistant who may not be sure of which services were or were not actually provided.

If one finds that mistakes have indeed been made in the preparation of any bill regarding one's medical care, one must contact the hospital billing office or the physician office in question. If one isn't sure a mistake has been made, or one is confused by the cost of an item, the description of an item or the coding of an item, one should contact one's quarterback doctor or one's primary caregiver for additional clarification. One also may choose to consult the facility's patient representative or medical social worker.

In addition, if the inaccurate bill has already been sent to one's insurer, one will need to contact her or his insurance broker or agent as well as perhaps the customer service department of one's insurer. If, however, one follows these steps and fails to find a satisfactory solution or still has questions about the accuracy of a bill, one may need to engage the services of a private consultant or company that specializes in medical bill auditing. Should this be the case, the hospital patient representative or medical social worker can be instrumental in helping one find the right individual or company to address one's specific needs.[571]

Yes, the task of reviewing one's medical bills to insure each and every charge is justified and has been calculated properly is formidable. It takes diligence and patience to keep a medical diary, and it takes time and energy to sort through all one's bills and review each charge. By knowing, however, how the system works, what to look for and where to find help, this task becomes do-able. It remains an essential part of the overall game plan for anyone who wishes to protect her or himself from billing improprieties and survive the financial demands that accompany cancer recovery.

Personal Note

In addition to a medical diary, one also should begin a file for medical bills as quickly as possible. Facilities often send "reminder" bills for the same procedure, and it's essential to know which bills are duplicates. One also needs to know which bills have been grouped together and which have been billed separately from different departments. Furthermore, cancer is expensive and the bills add up quickly. For example, my "minimal" cancer, which was treated over a period of two months on an out-patient basis with no hospital stay, resulted in the following expenses:

1) Second mammogram and ultrasound: $ 884.75
2) Biopsy:

Imaging	866.00
Operating Room	2400.07
Pathology	1967.90
Supply	494.41

3) Pre-surgery MRI:

Clinic	125.40
Imaging	660.00
Laboratory	1514.62
MRI	4700.96
Pharmacy	423.60

4) Lumpectomy Surgery:

Initial Consultation	250.00
Anesthesia Services	1302.00
Clinic	125.40
Imaging	851.00

	Operating Room	16257.18
	Pathology	5765.20
	Pharmacy	1685.05
	Physician Fee	2500.00
	Supply	2952.31
5)	Post-surgery MRI:	
	Imaging	660.00
	MRI	3823.22
	Pharmacy	423.60
6)	Pre-mammocyte Exam:	
	Clinic	125.40
	Consult	125.40
	Imaging	617.76
	Ultrasound	617.76
7)	Mammocyte Surgery:	
	Anesthesia Services	837.00
	Implant	9625.00
	Operating Room	9183.80
	Pharmacy	1858.20
	Supply	1504.81
8)	Radiation:	
	Clinic	125.40
	Five-Day Treatment/Follow-up	20000.00
	Total	90,721.44

Yes, these figures are accurate. Even for a "minimal" cancer treated on an out-patient basis, the medical bills totaled nearly $100,000. Fortunately, I had excellent insurance coverage through Blue Cross of California. As a result, my out-of-pocket expense for this "minimal" cancer also remained minimal. Unfortunately, forty-seven million American citizens have no medical insurance coverage whatsoever. And knowing this, it's easy to see why medical debt is the second leading cause of personal bankruptcy in America. One serious illness, such as cancer, literally can wipe out the life savings of an individual and destroy the financial security of an entire family.

Choice of Facility

In the world's developed countries, the facility in which a patient receives her or his treatment more often has less to do with personal choice than with circumstance. Typically, cancer is first suspected when an individual experiences specific symptoms or when an individual undergoes a normal routine procedure or check up that produces abnormal results. At this point, the individual will undergo a battery of additional tests that generally will take place under the guidance of one's family or primary care physician.

Now, if these additional tests confirm the existence of a malignancy, this physician will then refer the individual to another physician who specializes in oncology. In many cases, this referral will reflect a decision made solely by the physician. The referred oncologist may be a personal friend of the physician or may work in the same clinic or share "privileges" in the same hospital.

The oncologist may be chosen because she or he works nearby and is geographically close to the diagnosed individual. The oncologist may be chosen based upon her or his reputation or the fact that she or he specializes in a particular type of cancer or cancers that affect a certain segment of the population such as pediatric or AIDs-related cancers. The oncologist may be chosen because she or he is on an insurer's approved list of physicians.

In some cases, however, the oncologist may be chosen in part because of the individual's input. The individual may have been through cancer before and may choose to stay with the same oncologist. Or the individual may choose an oncologist who previously treated a family member or friend with cancer. In any event, the oncologist who's ultimately chosen will have a medical center or hospital with which she or he is associated. Each physician, regardless of her or his specialty, is employed by or has the privilege of working in, a specific facility or facilities and as such, the choice of one's oncologist will determine the facility in which one's treatment will take place. Of course, there will always be individuals who are unencumbered by insurance, geographic or financial limitations and remain free to receive treatment from any facility of their choice. This remains the exception, however, and in most cases the location of one's treatment generally will depend upon the choice of one's oncologist.

There are many types of facilities whose purpose is to provide medical care to individuals either on an in-patient or out-patient basis. Some are referred to as hospitals, some as medical centers and some as hospital medical centers. Some are called institutions, some are called clinics and some are hospices. More specifically, some are called cancer hospitals, Cancer Centers, Clinical Cancer Centers and Comprehensive Cancer Centers. So, how are these facilities similar and how do they differ? Is there really one type of facility that provides treatment for cancer that's better than another?

To answer these questions, let's begin by defining the term "hospital." This definition remains basically the same around the world in that it's a health facility or medical institution where sick or injured individuals receive treatment in the form of medical or surgical care. In the United States, "hospital" is the only one of the above terms to be defined by legislative statute. Although the definition will vary slightly depending upon the state in which one resides, hospital generally is defined as a building in which the sick, injured or infirm are received or treated; a public or private institution founded for reception and care of persons diseased, disabled, dependent or infirm where patients are treated at their own expense or through charity.[572]

A "general" hospital usually refers to one maintained for the purpose of providing medical care for a broad range of injuries and illnesses. A "specialized" hospital refers to one maintained for the purpose of providing medical care in one category, or a limited number of categories, of injury and illness such as a children's or pediatric hospital, a mental hospital or a cancer hospital. Further, hospitals are designed to offer medical services on either an in-patient or an out-patient basis.[573]

Let's compare this to the term "medical center," which typically is defined as a part of a city in which medical facilities are centered. According to the definition, therefore, medical center may be used to describe a collection of health facilities, including physician offices, imaging centers, specialty clinics and out-patient surgical facilities. Some also may include a hospital, although this isn't always the case.[574]

Those complexes that do include a hospital typically will still be called a medical center or, in some cases, a hospital medical center. Usually found in the world's larger cities, these generally are huge complexes that, in essence, are self-contained cities in which every type of medical care may be found. Medical centers that include a hospital also are equipped to offer medical services on an in-patient or an out-patient basis while those that don't include a hospital generally are only equipped to offer medical services on an out-patient basis.[575]

The term "institution" is usually reserved for a facility or organization that provides limited medical or surgical care to the injured or ill on a temporary basis. An example of this might be a birthing center or a facility in which one undergoes rehabilitation for a physical injury or is treated for a mental illness. The term also may apply to a facility or organization that focuses on medical research and conducts clinical trials in lieu of treating patients on a daily basis.

An institute also may refer to a business group that oversees hospitals and medical centers, helps set guidelines for the functioning of each and is devoted to the promotion of a particular objective.[576] A "clinic" usually refers to a smaller medical facility that treats individuals on an out-patient basis only.[577] This type of facility offers basic medical care, including examinations, blood testing, vaccinations and inoculations. Finally, a "hospice" is a facility that offers care and support to terminally ill patients and their families.[578]

Personal Note
A Word on Hospice

Hospice emphasizes palliative rather than curative treatment, offers support based upon the patient's wishes as well as the family's needs and emphasizes the quality of life in cases when quantity is limited. It is, however, beyond the scope of this book to address the numerous additional issues that confront the terminal cancer patient. As a cancer survivor, my own experience forces me to focus upon the tools one needs to prevent, detect, treat and survive this disease.

True, every individual who has ever been diagnosed with cancer finds her or himself wondering if their time in this world is up. We wonder if we'll see another year, another birthday, another holiday season. We wonder if all our unrealized dreams and goals will remain unrealized. We worry about our families and our friends and we wonder if the time to say our goodbyes is upon us. For while each human being must eventually face this unavoidable fact of life, for those diagnosed with cancer this confrontation shifts from the realm of the inevitable to that of the imminent. And, until our prognosis is determined, we remain in a limbo of doubt and numb paralysis.

My hope, however, is that many of the issues addressed within these pages will help guide the terminal patient, as well as the non-terminal patient, through many of the obstacles common to both. For this book is about the fight. While we must be realistic in our expectations, medical texts around the world are filled with case studies in which terminal patients who have been told they have a few weeks or months to live overcome the illness and go on to survive for decades. Having so stated, I'll respectfully defer further discussions that focus upon death and dying to the many medical professionals who specialize in this topic. As for this author, additional comments on that particular subject will be reserved for a future book.

The above are universal terms for facilities recognized around the world. In addition to these, however, there are specific facilities within the United States known which are known by the formal terms of Cancer Centers, Clinical Cancer Centers and Comprehensive Cancer Centers. These particular facilities are those recognized by the National Cancer Institute as possessing certain characteristics and capabilities in the field of cancer research.

Prior to 1970, several facilities known as "cancer centers" existed in the United States. It was the National Cancer Act of 1971 that greatly strengthened this program when it authorized continued support for the existing centers and the establishment of fifteen additional ones. The Act also significantly changed the structure of the centers and broadened their goal to encompass all aspects of clinical, basic and cancer control research.[579]

Emerging from the Act were three distinct types of centers all of which today are overseen and supported by grants from the NCI's Cancer Centers Support Program. Under this program, facilities designated as Cancer Centers concentrate upon basic or cancer control research. These Centers don't have clinical oncology programs and most of them focus almost exclusively on conducting research rather than providing patient care. [580]

Clinical Cancer Centers are facilities that also may conduct basic research as well as control, prevention and population based research. They're distinguished, however, by their additional efforts to conduct both laboratory and clinical research within the same facility or institution. This combined focus creates a setting of continual interaction between the Center's on-site research programs, the related clinical trials and the patients who participate in those trials.[581]

To be recognized as a "Comprehensive" Cancer Center by the NCI, a two-step process is used. First, peer review must determine that the center fulfills the broad scientific and interactive requirements for comprehensiveness. A facility must conduct research in the major categories including basic research, control, prevention and population-based research as well as clinical research. Second, these centers must demonstrate a significant body of interactive research that bridges the major categories and must provide educational and informational programs for the benefit of both medical professionals and the community it serves. Regardless of the type of center, however, each must pass a rigorous procedure of peer review to maintain its formal designation and receive its NCI research grants. An "NCI-designated Comprehensive Cancer Center" also is authorized to use a copyrighted logo developed by the NCI that signifies this particular recognition.[582]

Clearly, there are many qualified facilities around the world that have the capability to treat cancer patients with the newest technologies in a comfortable setting. There also are many qualified physicians and oncologists around the world who can offer cancer patients top-notch medical care in a competent and compassionate manner. Having said this, it also is true that the better facilities and better physicians generally will be found together in the same geographical locations.

Specifically, the best cancer care in terms of facility and physician typically will be found in the larger cities and urban areas of the world. Large cities have great populations that must be served. To serve these populations, large cities must concentrate on urban development, which in itself attracts money. This enables large cities to build major medical facilities that become magnets for additional monies used to purchase equipment, laboratories and state of the art research centers. Exceptional facilities, in turn, attract exceptional physicians. They offer physicians a work environment rich in intellectual stimuli, vast resources, career advancement opportunities, occupational recognition and, in many cases, higher salaries.

Accordingly, it's advisable for those diagnosed with cancer and who live in a rural area to seek help in a major urban facility close to her or his home. Similarly, a facility that specializes in treating the type of cancer with which one is diagnosed may be advisable, such as a facility specializing in pediatric cancers for child patients.

It's just as important, however, for one to discern the actual and established differences among facilities from those that are merely the result of creative marketing. Every public and private hospital, medical center and clinic is first and foremost a business. All businesses exist to make money and earn profits. Medical facilities are no different, and while their goal to treat and comfort the injured and ill remains fundamentally altruistic, they're governed by the same laws of economics as any other business.

Success in business is not the result of good luck. It's the result of diligent efforts to create and follow a well-designed business plan that takes into account every aspect of the business. Success requires an accurate assessment of the current market as well as an accurate understanding of future market movements and trends. Success requires the research and incorporation of leading industry data and analytical resources in forming comprehensive tactical and strategic objectives. Success requires a sophisticated understanding of the relevant customer base and the ability to identify realistic opportunities to increase that customer base and improve customer relations.

In addition to developing positive customer relations, success in business also demands the development of positive relations with the media and the local populace. It demands continued involvement with the community and co-sponsored activities such as fund-raisers and charity auctions that create goodwill and measurable financial gains.

Success also requires that each business create an identity that differentiates itself from its competitors. In the increasingly competitive health care industry, this particular requirement may be the most important. Medical facilities are constantly trying to find new ways to distinguish their abilities and services from those of other facilities. To succeed, they must generate third party endorsements and credibility from public organizations and private industries. They must engage in competitive efforts to align their names and reputations with those of other successful and recognized businesses.[583]

Many form partnerships with industry giants to sell specific products, the profits of which are shared with organizations dedicated to fighting a specific disease or illness. Known as "cause-related marketing," such partnerships are powerful tools that create positive publicity for a facility while raising much needed funds for a well known cause. The need to increase a facility's "brand recognition" within the health care environment and the community it serves and attract new patients and increase revenues remains a necessary and on-going reality.[584]

To this end, health care marketing and strategic planning has become a multibillion-dollar a year industry. An enormous amount of a medical facility's annual budget is allotted to marketing as well as to the operational, financial and quality assurance aspects of the business. Marketing in health care has the same purpose as marketing conducted for any other business. The goal is to emphasize a facility's uniqueness and distinguish it from its competitors.[585] Marketing always has an agenda, and the company in charge is paid to fulfill that agenda and make the facility look good. It isn't paid to be objective.

When comparing cancer facilities, therefore, it's important to analyze the relevant information carefully and exercise common sense. One must be realistic in one's assessment. For instance, a facility that specializes in pediatric cancers will differ in some ways from a facility that does not. Similarly, a facility that specializes in treating women's cancers will differ in some ways from those that do not. Such facilities may have more of the equipment needed to treat the specific cancers in which they specialize. Some may employ more physicians who specialize in these particular cancers. And, some may employ physicians who have more experience in treating the specific cancers in which the facility specializes.

In these ways, facilities may differ, and in some cases depending upon the circumstances, one facility may be a better choice for an individual than another. On the other hand, a facility isn't different from or better than another just because its name appears on one's favorite box of crackers. Nor is a facility different from or better than another because it co-sponsors a community event or raises funds for a local cause. While these endeavors are commendable and necessary, they don't signify a facility or health care community superior in medical sophistication or ability.

Most important of all perhaps is the need to understand the marketing efforts to distinguish a medical facility based upon its "cutting edge" technology or research. Many facilities claim to have the most advanced techniques in cancer treatment or the most comprehensive research. Such claims are largely misleading and create an inaccurate picture of the way in which cancer research is conducted.

To explain, cancer research is conducted in numerous hospitals, medical centers and institutions around the world. Not all of these facilities conduct the same type of research, and while some concentrate their research in one area, others concentrate in another. As a result, some facilities may have more experience in researching certain cancers than other facilities. And, some facilities actually may reach breakthroughs in their research or develop an improved technology before another facility.

When research, however, results in a wonderful new discovery or an innovative technique, the information is quickly disbursed throughout the entire cancer community. No one facility hoards a discovery or licenses new techniques for the facility's sole use. Such information is shared by the world for the benefit of all cancer researchers and cancer patients alike. Moreover, all facilities conduct research that's cutting edge. The very nature of research is to investigate and experiment with new theories and ideas.

No facility engages in research that is passé or obsolete. Accordingly, the major medical facilities in the major cities of the world typically will be comparable in their ability to offer the best treatment modern research can provide.

The exception to this rule, of course, may be treatment received in a clinical trial setting. Clinical trials, as discussed, are research programs that develop and test new medications, treatments and techniques. Clearly, one participating in such a trial will be receiving care not yet available to the general public. These trials also typically are one of a kind and, if so, the care they provide will only be available at the facility in which the trial is being conducted. Under these circumstances, a facility may realistically distinguish itself from others based upon its clinical trial and the related area of research.

The duration of this distinction, however, is limited and will dissipate when the trial is concluded and the results of its research are released. Otherwise, one must remember that statements claiming that new research and techniques are only available in a specific facility and no other are simply marketing tools, and should be recognized as such.

Headline:

Raspberries May Help Prevent Oral Cancers

This statement was issued in the United States by a facility in the State of Ohio in January of 2005. The facility was conducting a clinical trial in which black raspberry extract was given to participants in the form of a lozenge. Indeed, ingesting this concentrated form of the berry in this way appeared to be helpful in slowing or preventing the development of oral malignancies in the trial participants, and at the time this particular treatment was only available at the facility in which the clinical trial was being conducted.[586]

Finding Help

Finding help can be fairly easy if one anticipates the potential problems that may arise and knows the proper questions to ask. In the preceding pages, we've tried to identify many of the obstacles and difficulties that often accompany a diagnosis of cancer. We've discussed a variety of ways in which many of those obstacles and difficulties can be faced and overcome. We've tried to make it abundantly clear that cancer isn't a disease with which any individual should have to suffer through or experience alone. For virtually every problem that's consistent with a diagnosis of cancer, help is available from a number of reliable and responsible sources.

Not surprisingly, some of the best sources of help will often be found within one's own community of family and professional acquaintances. One's appointed quarterback doctor may be in the best position to help guide one's choices and direct one toward additional appropriate resources. Other medical specialists, nurses and medical social workers assigned to one's case can be instrumental in helping one answer questions and formulate necessary strategies. Remember, these are the professionals who have first hand knowledge of one's case and circumstances and, as such, may be in the best position to affect immediate and personalized help.

For those who wish to use computers, however, the Internet can provide names and websites for many useful organizations around the world, and for those who wish to speak directly to a representative of an organization telephone directories and information lines can provide toll free access numbers. Yet, just as one must exercise caution and common sense when seeking information on any other aspect of cancer, one must do likewise when seeking help. While numerous respectable resources exist, others often lack integrity or objectivity. Some may have personal agendas and some may advocate a specific course of action without consideration for the specific needs of the individual.

Internet searches in particular may prove troublesome when looking for reliable general consumer information. Many websites simply serve as advertisements for specific medical clinics or organizations and some merely promote books and merchandise for purchase. Some offer reprints of specifically chosen articles, personal endorsements, online chat rooms or information log-ins for members only. Accordingly, the following contact list includes several well known and consumer friendly resources that do provide basic, balanced and well researched general consumer information. It's by no means complete and includes only a few of the numerous and reliable resources throughout the world. It's limited for practical reasons and is offered simply as a starting point for one seeking help.

These resources are divided into categories for the purpose of organization, yet several provide a variety of information on a number of different topics. These resources also are familiar with one another and won't hesitate to direct an individual to the source that may best serve that individual should it be necessary. Furthermore, while most of the following contacts focus upon resources located within the United States, many will nevertheless be able to direct an individual to an appropriately similar resource within her or his own country of citizenship or residency.

Basic Cancer Information:

American Cancer Society:
    www.cancer.org   1-800-227-2345

International Agency for Research on Cancer:
    www.iarc.fr   +33 47 273 8485

International Cancer Foundation:
    www.uicc.org   +41 22 809 1811

International Union Against Cancer:
    www.uicc.org   +41 22 809 1811

National Cancer Institute:
    www.cancer.gov   1-800-422-6237

National Childhood Cancer Foundation:
    www.nccf.org   1-800-458-6223

National Comprehensive Cancer Network:
    www.nccn.org   1-800-909-6226

National Women's Health Information Center:
    www.4women.org   1-800-994-9662

Office of Minority Health Resource Center:
    www.omhrc.gov   1-800-444-6472

World Health Organization:
    www.who.int   +41 22 791 2111

Complementary and Alternative Medicine:

National Center for Complementary & Alternative Medicine:
    info@nccam.nih.gov   1-888-644-6226

Emotional Support:

Cancer Care, Inc.:
    www.cancercare.org   1-800-813-4673

Cancer Hope Network:
www.cancerhopenetwork.org   1-800-552-4366

Cancer Information and Counseling Line:
www.amc.org   1-800-525-3777

HOSPICELINK:
www.hospiceworld.org   1-800-331-1620

The Wellness Community:
www.thewellnesscommunity.org 1-888-793-9355

Financial Assistance:

AVONCares:
www.cancercare.org   1-800-813-4673

Candlelighters Childhood Cancer Foundation:
www.candlelighters.org   1-800-366-2223

US Department of Health and Human Services:
www.hhs.gov   1-877-696-6775

Hill-Burton:
www.hrsa.gov   1-800-638-0742

Major Risk Medical Insurance Program:
www.mrmib.gov   1-800-255-4472

National Foundation for Credit Counseling:
www.nfcc.org   1-800-388-2227

National Patient Travel Center:
www.patienttravel.org   1-800-296-1217

Patient Advocate Foundation:
www.patientadvocate.org   1-800-532-5274

Pharmaceutical Research and Manufacturers of America:
www.phrma.org   1-800-762-4636

Social Security Administration:
    www.ssa.gov   1-800-772-1213

State Prescription Drug Assistance Programs:
    www.medicare.gov   1-800-medicare

The Leukemia and Lymphoma Society:
    www.leukemia-lymphoma.org   1-800-955-4572

Genetic Counseling:

Cancer Genetics Services Directory:
    www.cancer.gov   1-800-422-6237

Geriatric and Aging Issues:

AARP:
    www.aarp.org   1-800-424-3410

National Institute on Aging:
    www.nih.gov/nia   1-800-222-2225

Health Insurance Matters:

Children's Health Insurance Program (CHIP):
    www.insurekidsnow.gov   1-877-543-7669

Medicare:
    www.medicare.gov   1-800-633-4227

Medicaid:
    www.cms.gov   1-800-633-4227

Medigap:
    www.cms.gov   1-800-633-4227

Department of Veteran Affairs:
    www.va.gov
    VA Benefits: 1-800-827-1000
    Pension Benefits: 1-877-294-6380

Health Care Benefits: 1-877-222-8387
Mammography Helpline: 1-888-492-7844
Special Issues: 1-800-749-8387
    Gulf War
    Agent Orange
    Mustard Agents
    Ionizing Radiation

Indian Health Service:
    www.ihs.gov   1-301-443-1083

State Health Insurance Counseling and Assistance Program:
    www.medicare.gov   1-800-633-4227

Legal and Employment Rights:

Equal Employment Opportunity Commission:
    www.eeoc.gov   1-800-669-6820

National Employment Lawyers Association:
    www.nela.org   1-415-296-7629

United States Department of Labor:
    www.dol.gov   1-202-376-6200

Rehabilitation:

National Rehabilitation Information Center:
    www.naric.com   1-800-346-2742

Survivorship and Follow-Up Care:

American Society of Clinical Oncology:
    www.asco.org   1-888-282-2552

Cancer Survivors Network:
    www.acscsn.org   1-877-333-hope

National Coalition for Cancer Survivorship:
    www.canceradvocacy.org   1-888-650-9127

Personal Note

While conducting my own online cancer research, the top fifteen picks for one particular subject included ten advertisements and sites promoting the same medical guidebook for sale. In another search, ten of the top fifteen picks promoted books and merchandise for sale and five were article reprints. In yet another search the top fifteen picks included two ads for organizations, two promotions for the same clinic, two article reprints, two sites promoting specific books and merchandise, one promoting another website that sold books and merchandise, one members only log in site and one chat room. Now, while all of these sites are valuable in their own way, only four of the fifteen provided objective, balanced, comprehensive and practical consumer information about the subject at hand. As with any subject, when searching the internet for reliable information on cancer, it's important to exercise caution.

Part 5:
Hope for the Future

*Discovery consists of seeing what everybody
has seen and thinking what nobody has thought.*
Albert Szent-Gyorgyi

Will we ever have a cure for cancer? More than any other, this is the question that occupies the minds of all who have been directly or indirectly affected by the disease, all who treat those with the disease and all who have devoted their lives to researching it. Yet, to respond to this question in a meaningful way, we need to put the question itself in the proper perspective.

If we ask whether a cure for cancer will ever be available at some time in the future, the answer is maybe. We live in a world in which everyday reality is constantly changing and evolving, and within that structure, anything is possible. Someday, our understanding of cancer just may provide us with a method of preventing or curing all cancers. If, however, we ask if a cure is likely within the foreseeable future, the answer is probably no.

To understand the difficulty of the task, it's helpful to remember that the term cancer doesn't really describe one disease. Rather, it's a general term used to describe a variety of cellular mutations that can occur in any of the tissues of the human body. We know that the adult human body is composed of approximately six trillion cells, and each cell is unique. As a unique, living and growing physical entity, each cell embodies the potential to act and react to stimuli in ways that may differ from other cells.

True, cancers typically are named for the body part in which the disease originates, such as breast cancer or lung cancer. Moreover, a cell within specific body tissue typically will behave similarly to the other cells within the same body tissue. This, however, isn't always the case, and it isn't always possible to accurately predict the behavioral pattern of a cell by comparing it to the behavior of similar cells. Cells said to be cancerous may follow a specific pattern of mutation or they may mutate in unexpected and unusual ways. And, within each type of cancer there can be numerous sub-types in which the cells behave and further distort the tissue in different ways.

Blood cells, for example, can be altered and mutated in many different ways on many different levels, and when a new type of mutation is detected, a new type of leukemia is born. In theory, therefore, it might be possible to have as many different types of mutations, or cancers, as there are cells within the human body. Indeed, while we're making significant gains in understanding some cancers, new cancers about which we know little or nothing are constantly being discovered. At present, it simply isn't within our grasp to fully understand and predict the origin and progression of cancer mutation within every cell of the human body, as the number of variables is far too great.

We are, however, making significant progress toward our goal to eliminate the suffering and death caused by cancer even if we cannot eliminate all forms of the disease itself. Over the last few decades cancer research has advanced exponentially in its quest to identify and define the many aspects that influence the process of cancer development and growth. We do have within our grasp a solid working knowledge of the molecular, cellular and genetic factors associated with the disease and its progression.

We also have the ability to translate this knowledge into new and effective strategies and treatments that will help prevent cancer from developing and detect it earlier and treat it more efficiently should it develop. We are making great strides in perfecting new procedures that are minimally invasive and new tailored therapies that are well tolerated and target only diseased cells while preserving healthy tissues.

Our first line of defense, of course, remains prevention, as preventing something from occurring in the first place is always preferable to finding a cure for it after the fact. In this respect researchers the world over continue to make great advances. We've identified behaviors that increase one's risk for certain cancers, such as tobacco use, physical inactivity and improper diet. We've documented the potential risks of specific environmental factors and have substantiated the relationship between genetics and cancer development.[587]

We've also recognized the need for all individuals to maintain an "energy balance" in which factors that contribute to the risk of cancer are offset by factors that help modify and reduce that risk. For cancer prevention relies upon the modification of risky behaviors, the mitigation of genetic and environmental risk factors and the early intervention of medical technologies.[588]

Today, food compounds, vitamins and medicines are being used to stop or inhibit the development of cancer in individuals who have precancerous conditions or are at risk for certain cancers. New drugs and experimental vaccines are leading the way in cancer prevention efforts and promise to suppress the carcinogenic process at its inception or its early stages of development.[589] For example, drugs that to date have been used primarily to treat benign enlargements of the prostate may now be used to prevent prostate cancer.[590]

Research also is being conducted on prostate cancer and the preventative properties of micronutrients, selenium, vitamin E as well as anti-inflammatories, anti-androgens and anti-estrogen drugs. Similarly, new combinations of anti-inflammatory drugs and vaccinations may provide help in the prevention of colorectal cancer. This is extremely noteworthy as anti-inflammatories act in part by suppressing the immune system and vaccines work by stimulating the immune system. Yet, despite their apparently opposite effects upon the immune system, new studies indicate a great potential for these agents to work together in a synergistic fashion when applied in combination.[591]

Additional studies are documenting the positive effect of diarrhea and the fact that some of the bacterial toxins that cause this condition may actually inhibit the growth of malignant cells and protect one from colorectal cancer as well.[592] Newly developed chicken eggs high in cancer fighting proteins are under study.[593] A soy derivative that inhibits the production of certain enzymes that can prompt cells to become cancerous is the subject of study in the prevention of oral cancers, and a new lotion that appears to repair mutant skin cells before they turn cancerous may help prevent skin cancers.[594] These are just a few examples of the many ways in which science has been advancing in this area.

In the pursuit of early detection, a firm understanding of risk factors and existing technologies have resulted in established practices that outline the necessary procedures one must undergo and the frequency with which each should be conducted. New and improved technologies such as Oncotype DX combine to enhance the early detection process by incorporating molecularly based diagnostics that can actually predict the recurrence of certain cancers, such as that of the breast and lung, as well as predict which individuals will benefit from chemotherapy.[595]

By rearranging atoms through nanotechnology, we'll improve cancer imaging in the future by identifying the specific molecular properties of cancer that to date have been extremely difficult to detect.[596] The field of proteomics is enabling researchers to identify the proteins associated with the development and progression of certain cancers. Indeed, this new field may provide the key to early detection of an initial cancer as well as pinpointing recurrences before they become a threat.[597]

Innovative biomarkers are paving the way for new applications in early diagnostic testing and the monitoring of individual responses to treatments. Protein-based biomarkers, for example, one day will provide early cancer detection based upon an analysis of protein patterns in a single drop of blood and an analysis of simple mucous will help detect early breast, colorectal and lung cancers.[598]

Researchers continue their work with "cancer sniffing" dogs trained to detect cancer cells in the same way they're trained to detect illegal drugs and explosive devices. In theory, dogs may possess the ability to discern in breath or urine samples cancers of the skin, prostate, breast and lung by detecting an odor that isn't present in healthy cells.[599] Innovative imaging technologies continue to provide more accurate diagnoses while subjecting one to less physical intrusion.[600]

As the significant advances continue in the area of early detection, so too do the significant advances in successful treatment. In addition to their role in early detection and diagnostic testing, biomarkers also possess a potential application in creating "designer" therapies and monitoring the individual responses to those therapies and treatments. Biomarkers also will help scientists develop new drugs as well as help them identify the patients who will respond to those new drugs and therapeutic interventions. In this way, therapies themselves will become more streamlined and increasingly tailored to the needs of the individual so that "personalized" medicine will, indeed, become a reality.[601]

Physicians will someday be able to analyze the DNA in a patient's tumor, then administer a cocktail of customized drugs that attack the tumor's specific genetic anomalies. Cancer tumors of the future may not be treated as a collection of mutated cells, but may be treated by targeting only the few genes responsible for the specific mutation. Further, specific genes inserted into hair follicles may prevent hair from falling out during aggressive chemotherapies, and new chemotherapy drugs may not be used only to treat current cancers, but also to prevent the recurrence of some types of metastic cancers.[602]

Indeed, chemotherapy itself may become a tool to prevent rather than treat certain cancers. Known as "chemoprevention," the roles of specific drugs and their ability to treat potential pre-cancerous conditions are an active area of research. For example, the drugs finasteride and dutasteride are now being used to prevent prostate cancer. By reducing the amount of male hormones, these drugs treat the symptoms of an enlarged prostate thereby lowering the risk for developing cancer of the prostate.[603]

Seaweed is already being used to fight lymphoma and hormone-related cancers, and brain tumors are being effectively treated and reduced in size as the patient lies comfortably in a hyperbaric oxygen chamber.[604] Toxic compounds such as one derived from poisonous mushrooms are showing promise in fighting certain forms of cancer.[605] Other toxins such as thalidomide, a substance responsible for birth defects in the 1950s, may help fight cancer indirectly by interrupting the blood supply to malignant cells and literally starving them to death.[606]

Additional drugs that block the pathways of cancer cell growth in various ways such as **Avastin**, **Tarceva** and **Tykerb** continue to be developed. Blood from the human umbilical cord that has been used to treat children with leukemia in the past is now being used to treat and save thousands of adults with leukemia who cannot find bone marrow donors, and stem cell research may find a way to deliver cancer treatments directly to a tumor.[607]

The indiscriminate sciences of chemotherapy and radiation are undergoing changes that will transform them into new "smart" therapies capable of discerning healthy cells from malignant cells, preserving one while eliminating the other. Tiny, sponge-like nanoparticles laced with chemotherapy drugs may be used to target human cancer cells and gene therapy will enable cells in the human immune system to seek and destroy malignant tumors.

For our understanding of the human genome will usher in an era of molecular medicine and genetically geared therapies that will push our current ability to identify and treat cancers into a new realm of possibilities that as yet remains virtually unexplored.[608]

More often than not, innovative technologies and miracle life-saving drugs are the result of years of meticulous and painstaking concentration, rarely do they result from a flash of inspiration or a "light bulb" moment of clarity. Success in the field of cancer research depends upon the relentless pursuit by those champions dedicated to conquering the disease and eradicating its powerful hold on humankind. Gifted individuals the world over continue to focus their immense energies and intellects on this pursuit and cancer prevention, early detection and improved treatment are at the heart of the world's public health agenda.

As some cancers are being eliminated, others are being controlled. Highly lethal cancers are becoming less threatening, others are being transformed into well managed chronic diseases and the quality of life for survivors continues to dramatically improve. Moreover, the disbursement of these new medical technologies will be facilitated by the increasing power of the world's information technology.[609]

Analytical tools and cancer data essential to research can now be efficiency transmitted around the globe in a matter of minutes. Medical researchers and investigators will be able to communicate easily with one another and will be connected not only to each other, but also to health care providers and patient communities around the world. Joint efforts by the world's medical communities, governmental agencies and social welfare programs promise to provide universal access to screening, detection and treatment for all individuals regardless of where they live or what their economic or social status may be.

For the overall goal of cancer research is, of course, to not only insure that all people have knowledge of the medical realities associated with cancer, but have the means to detect and successfully fight the disease as well. Balance must be achieved among the world's populations to insure that no one segment needlessly suffers a higher rate of cancer mortality due to geographical location, socioeconomic status, education, race or ethnicity.

No population or individual should die from preventable cancers or those that are typically curable. No population or individual should suffer from late stage cancers that are easily detectable at the earliest stage of development through proper screening procedures. No population or individual should lack for proper cancer treatment or endure lethal cancers without adequate pain control or the benefit of palliative care. As our knowledge of the disease increases, so too must our determination to eliminate the health disparities that create an unnecessary cancer burden for so many of the world's inhabitants. True, we may never eradicate the presence of cancer from the earth. The probability of finding a way to insure that every dividing cell within every human body does so according to the rules of scientific protocol is highly unlikely. We may never harness the ability to prevent all forms of the disease or to completely remove the negative impact the disease has had upon the human race.

Yet, we continue to move forward in the creation of new cancer diagnostic tools and innovative cancer treatments. We continue to improve our understanding of molecular biology and molecular genetics and the role each plays in the prevention or development of cancer. We continue to increase our working knowledge of the mechanisms that trigger the disease and of the humane genome and its significance to individualized patient care. And, we'll continue to save lives, reduce suffering and preserve the quality of life for each cancer survivor.

It's often the existence of a common threat or a common disaster that brings human beings, otherwise often distant, disinterested and differentiated, together in pursuit of a common goal and a common cause. Cancer is one such threat. In response to this threat and the disastrous effect it can wreck upon the human race, the human race has come together. As in centuries past, the world today is filled with teams of dedicated cancer researchers and scientists who hail from every country on the planet. The world is home to numerous cancer foundations, institutes and educational programs. The state of cancer research today is a constantly evolving and changing process of discovery, a commonly recognized goal distinguished by one common quest for knowledge.

Are the odds against us in this quest? Quite possibly. Are we likely to give up as a result? Not a chance. The world will continue to spend vast amounts of time, money and energy fighting this common foe. It will continue to pool its accumulated intellectual resources in an effort to subdue and eliminate this disease that for ages has plagued humanity. The human spirit itself, the essence of which is so often at its best when circumstances are at their worst, will triumph. In this respect, we and the world in which we live are indeed fortunate.

Success is not final, failure is not fatal:
it is the courage to continue that counts.
Winston Churchill

END OF VOLUME 2

REFERENCES

(Endnotes)

1   Mayo Clinic Family Health Book 810-814 (4th ed. 2009); NATIONAL CANCER INSTITUTE, WHAT YOU NEED TO KNOW ABOUT BREAST CANCER, NIH PUBLICATION NO. 03-1556 (2009).

2   Linda Marsa, *Breast cancer's cold war,* LOS ANGELES TIMES, July 19, 2004, at F3.

3   Paul D. Friedman et al: Breast MRI: The importance of bilateral imaging, *American J of Roentgenology*, 187:345-349, 2006.

4   NATIONAL CANCER INSTITUTE, WHAT YOU NEED TO KNOW ABOUT BREAST CANCER, NIH PUBLICATION NO. 03-1556 (2009).

5   Mosby's Medical, Nursing, & Allied Health Dictionary 1091 (2nd ed. 2002).

6   Mayo Clinic Family Health Book 810-812 (4th ed. 2009); NATIONAL CANCER INSTITUTE, WHAT YOU NEED TO KNOW ABOUT BREAST CANCER, NIH PUBLICATION NO. 03-1556 (2009).

7   Id.

8   Id.

9   Id.

10 http://wwwfda.gov/MedicalDevices/ProductsandMedicalProcedures/ ImplantsandProsthetics/Breast.

11 NATIONAL CANCER INSTITUTE, WHAT YOU NEED TO KNOW ABOUT BREAST CANCER, NIH PUBLICATION NO. 03-1556 (2009).

12 NATIONAL CANCER INSTITUTE, STUDY SHOWS LINK BETWEEN ANTIBIOTIC USE AND INCREASED RISK OF BREAST CANCER (2004); Rob Stein, *Antibiotics may raise risk for breast cancer*, WASHINGTON POST, Feb. 17, 2004.

13 Mosby's Medical, Nursing, & Allied Health Dictionary 1488 (6th ed. 2002).

14 Id. at 974.

15 Id. at 1516.

16 Mayo Clinic Family Health Book 844 (4th ed. 2009).

17 NATIONAL CANCER INSTITUTE, WHAT YOU NEED TO KNOW ABOUT LUNG CANCER, NIH PUBLICATION NO. 07-1553 (2007).

18 Mayo Clinic Family Health Book 1006 (4th ed. 2009).

19 www.merck.com/mmpe/print/sec05/ch047/cho47e.html.

20 Mayo Clinic Family Health Book 1220 (4th ed. 2009); Mosby's Medical, Nursing, & Allied Health Dictionary 860-861 (6th ed. 2002).

21 Mosby's Medical, Nursing, & Allied Health Dictionary 1222 (6th ed. 2002); http://mayo-clinic.com/health/breast-cancer/WO00095/METHOD.

22 REUTERS, SURGERY MAY LOWER CANCER RISK (2009).

23 NATIONAL CANCER INSTITUTE, WHAT YOU NEED TO KNOW ABOUT PROSTATE CANCER, NIH PUBLICATION NO. 08-1576 (2008).

24 Id.; Timothy Gower, *A man's tough choice*, LOS ANGELES TIMES, Nov. 8, 2004, at F1, F8.

25 Timothy Gower, *A man's tough choice*, LOS ANGELES TIMES, Nov. 8, 2004, at F1, F8.

26 Id.

27 Id.

28 MIRANDA HITTI, WEBMD, INC., PROSTATE CANCER VACCINE MEETS GOAL (2009).

29 NATIONAL CANCER INSTITUTE, WHAT YOU NEED TO KNOW ABOUT SKIN CANCER, NIH PUBLICATION NO. 95-1564 (1995); NATIONAL CANCER INSTITUTE, WHAT YOU NEED TO KNOW ABOUT MELANOMA, NIH PUBLICATION NO. 02-1563 (2003).

30 Id.; Mayo Clinic Family Health Book 1104-1109 (4th ed. 2009).

31 Mayo Clinic Family Health Book 1104-1109 (4th ed. 2009).

32 ROBERT BAZELL, MSNBC.COM, MELANOMA DRUG A SEISMIC SHIFT IN CANCER (2010).

33 Jane E. Allen, *A window into treatments*, LOS ANGELES TIMES, May 20, 2002, at S6.

34 Mayo Clinic Family Health Book 421 (4th ed. 2009).

35 NATIONAL CANCER INSTITUTE, WHAT YOU NEED TO KNOW ABOUT BREAST CANCER, NIH PUBLICATION NO. 03-1556 (2009).

36 Id.

37 NATIONAL CANCER INSTITUTE, WHAT YOU NEED TO KNOW ABOUT CANCER OF THE COLON AND RECTUM, NIH PUBICATION NO. 06-1552 (2006).

38   Mayo Clinic Family Health Book 421 (4th ed. 2009).

39 David M. Prescott, The Cancer Reference Book 45-46 (1978).

40 Mayo Clinic Family Health Book 425-426 (4th ed. 2009).

41 Id.

42 NATIONAL CANCER INSTITUTE, CHEMOTHERAPY AND YOU, NIH PUBLICATION NO. 02-1136 (2002).

43 Id.

44 Mayo Clinic Family Health Book 1219 (4th ed. 2009).

45 http://www.medical-dictionary.thefreedictionary.com/butterfly+needle.

46 NATIONAL CANCER INSTITUTE, CHEMOTHERAPY AND YOU, NIH PUBLICATION NO. 02-1136 (2002).

47 Id.

48 http://www.who.int/mediacentre/factsheets/fs297/en/index.html.

49 NATIONAL CANCER INSTITUTE, CANCER RATES AND RISKS 191-192 (4th ed. 1996).

REFERENCES

50 NATIONAL CANCER INSTITUTE, CHEMOTHERAPY AND YOU, PUBLICATION NO. 02-1136 (2009).

51 Id.

52 Id.

53 Mayo Clinic Family Health Book 1048-1049 (4th ed. 2009).

54 NATIONAL CANCER INSTITUTE, CHEMOTHERAPY AND YOU, PUBLICATION NO. 02-1136 (2009).

55 http://www.leiomyosarcoma.information/chemo30cocktail.htm.

56 Mayo Clinic Family Health Book 1110-1111 (4th ed. 2009).

57 Id.

58 Id.

59 Id. 427-428; NATIONAL CANCER INSTITUTE, CHEMOTHERAPY AND YOU, PUBLICATION NO. 02-1136 (2002).

60 NATIONAL CANCER INSTITUTE, CHEMOTHERAPY AND YOU, PUBLICATION NO. 02-1136 (2002); LILLIAN NAIL, PHD, RN, SIDE EFFECTS – MANAGING YOUR LIFE ON CHEMOTHERAPY (2002).

61 Mayo Clinic Family Health Book 1114-1116 (4th ed. 2009); SKINBIO.COM, BETTER FINGER NAIL HEALTH TO STOP NAIL BREAKS, TEARS AND HANGNAILS (2004).

62 Id.

63 Id.

64 SKINBIO.COM, BETTER FINGER NAIL HEALTH TO STOP NAIL BREAKS, TEARS AND HANGNAILS (2004).

65 Id.

66 Id.

67 Id.

68 Id.

69 SKINBIO.COM, BETTER FINGER NAIL HEALTH TO STOP NAIL BREAKS, TEARS AND HANGNAILS (2004).

70 NATIONAL CANCER INSTITUTE, CHEMOTHERAPY AND YOU, PUBLICATION NO. 02-1136 (2002).

71 Id.

72 Id.

73 Id.

74 Lindsey Tanner, *Cancer study yields new tea theory*, LOS ANGELES TIMES, Dec. 19, 2005, at 427.

75 NATIONAL CANCER INSTITUTE, CHEMOTHERAPY AND YOU, PUBLICATION NO. 02-1136 (2002); LILLIAN NAIL, PHD, RN, SIDE EFFECTS-MANAGING YOUR LIFE ON CHEMOTHERAPY (2002).

76 Id.

77 Id.

78 Id.

79 Id.

80 NATIONAL CANCER INSTITUTE, CHEMOTHERAPY AND YOU, PUBLICATION NO. 02-1136 (2002); LILLIAN NAIL, PHD, RN, SIDE EFFECTS-MANAGING YOUR LIFE ON CHEMOTHERAPY (2002).

81 NATIONAL CANCER INSTITUTE, CHEMOTHERAPY AND YOU, PUBLICATION NO. 02-1136 (2002).

82 LILLIAN NAIL, PHD, RN, SIDE EFFECTS-MANAGING YOUR LIFE ON CHEMOTHERAPY (2002).

83 Mosby's Medical, Nursing, & Allied Health Dictionary 883 (6th ed. 2002).

84 http://www.medical-dictionary.thefreedictionary.com/condom+catheter.

85 NATIONAL CANCER INSTITUTE, CHEMOTHERAPY AND YOU, PUBLICATION NO. 02-1136 (2002).

86 Id.; Mayo Clinic Family Health Book 1039-1041 (4th ed. 2009).

87 MAYOCLINIC.COM, CHEMO BRAIN, DEFINITION (2008).

88 http://www/medical-dictionary.thefreedictionary.com/blood-brain+barrier; Linda Marsa, *Brain cancer in its sights*, LOS ANGELES TIMES, Aug. 15, 2005.

89 Mosby's Medical, Nursing, & Allied Health Dictionary 626 (6th ed. 2002).

90 NATIONAL CANCER INTITUTE, CHEMOTHERAPY AND YOU, PUBLICATION NO. 02-1136 (2002); LILLIAN NAIL, PHD, RN, SIDE EFFECTS-MANAGING YOUR LIFE ON CHEMOTHERAPY (2002).

91 Id.

92 NATIONAL CANCER INSTITUTE, CHEMOTHERAPY AND YOU, PUBLICATION NO. 02-1136 (2002).

93 Id.

94 Id.

95 Id.

96 Id.

97 NATIONAL CANCER INSTITUTE, CHEMOTHERAPY AND YOU, PUBLICATION NO. 02-1136 (2002).

98 Id.; LILLIAN NAIL, PHD, RN, SIDE EFFECTS-MANAGING YOUR LIFE ON CHEMOTHERAPY (2002).

99 Id.

100 Id.

101 NATIONAL CANCER INSTITUTE, RADIATION THERAPY AND YOU, PUBLICATION NO. 01-2227 (2002); Mayo Clinic Family Health Book 425 (4th ed. 2009).

102 NATIONAL CANCER INSTITUTE, RADIATION THERAPY AND YOU, PUBLICATION NO. 01-2227 (2002).

103 Id.

REFERENCES

104 Id.

105 Id.

106 Id.

107 NATIONAL CANCER INSTITUTE, RADIATION THERAPY AND YOU, PUBLICATION NO. 01-2227 (2002).

108 Id.

109 Id.

110 Id.

111 Id.

112 NATIONAL CANCER INSTITUTE, RADIATION THERAPY AND YOU, PUBLICATION NO. 01-2227 (2002).

113 Id.

114 Mosby's Medical, Nursing, & Allied Health Dictionary 928-929 (4th ed. 2002).

115 Id. at 1457, 1461-1462.

116 http://www.who.int/ionizing_radiation/about/what_is_ir/en/index.html.

117 Id.

118 Mosby's Medical, Nursing, & Allied Health Dictionary 1457 (6th ed. 2002).

119 NATIONAL CANCER INSTITUTE, RADIATION THERAPY AND YOU, PUBLICATION NO. 01-2227 (2002).

120 Id.

121 Id.

122 Id.

123 Id.

124 Mosby's Medical, Nursing, & Allied Health Dictionary 1456-1457 (6th ed. 2002).

125 NATIONAL CANCER INSTITUTE, RADIATION THERAPY AND YOU, PUBLICATION NO. 01-2227 (2002).

126 Mosby's Medical, Nursing, & Allied Health Dictionary 1456 (6th ed. 2002).

127 NATIONAL CANCER INSTITUTE, RADIATION THERAPY AND YOU, PUBLICATION NO. 01-2227 (2002).

128 Elena Conis, *Tropical fruit has reputation as a cancer fighter*, LOS ANGELES TIMES, Jan. 23, 2006, at 472.

129 NATIONAL CANCER INSTITUTE, RADIATION THERAPY AND YOU, PUBLICATION NO. 01-2227 (2002).

130 Id.

131 Mosby's Medical, Nursing, & Allied Health Dictionary 1246 (6th ed. 2002).

132 NATIONAL CANCER INSTITUTE, WHAT YOU NEED TO KNOW ABOUT PROSTATE CANCER, PUBLICATION NO. 08-1576 (2008).

133 Mosby's Medical, Nursing, & Allied Health Dictionary 1456 (6th ed. 2002).

134   NATIONAL CANCER INSTITUTE, RADIATION THERAPY AND YOU, PUBLICATION NO. 01-2227 (2002).

135   Mosby's Medical, Nursing, & Allied Health Dictionary 1456 (6th ed. 2002).

136   DANIEL CUKIER, MD AND VIRGINIA MCCLLOUGH, DIET AND LIFESTYLE DURING RADIATION THERAPY (1996); NATIONAL CANCER INSTITUTE, RADIATION THERAPY AND YOU, PUBLICATION NO. 01-2227 (2002).

137   Mosby's Medical, Nursing, & Allied Health Dictionary 1457 (6th ed. 2002).

138   http:/www.mayoclinic.com/health/cancer-treatment/CA00066.

139   Mosby's Medical, Nursing, & Allied Health Dictionary 775-776, 573 (6th ed. 2002).

140   Id. at 1689.

141   http:/www.medicaldictionary.the freedictionary.com/tenesmus.

142   Mosby's Medical, Nursing, & Allied Health Dictionary 1407 (6th ed. 2002).

143   http:/www.p-therapie.web.psi.ch/e/wirkung/html.

144   5000 RADS is the typical or estimated dose of radiation recommended for many cancers; http:/www.ANworld.com/radiation.

145   ONCOLINK.COM, ASK THE EXPERTS, RADIATION RECALL PHENOMENON (2001).

146   Id.

147   NATIONAL CANCER INSTITUTE, CANCER RATES AND RISKS 90-91 (4th ed. 1996).

148   NATIONAL CANCER INSTITUTE, RADIATION THERAPY AND YOU, PUBLICATION NO. 01-2227 (2002).

149   http://www.netwellness.org/healthtopics/menopause/faq1.cfm.

150   NATIONAL CANCER INSTITUTE, CHEMOTHERAPY AND YOU, PUBLICATION NO. 02-1136 (2002).

151   http://www.medicinenet.com/cyclophosphamide/article.htm.

152   AMERICAN CANCER SOCIETY, RADIATION PRINCIPLES, POSSIBLE SIDE EFFECTS OF RADIATION THERAPY (2009).

153   Mayo Clinic Family Health Book 1187 (4th ed. 2009).

154   THE AMERICAN SURROGACY CENTER, INC., WHAT HAPPENS AT EGG RETRIEVAL (1996); IVF.COM, OVULATION INDUCTION (2003).

155   http:/www.follistim.com/Consumer/TreatmentOptions/Ovulationinduction/ ClomipheneCitrate/index.asp?guid={EDFDCED2-59DF-402C-B534-DCF 14A9A3AC3}&SID=384649981; http:/www.webmd.com/infertility-and-reproduction/ clomiphene-citrate-for-infertility.

156   Id.

157   Manipalviratn S. Decherney. Clinical application of human oocyte cryopreservation. *Rev Recent Clin Trials*, 2008 May;3 (2): 104-110; Ruthann Richter, *Cancer patients may preserve fertility through egg-freezing program*, STANFORD REPORT, Feb. 23, 2000; Linda Marsa, *Frozen eggs yield promising results*, LOS ANGELES TIMES, Sept. 20, 2004, at F2.

REFERENCES

158 Id.

159 Id.

160 Id.

161 IVF.COM, OVULATION INDUCTION (2003); IVF.COM, IVF MEDICATIONS (2003).

162 http://www.infertility.about.com/od/infertilitytreatments/a/ohss_symptoms.htm.

163 http://www.medical-dictionary.thefreedictionary.com/superovulation.

164 Porcu E et al: Oocyte cryopreservation in oncological patients, *Eur J Obstet Gynecol Reprod Biol*, 2004 Apr 5: 113 Suppl 1:S14-16; Porcu E et al: Human oocyte creopreservation in infertility and oncology, *Curr Opin Endocrinol Diabetes Obes*, 2008 Dec. 15(6): 529-535.

165 Id; Linda Marsa, *Frozen eggs yield promising results*, LOS ANGELES TIMES, Sept. 20, 2004, at F2.

166 SHERMAN J. SILBER, MD, OVARIAN TISSUE FREEZING (2004).

167 Id.

168 THE CLEVELAND CLINIC, BREAST CANCER DURING PREGNANCY (2004).

169 Id.; NATIONAL CANCER INSTITUTE, HODGKIN'S LYMPHOMA DURING PREGNANCY (2003).

170 Mayo Clinic Family Health Book 112-114 (4th ed. 2009).

171 Id.

172 REUTERS LIMITED, MORE EVIDENCE CHEMO DURING PREGNANCY CAN BE SAFE (2003).

173 NATIONAL CANCER INSTITUTE, HODGKIN'S LYMPHOMA DURING PREGNANCY (2003).

174 CLEVELAND CLINIC, BREAST CANCER DURING PREGNANCY (2004); MOTERISK.ORG, MANAGEMENT OF COMPLICATIONS ASSOCIATED WITH CANCER OR ANTINEOPLASTIC TREATMENT DURING PREGNANCY (2004).

175 Id.; NATIONAL CANCER INSTITUTE, RADIATION THERAPY AND YOU, PUBLICATION NO. 01-2227 (2002); NATIONAL CANCER INSTITUTE, CHEMOTHERAPY AND YOU, PUBLICATION NO. 02-1136 (2002).

176 NATIONAL CANCER INSTITUTE, RADIATION THERAPY AND YOU, PUBLICATION NO. 01-2227 (2002).

177 Claudia Kalb, *What's a woman to do?*, NEWSWEEK, July 25, 2002; Susan Pierres, *The hormone replacement dilemma, so what's a woman to do?*, HEALTH, at 134.

178 NATIONAL CANCER INSTITUTE, RADIATION THERAPY AND YOU, PUBLICATION NO. 02-1136 (2002).

179 http://www.uwhealth.org/healthfacts/B_EXTRANET_HEALTH_INFORMATION-FlexMember.

180 http://www.health.yahoo.com/women-menopause/low-dose-vaginal-estrogen.

181 Http:/www.breastcancer.org/treatment/hormonal/serms.

182 *To ease your next pelvic exam*, WOMEN'S HEALTH, Jan/Feb. 2006, at 75.

183 Susan Pierres, *The hormone replacement dilemma, so what's a woman to do?*, HEALTH, at 134; Jane E. Allen, *Bone study gives estrogen therapy another chance*, LOS ANGELES TIMES, Sept. 1, 2003, at F5.

184 Id.

185 http://www.spaceref.com/news/viewpr.html.

186 NATIONAL CANCER INSTITUTE, CHEMOTHERAPY AND YOU, NIH PUBLICATION NO. 02-1135 (2002).

187 MALE REPRODUCTIVE CLINIC, PA, INFERTILITY ENCYCLOPEDIA, ASSISTED REPRODUCTIVE TECHNOLOGIES (ART) (2002).

188 Id.

189 Id.

190 Id.

191 Id.

192 MALE REPRODUCTIVE CLINIC, PA, INFERTILITY ENCYCLOPEDIA, ASSISTED REPRODUCTIVE TECHNOLOGIES (ART) (2002).

193 Id.

194 Id.

195 NATIONAL CANCER INSTITUTE, U.S. NATIONAL INSTITUTE OF HEALTH, CANCER TOPICS, BIOLOGICAL THERAPY (2004).

196 http://www.medical-dictionary.thefreedictionary.com/interferon-alpha.

197 KAREN PALLARITO, HEALTHDAY, HERCEPTIN PROVES A WONDER DRUG FOR BREAST CANCER (2005).

198 Id.

199 NATIONAL CANCER INSTITUTE, WHAT YOU NEED TO KNOW ABOUT HODGKIN'S DISEASE, NIH PUBLICATION NO. P022 (2007).

200 Mayo Clinic Family Health Book 967 (2nd ed. 1991).

201 Id.

202 NATIONAL CANCER INSTITUTE, WHAT YOU NEED TO KNOW ABOUT LEUKEMIA, NIH PUBLICATION NO. P832 (2008).

203 MARY KUGLER, R.N., ABOUT.COM RARE DISEASES, WHAT IS A BONE MARROW TRANSPLANT? PROCEDURE REPLACES UNHEALTHY CELLS WITH HEALTHY CELLS (2009).

204 NATIONAL CANCER INSTITUTE, WHAT YOU NEED TO KNOW ABOUT LEUKEMIA, NIH PUBLICATION NO. 08-1576 (2008).

205 DANIEL DENOON, NEW BREAST CANCER DRUGS MAY BEAT TAMOXIFEN (March 15, 2004); Jane E. Allen, *New drugs may rival tamoxifen*, LOS ANGELES TIMES, March 22, 2004, at F3.

206 Id.

207 Id.

REFERENCES

208 NATIONAL CANCER INSTITUTE, WHAT YOU NEED TO KNOW ABOUT BREAST CANCER, NIH PUBLICATION NO. 03-1556 (2009); NATIONAL CANCER INSTITUTE, WHAT YOU NEED TO KNOW ABOUT PROSTATE CANCER, NIH PUBLICATION NO. 08-1576 (2008).

209 NATIONAL CANCER INSTITUTE, WHAT YOU NEED TO KNOW ABOUT PROSTATE CANCER, NIH PUBLICATION NO. 08-1576 (2008).

210 Thomas H. Maugh II, *Researchers open several new fronts on prostate cancer*, LOS ANGELES TIMES, June 14, 2004; Sally Lehman, *Concerns rise as more men use hormone therapy*, LOS ANGELES TIMES, Nov. 3, 2003, at F1, F4.

211 Id.

212 Id.; http://www.health.usnews.com/usnews/health/cancer/prostate/pros.treat.hormone.block.html.

213 Mayo Clinic Family Health Book 1254 (4th ed. 2009).

214 NATIONAL CANCER INSTITUTE, WHAT YOU NEED TO KNOW ABOUT PROSTATE CANCER, NIH PUBLICATION NO. 08-1576 (2008).

215 Id.

216 Id.

217 http://www.skinsite.com/info_puva_phototherapy.htm.

218 Id.

219 PUVA is an abbreviation for psoralens ultraviolet A; NATIONAL CANCER INSTITUTE, CANCER RATES AND RISKS 88 (4th ed. 1996).

220 Id.

221 *The real stats for cancer risk*, LOS ANGELES TIMES, HEALTH, May 22, 2006.

222 ADAMS COUNTY MEMORIAL HOSPITAL, PATIENT RIGHTS & RESPONSIBILITY (2004).

223 Id.

224 OHIO DEPARTMENT OF AGING, OHIO STATE UNIVERSITY EXTENSION SENIOR SERIES, LEGAL RIGHTS OF MEDICAL PATIENTS, SS-107-96 (2004).

225 Id.

226 Id.

227 Id.

228 Id.

229 ADAMS COUNTY MEMORIAL HOSPITAL, PATIENT RIGHTS & RESPONSIBILITY (2004).

230 Mayo Clinic Family Health Book 343-345 (4th ed. 2009).

231 Tom Clavin, *How you can protect yourself*, PARADE, May 23, 2004, at 4-6.

232 HARVARD CLASSICS, VOLUME 38, *Oath of Hippocrates, cerca 400 B.C.*, P.F. Collier and Son (1910).

233 U.S. DEPARTMENT OF HEALTH AND HUMAN SERVICES, HHS FACT SHEET, PROTECTING THE PRIVACY OF PATIENTS' HEALTH INFORMATION (2001).

234 Id.

235 Id.

236   HEALTH INSURANCE PORTABILITY AND ACCOUNTABILITY ACT OF 1996, [45 CFR 160, 164], Revised 2003.

237   Id. at [45 CFR 164.502(a)(1)(iii)].

238   Legal-dictionary.thefreedictionary.com/reasonable.

239   HEALTH INSURANCE PORTABILITY AND ACCOUNTABILITY ACT OF 1996, [45 CFR 164.502(a)(1)(iii)], Revised 2003.

240   Id.

241   Id.

242   Id.

243   Id.

244   HEALTH INSURANCE PORTABILITY AND ACCOUNTABILITY ACT OF 1996, [45 CFR 164.502(a)(1)(iii)], Revised 2003.

245   U.S DEPARTMENT OF HEALTH AND HUMAN SERVICES, HHS FACT SHEET, PROTECTING THE PRIVACY OF PATIENTS' HEALTH INFORMATION (2001).

246   HEALTH INSURANCE PORTABILITY AND ACCOUNTABILITY ACT OF 1996, [45 CFR 160, 164], Revised 2003.

247   Id.

248   Id.

249   Id. at [42 CFR, Part 2].

250   HEALTHCARE TRAINING INSTITUTE, EXPLORING PRIVACY & CONFIDENTIALITY, BIOETHICS AND HIV/AIDS PATIENTS COURSE.

251   Id.

252   HEALTH INSURANCE PORTABILITY AND ACCOUNTABILITY ACT OF 1996, [45 CFR 164.512(b)(1)(iv)], Revised 2003.

253   Id.

254   http://www.epic.org/privacy/medical/Genetics Nondiscrimination Act of 2003, S.1053, HR. 1910.

255   HARVARD CLASSICS, VOLUME 38, *Oath of Hippocrates, cerca 400 B.C.*, P.F. Collier and Son (1910).

256   AMERICAN ACADEMY OF FAMILY PHYSICIANS, CONFIDENTIALITY, PHYSICIAN/ PATIENT COMMUNICATIONS (2004).

257   Id.

258   Id.

259   ACOR, INC., KNOWLEDGE FOR ACTION, UNDERSTANDING CANCER PAIN (2000-2001).

260   Id.

261   Id.

262   Id.

263   ACOR, INC., KNOWLEDGE FOR ACTION, FIRST-LINE PAIN MEDICATIONS (2000).

REFERENCES

264   Shawn Le, *Duo of drugs pair up to battle lung cancer*, CITY OF HOPE, VOL. 8, ISSUE 6, June 25, 2009.

265   ADDICTION SCIENCE NETWORK, DRUG CLASSIFICATION (2000).

266   Id.

267   Mayo Clinic Family Health Book 1313 (4th ed. 2009).

268   Id.

269   ACOR, INC., KNOWLEDGE FOR ACTION, FIRST-LINE PAIN MEDICATIONS (2000).

270   Id.

271   ACOR, INC., KNOWLEDGE FOR ACTION, THE MYTH OF ADDICTION (2000).

272   Id.

273   Id.

274   Id.

275   ADDICTION SCIENCE NETWORK, DRUG CLASSIFICATION (2000).

276   Id.

277   Id.; DRUG ENFORCEMENT AGENCY, U.S. DRUG ENFORCEMENT ADMINISTRATION, DRUG SCHEDULING (2004).

278   DRUG ENFORCEMENT AGENCY, U.S. DRUG ENFORCEMENT ADMINISTRATION, DRUG SCHEDULING (2004).

279   JANA RAY, MARIJUANA – A MEDICINAL MARVEL (1996).

280   Id.

281   Id.

282   U.S. DRUG ENFORCEMENT AGENCY, MEDICAL MARIJUANA – THE FACTS (2004).

283   JANA RAY, MARIJUANA – A MEDICINAL MARVEL (1996).

284   David G. Savage, *Justices rule U.S. can ban medical pot*, LOS ANGELES TIMES, June 7, 2005; Ryan Grim, *Supreme court hands medical marijuana major victory*, HUFFPOST REPORTING, May 18, 2009.

285   ProCon.org. 14 LEGAL MEDICAL MARIJUANA STATES, LAWS, FEES, AND POSSESSION LIMITS. Jan. 26, 2010.

286   U.S. DRUG ENFORCEMENT AGENCY, MEDICAL MARIJUANA – THE FACTS (2004).

287   Id.

288   Id.

289   Id.

290   U.S. DRUG ENFORCEMENT AGENCY, MEDICAL MARIJUANA – THE FACTS (2004).

291   Id.

292   ACOR, INC., KNOWLEDGE FOR ACTION, CANCER PAIN TREATMENTS (2000); Mayo Clinic Family Health Book 1326-1327 (4th ed. 2009).

293   Id.

294   ACOR, INC., KNOWLEDGE FOR ACTION, CANCER PAIN TREATMENTS (2000).

295   Id.; Mosby's Medical, Nursing, & Allied Health Dictionary (6th ed. 2002).

296 ACOR, INC., KNOWLEDGE FOR ACTION, CANCER PAIN TREATMENTS (2000).

297 Id.

298 Id.

299 Mosby's Medical, Nursing, & Allied Health Dictionary (6th ed. 2002).

300 ACOR, INC., KNOWLEDGE FOR ACTION, CANCER PAIN TREATMENTS (2000).

301 Id.

302 Id.

303 Id.

304 Id.

305 ACOR, INC., KNOWLEDGE FOR ACTION, CANCER PAIN TREATMENTS (2000).

306 Id.

307 Id.; MAHARISHI VEDIC EDUCATION DEVELOPMENT CORPORATION, SCIENTIFIC RESEARCH ON TRANSCENDENTAL MEDITATION AND TM-SIDHI PROGRAMS (2002).

308 ACOR, INC., KNOWLEDGE FOR ACTION, CANCER PAIN TREATMENTS (2000); UAB HEALTH SYSTEM, COMPLEMENTARY AND ALTERNATIVE MEDICINE? (2004).

309 HEALTHWISE, INCORPORATED, ACUPUNCTURE (2004).

310 Id.

311 ACUPUNCTURE TODAY, MOXIBUSTION (2004).

312 Id.

313 B. EICHELBERGER, A CHI KUNG (QI GONG) PRIMER (1995); MTSU.EDU, TAI CHI CHUAN (2004).

314 Id.

315 ACOR, INC., KNOWLEDGE FOR ACTION, CANCER PAIN TREATMENTS (2000).

316 UAB HEALTH SYSTEM, WHAT IS CHIROPRACTIC MEDICINE? (2004).

317 MICHAEL KERN, INRODUCTION TO BIODYNAMIC CRANIOSACRAL THERAPY (2003).

318 UAB HEALTH SYSTEM, WHAT IS AYURVEDA? (2004).

319 http:// www.cancer.gov/cancertopics/pdq/cam/laetrile.

320 Kenneth L. Milstead, Quackery in the medical device field, DEVICE WATCH, Oct. 25, 1963.

321 AMERICAN CANCER SOCIETY, CANCER FACTS AND FIGURES (2009).

322 Delthia Ricks, Night-shift link to cancer suggested in new study, THE DENVER POST; Judy Foreman, Putting cancer cells to sleep, LOS ANGELES TIMES, Oct. 31, 2005, at F3.

323 Id.

324 Marianne Szegedy-Maszak and Katherine Hobson, Beating a killer, US NEWS AND WORLD REPORT, April 5, 2004, at 56.

325 Id.

326 Id.

327 Mayo Clinic Family Health Book 327 (4th ed. 2009).

328 Id. at 1033, 1258-1260; ALLHEALTH.ORG, BLOOD TESTS (2004); BREAST CANCER.ORG, BLOOD TESTS (2004).

REFERENCES

329 Id.

330 Id.

331 WEBMD, CANCER HEALTH CENTER, CARCINOEMBRYONIC ANTIGEN (CEA) (2009).

332 WEBMD, HEALTH & PREGNANCY, ALPHA-FETOPROTEIN (AFP) IN BLOOD (2008).

333 Marianne Szegedy-Maszak and Katherine Hobson, *Beating a killer*, US NEWS AND WORLD REPORT, April 5, 2004, at 56.

334 THE INSTITUTE OF FOOD AND SCIENCE TECHNOLOGY, IFST: CURRENT HOT TOPICS, ORGANIC FOOD (2003); ABOUT, INC., GOING ORGANIC, NATIONAL STANDARDS SET BY THE USDA (2004).

335 Id.

336 ORGANIC CONSUMERS ASSOCIATION, SAFEGUARD ORGANIC STANDARDS CAMPAIGN (2004).

337 Id.

338 THE ORGANIC EXPLAINER, CNN.COM (2004).

339 STEPHEN BARRETT, MD, ORGANIC FOODS: CERTIFICATION DOES NOT PROTECT CONSUMER (2004).

340 Id.

341 Melinda Lee, *Food News*, KNX 10.70 NEWS RADIO, Los Angeles, California.

342 ALAN GREENE, MD, FAAP, CLEAN HANDS (2005).

343 ALAN GREENE, MD, FAAP, HANDWASHING NO LONGER NECESSARY? (2001).

344 Tom Clavin, *How you can protect yourself*, PARADE, May 23, 2004, at 4-6.

345 VAN.HEP.UIUC.EDU, ANTIBACTERIAL SOAPS (2005).

346 DR. JOSEPH MERCOLA WITH RACHEL DROEGE, THE TRUTH ABOUT ANTIBACTERIAL SOAPS – AND WHY YOU SHOULD AVOID THEM (2005).

347 SOAP AND DETERGENT ASSOCIATION, ANTIBACTERIAL PRODUCTS AND ANTIBIOTIC RESISTANCE (2004).

348 VAN.HEP.UIUC.EDU, ANTIBACTERIAL SOAPS (2005).

349 ALAN GREENE, MD, FAAP, HANDWASHING NO LONGER NECESSARY? (2001).

350 Id.

351 Id.

352 Mayo Clinic Family Health Book 625 (4th ed. 2009).

353 Mosby's Medical, Nursing, & Allied Health Dictionary 96 (6th ed. 2002).

354 TOPCONDITION.COM, ANGER MANAGEMENT (2004).

355 Mosby's Medical, Nursing, & Allied Health Dictionary 117 (6th ed. 2002).

356 ALLREFER.COM, HEALTH, SYMPTOMS GUIDE, STRESS AND ANXIETY (2005); CANCERCARE.ORG, EMOTIONAL ISSUES FOR CAREGIVERS AND PATIENTS, ANXIETY (2004).

357 Id.

358 Mosby's Medical, Nursing, & Allied Health Dictionary 765 (6th ed. 2002).

359 CANCERCARE.ORG, EMOTIONAL ISSUES FOR CAREGIVERS AND PATIENTS, BEREAVEMENT AND GRIEF (2004).

360 Id.

361 ALLREFER.COM, HEALTH, DISEASES & CONDITIONS, GRIEF (2005).

362 DONALD J FRANKLIN, PSYCHOLOGY INFORMATION ONLINE, DIAGNOSTIC EVALUATION FOR DEPRESSION (2004).

363 Id.

364 THE UNIVERSITY OF TULSA, COUNSELING AND PSYCHOLOGICAL SERVICES CENTER, BEREAVEMENT (2003).

365 DONALD J FRANKLIN, PSYCHOLOGY INFORMATION ONLINE, DEPRESSION-INFORMATION AND TREATMENT (2004).

366 Mosby's Medical, Nursing, & Allied Health Dictionary 501 (6th ed. 2002).

367 DONALD J FRANKLIN, PSYCHOLOGY INFORMATION ONLINE, DEPRESSION-INFORMATION AND TREATMENT (2004).

368 Id.

369 Id.

370 Id.

371 Id.

372 DONALD J FRANKLIN, PSYCHOLOGY INFORMATION ONLINE, DEPRESSION-INFORMATION AND TREATMENT (2004); Mayo Clinic Family Health Book 1149-1152 (4th ed. 2009).

373 Id.

374 Id.

375 Id.

376 NATIONAL CANCER INSTITUTE, FACING FORWARD SERIES, YOUR SOCIAL RELATIONSHIPS AFTER CANCER TREATMENT (2002).

377 Random House Webster's Dictionary 723 (4th ed. 2001).

378 NATIONAL CANCER INSTITUTE, FACING FORWARD SERIES, YOUR SOCIAL RELATIONSHIPS AFTER CANCER TREATMENT (2002).

379 http://www.medical-dictionary.thefreedictionary.com/Avoidance+behavior.

380 http://www.answers.com/topic/pathophobia/panthophobia/carcinophobia.

381 http://www.answers.com/topic/self-preservation.

382 NATIONAL CANCER INSTITUTE, FACING FORWARD SERIES, YOUR SOCIAL RELATIONSHIPS AFTER CANCER TREATMENT (2002).

383 Id.

384 Marianne Szegedy-Maszak and Katherine Hobson, *Beating a killer*, US NEWS AND WORLD REPORT, April 5, 2004, at 56.

385 Id.

REFERENCES

386   SPACE COAST MEDICAL ASSOCIATIONS, LLP, INTIMACY AND SEXUALITY AFTER CANCER (2004).

387   Id.

388   Id.

389   Id.

390   PAULA J. WART, WELL SOURCE INC., SEX AFTER CANCER (2001).

391   SKY.COM, ORAL SEX LINKED TO MOUTH CANCER (2004).

392   DR. JOE GLICKMAN, JR., M.D., HPV MOUTH (2005).

393   SKY.COM, ORAL SEX LINKED TO MOUTH CANCER (2004).

394   NATIONAL CANCER INSTITUTE, FACING FORWARD SERIES, YOUR SOCIAL RELATIONSHIPS AFTER CANCER TREATMENT (2002).

395   COSMETIC EXECUTIVE WOMEN, CANCER AND CAREERS.ORG, HOW CAN A COWORKER HELP? (2003); MAYO CLINIC.COM, WORKING AFTER CANCER: TIPS TO MAKE YOUR TRANSITION EASIER (2004).

396   Id.

397   Id.

398   Barbara Hoffman, JD, *Cancer survivors' employment and insurance rights: A primer for oncologists*, ONCOLOGY, Vol. 13, No. 6, June 1999.

399   Id.

400   Id.

401   2008 amendments also extend the FMLA's protections for next of kin and adult children to military family members. US DEPARTMENT OF LABOR, COMPLICANCE ASSISTANCE – FAMILY AND MEDICAL LEAVE ACT (FMLA) (2004); US OFFICE OF PERSONNEL MANAGEMENT, FINAL REGULATIONS OF FAMILY AND MEDICAL LEAVE (1996).

402   Id.; COSMETIC EXECUTIVE WOMEN, CANCER AND CAREERS, FEDERAL LEGISLATION: OVERVIEW AND RELEVANCE TO THE PRINCIPLES (2003).

403   Id.; US DEPARTMENT OF LABOR, 29 CTR 825.110 – WHICH EMPLOYEES ARE "ELIGIBLE" TO TAKE LEAVE UNDER FMLA? (1995).

404   Id.

405   Id.

406   Id.

407   US DEPARTMENT OF LABOR, COMPLICANCE ASSISTANCE – FAMILY AND MEDICAL LEAVE ACT (FMLA) (2004).

408   Id.; US OFFICE OF PERSONNEL MANAGEMENT, FINAL REGULATIONS ON FAMILY AND MEDICAL LEAVE (1996).

409   Id.

410   http://www.nolo.com/legal-encyclopedia/faqEditorial-29086.html.

411 US EQUAL EMPLOYMENT OPPORTUNITY COMMISSION, FACTS ABOUT THE AMERICANS WITH DISABILITIES ACT (2008).

412 Id.

413 Barbara Hoffman, JD, *Cancer survivors' employment and insurance rights: A primer for oncologists,* ONCOLOGY, Vol. 13, No. 6, June 1999.

414 Id.

415 Id.

416 Id.; ALEXANDER, HAWES & AUDET, LLP, THE CONSUMER LAW PAGE, THE AMERICAN WITH DISABILITIES ACT QUESTIONS AND ANSWERS (2004).

417 Id.

418 Barbara Hoffman, JD, *Cancer survivors' employment and insurance rights: A primer for oncologists,* ONCOLOGY, Vol. 13, No. 6, June 1999.

419 Id.

420 Id.

421 Id.

422 Id.

423 Barbara Hoffman, JD, C*ancer survivors' employment and insurance rights: A primer for oncologists,* ONCOLOGY, Vol. 13, No. 6, June 1999.

424 Id.

425 Id.

426 Id.

427 Id.

428 US DEPARTMENT OF JUSTICE, CIVIL RIGHTS DIVISION, A GUIDE TO DISABILITY RIGHTS LAWS (2005).

429 Id.

430 Id.

431 Barbara Hoffman, JD, C*ancer survivors' employment and insurance rights: A primer for oncologists,* ONCOLOGY, Vol. 13, No. 6, June 1999.

432 Id.

433 COMPASSION RESPONSE NETWORK, FUTURE CHALLENGE FOR THIRD WORLD COUNTRIES IN AFRICA (2005).

434 Id.

435 Id.; LOWELL GREENBERG, HEALTH CARE IN "THIRD WORLD" COUNTRIES (2004).

436 DISCOVERFRANCE.NET, HEALTH CARE IN FRANCE (2004).

437 JAPAN'S UNIVERSAL AND AFFORDABLE HEALTH CARE: LESSONS FOR THE UNITED STATES?

438 US CENSUS BUREAU, HEALTH INSURANCE DATA, TYPES OF HEALTH INSURANCE COVERAGE (2004).

REFERENCES

439 NATIONAL CANCER INSTITUTE, CHEMOTHERAPY AND YOU: A GUIDE TO SELF-HELP DURING CANCER TREATMENT, PAYING FOR CHEMOTHERAPY (1999).

440 Id.; US MEDICAL, LLC, CHEMOTHERAPY: WHAT QUESTIONS SHOULD I BE ABLE TO ANSWER ABOUT MY INSURANCE (2004).

441 http://www.census.gov/hhes/www/hlthins/hlthin07/hlth07asc.html.

442 http://www.census.gov/hhes/www/hlhins/hlthin07/fig07.pdf.

443 Medicare Part B covers out-patient care. WEBMD, MEDICARE HEALTH CENTER, MEDICARE ELIGIBILITY AND ENROLLMENT (2009).

444 Id. The MMA also is known as the Medicare Prescription Drug, Improvement, and Modernization Act.

445 Id.

446 Id.

447 DEPARTMENT OF PUBLIC HEALTH & HUMAN SERVICES, MEDICAID ELIGIBILITY, MEDICAID: ARE YOU ELIGIBLE? (2009).

448 Figures as of 2008. http://www.statehealthfacts.org/comparetable.jsp?typ=1+ind=184&cat=4&sub+47.

449 US CENSUS BUREAU, TYPES OF HEALTH INSURANCE COVERAGE (2004); ROD POWERS, YOUR GUIDE TO U.S. MILITARY, UNDERSTANDING MILITARY MEDICAL CARE (2004).

450 DEPARTMENT OF VETERANS AFFAIRS, HEALTH ADMINISTRATION CENTER, CHAMPVA (2004).

451 US CENSUS BUREAU, HEALTH INSURANCE DATA, TYPES OF HEALTH INSURANCE COVERAGE (2004).

452 US DEPARTMENT OF HEALTH AND HUMAN SERVICES, NATIONAL CONFERENCE OF STATE LEGISLATURES, CHILDREN'S HEALTH INSURANCE PROGRAM (CHIP) (2009). CHIP was formerly known as the State Children's Health Insurance Program (SCHIP).

453 DANIAL FORTUNO AND KEREN STRONACH, UCSF COMPREHENSIVE CANCER CENTER, HEALTH INSURANCE AND DISABILITY BENEFITS (2004).

454 NEW YORK STATE OFFICE FOR THE AGING, THINGS TO KNOW ABOUT MEDIGAP INSURANCE (2004).

455 NEW YORK STATE OFFICE FOR THE AGING, HELP IN OTHER STATES, STATE HEALTH INSURANCE ASSISTANCE PROGRAMS (2004).

456 Id.

457 Id.

458 http://www.census.gov/hhes/www/hlthins/hlthin07/fig07/pdf.

459 US CENSUS BUREAU, TYPES OF HEALTH INSURANCE COVERAGE, FIG. 1 (2002).

460 DANIAL FORTUNO AND KEREN STRONACH, UCSF COMPREHENSIVE CANCER CENTER, HEALTH INSURANCE AND DISABILITY BENEFITS (2004).

461 Id.

462 Id.

463 Id.

464 Id.

465 DANIAL FORTUNO AND KEREN STRONACH, UCSF COMPREHENSIVE CANCER CENTER, HEALTH INSURANCE AND DISABILITY BENEFITS (2004).

466 Id.

467 DARTMOUTH-HITCHCOCK MEDICAL CENTER, PATIENT ACCOUNTS CUSTOMER SERVICE, REFERRALS/PRECERTIFICATIONS (2010); SOUTHEAST MISSOURI HOSPITAL, PATIENTS/VISITORS, PRE-CERTIFICATION (2009).

468 Id.

469 Id.

470 Id.

471 Id.

472 DARTMOUTH-HITCHCOCK MEDICAL CENTER, PATIENT ACCOUNTS CUSTOMER SERVICE, REFERRALS/PRECERTIFICATIONS (2010); SOUTHEAST MISSOURI HOSPITAL, PATIENTS/VISITORS, PRE-CERTIFICATION (2009).

473 DANIAL FORTUNO AND KEREN STRONACH, UCSF COMPREHENSIVE CANCER CENTER, HEALTH INSURANCE AND DISABILITY BENEFITS (2004).

474 Barbara Hoffman, MD, *Cancer survivors' employment and insurance rights: A primer for oncologists*, ONCOLOGY, Vol. 13, No. 6, June 1999; Drs Jason Madosakis and David T. Feinberg, *When your insurance won't pay*, PARADE, Sept. 19, 2004, at 10-11.

475 Id.

476 Id.

477 COBRAINS.COM, WHAT IS COBRA INSURANCE? (2004); COBRAINSINSURANCE.COM, COBRA QUESTIONS AND ANSWERS (2004).

478 Id.

479 Id.

480 http://www.dol.gov/ebsa/cobra.html.

481 COBRAINSINSURANCE.COM COBRA QUESTIONS AND ANSWERS (2004).

482 Id.

483 WORLD INSTITUTE ON DISABILITY, OBRA: FREQUENTLY ASKED QUESTIONS (2004).

484 Id.

485 DANIAL FORTUNO AND KEREN STRONACH, UCSF COMPREHENSIVE CANCER CENTER, HEALTH INSURANCE AND DISABILITY BENEFITS (2004).

486 Id.

487 Id.; http://www.ssa.gov/pubs/10029.html.

488 Id.

489 http://www.ssa.gov/ssi/text-resources-ussi.htm.

490 DANIAL FORTUNO AND KEREN STRONACH, UCSF COMPREHENSIVE CANCER CENTER, HEALTH INSURANCE AND DISABILITY BENEFITS (2004).

REFERENCES

491   Id.

492   Id.

493   ALLCARE INSURANCE INC., INSURANCE GLOSSARY, PRE-EXISTING CONDITION (2004).

494   Id.

495   MICHAEL BIHARI, MD, ABOUT.COM, HEALTH INSURANCE, PRE-EXISTING CONDITION EXCLUSION PERIOD (2010).

496   Id.

497   Id.

498   U.S. EQUAL EMPLOYMENT OPPORTUNITY COMMISSION, FACTS ABOUT THE AMERICANS WITH DISABILITIES ACT (2008).

499   Barbara Hoffman, MD, *Cancer survivors' employment and insurance rights: A primer for oncologists,* ONCOLOGY, Vol. 13, No. 6 (1999).

500   Id.

501   Id.

502   Crothers HM: Health insurance: Problems and solutions for people with cancer histories, in American Cancer Society: Proceedings of the Fifth National Conference on Human Values and Cancer, 100-109. San Francisco, California Division of the American Cancer society, 1987.

503   Vann JC et al: Health insurance access to young adult survivors of childhood cancer in North Carolina. *Med Pediatr Oncol* 25(5):389-393, 1999.

504   Barbara Hoffman, MD, *Cancer survivors' employment and insurance rights: A primer for oncologists,* ONCOLOGY, Vol. 13, No. 6 (1999).

505   DANIAL FORTUNO AND KEREN STRONACH, UCSF COMPREHENSIVE CANCER CENTER, HEALTH INSURANCE AND DISABILITY BENEFITS (2004).

506   Id.

507   Id.

508   Id.

509   Id.

510   John Leighty, *Financially strapped hospitals close doors, displace patients*, NURSEWEEK, Oct. 18, 2004.

511   FAMILIES USA, THE VOICE FOR HEALTH CARE CONSUMERS, WORKING WITHOUT A NET: THE HEALTH CARE SAFETY NET STILL LEAVES MILLIONS OF LOW-INCOME WORKERS UNINSURED, April 2004, updated from 2002 US Census Bureau figures.

512   Chris Isidore, *GM to cut 25,000 jobs by '08*, FORTUNE 500, June 7, 2005.

513   http://www.census.gov/hhes/www/hlthins/hlthin07/fig07.pdf.

514   THE McLAUGHLIN GROUP, KCET TELEVISION, LOS ANGELES, CALIFORNIA (2007).

515   http://www.census.gov/hhes/www/hlthins/hlthin07/hlth07asc.html.

516   FAMILIES USA, THE VOICE FOR HEALTH CARE CONSUMERS, WORKING WITHOUT A NET: THE HEALTH CARE SAFETY NET STILL LEAVES MILLIONS OF LOW-INCOME WORKERS UNINSURED, April 2004.

517   http://www.aspe.hhs.gov/poverty/08Poverty.shtml.

518   http://www.statehealthfacts.org/comparereport.jsp?rep=54&cat=4.

519   FAMILIES USA, THE VOICE FOR HEALTH CARE CONSUMERS, WORKING WITHOUT A NET: THE HEALTH CARE SAFETY NET STILL LEAVES MILLIONS OF LOW-INCOME WORKERS UNINSURED, April 2004.

520   http://www.statehealthfacts.org/comparereport.jsp?rep=54&cat=4.

521   Id.

522   H.R. 3590, Patient Protection and Affordable Care Act, March 23, 2010; H.R. 4872, Reconciliation Act of 2010, March 30, 2010.

523   Dan Roam and C. Anthony Jones, M.D., *American health care: a 4 napkin explanation* (2009).

524   Id.

525   H.R. 3590, Patient Protection and Affordable Care Act. Congressional Budget Office, March 11, 2010; Jeremy Binckes and Nick Wing, *Health reform bill summary: The top 18 immediate effects*, THE HUFFINGTON POST, March 22, 2010; Smriti Rao, *Health care reform passed. So what does it mean?*, DISCOVER, March 22, 2010.

526   UCSF COMPREHENSIVE CENTER, COMMUNICATIONS, WHAT ARE CLINICAL TRIALS? (2004).

527   Id.

528   Id.

529   Id.

530   Id.

531   COALITION OF NATIONAL CANCER COOPERATIVE GROUPS, INC., ABOUT CLINICAL TRIALS: ABCs OF CLINICAL TRIALS (2005).

532   Id.

533   COALITION OF NATIONAL CANCER COOPERATIVE GROUPS, INC., ABOUT CLINICAL TRIALS: INSURANCE (2005).

534   Id.

535   Id.

536   Id.

537   Id.

538   COALITION OF NATIONAL CANCER COOPERATIVE GROUPS, INC., ABOUT CLINICAL TRIALS: INSURANCE (2005).

539   US MEDICAL, LLC, GETTING MAXIMUM COVERAGE OF CLINICAL TRIALS COSTS (2002).

540   COALITION OF NATIONAL CANCER COOPERATIVE GROUPS, INC., ABOUT CLINICAL TRIALS: INSURANCE (2005).

541   Id.

542   Id.

543   US MEDICAL, LLC, GETTING MAXIMUM COVERAGE OF CLINICAL TRIALS COSTS (2002).

REFERENCES

544 Lori Oliwenstein, *The age of cancer*, USC HEALTH, Spring 2005, at 18-21.

545 Id.

546 Id.

547 EDWARD R. WAXMAN & ASSOCIATES, HOSPITAL BILL AUDITING, THE KINDS OF ERRORS HOSPITAL BILLS CONTAIN (2005).

548 Dina ElBoghdady, *Killer billing errors, duplicate charges, faulty totals. Your hospital's mistakes can ruin you*, WASHINGTON POST, June 27, 2004, at F01.

549 Id.

550 Id.

551 Id.

552 THE LEWIS GROUP, HOW TO CATCH HOSPITAL BILLING ERRORS (2006).

553 Id.

554 PETER DAVIDSON, MICROSOFT CORPORATION, 8 MOST COMMON HOSPITAL BILLING ERRORS (2005).

555 Id.

556 Id.

557 Id.

558 THE LEWIS GROUP, HOW TO CATCH HOSPITAL BILLING ERRORS (2006).

559 Id.

560 EDWARD R. WAXMAN & ASSOCIATES, HOSPITAL BILL AUDITING, THE KINDS OF ERRORS HOSPITAL BILLS CONTAIN (2005).

561 Id.

562 Id.

563 PETER DAVIDSON, MICROSOFT CORPORATION, 8 MOST COMMON HOSPITAL BILLING ERRORS (2005).

564 AMERICAN ACADEMY OF CHILD AND ADOLESCENT PSYCHIATRY, CPT CODES INFORMATION PAGE (2003).

565 PETER DAVIDSON, MICROSOFT CORPORATION, 8 MOST COMMON HOSPITAL BILLING ERRORS (2005).

566 THE LEWIS GROUP, HOW TO CATCH HOSPITAL BILLING ERRORS (2005); Dina Elboghdady, *Killer billing errors, duplicate charges, faulty totals: Your hospital's mistakes can ruin you*, WASHINGTON POST, June 27, 2004, at F01.

567 MARGIE PARENT, PAGEWISE, MEDICAL ISSUES: DETECTING BILLING ERRORS IN HOSPITAL BILLS (2002).

568 EDWARD R. WAXMAN & ASSOCIATES, HOSPITAL BILL AUDITING, THE KINDS OF ERRORS HOSPITAL BILLS CONTAIN (2005).

569 Dina ElBoghdady, *Killer billing errors, duplicate charges, faulty totals. Your hospital's mistakes can ruin you*, WASHINGTON POST, June 27, 2004, at F01.

570 Id.

571   EDWARD R. WAXMAN & ASSOCIATES, HOSPITAL BILL AUDITING, THE KINDS OF ERRORS HOSPITAL BILLS CONTAIN (2005).

572   WEBNOX CORP., MEANING OF HOSPITAL (2003).

573   Id.

574   WEBNOX CORP., MEANING OF MEDICAL CENTER (2003).

575   Id.

576   http://www.thefreedictionary.com/institution.

577   http://www.answers.com/topic/clinic.

578   HOSPICE.NET, THE HOSPICE CONCEPT (2005).

579   NATIONAL CANCER INSTITUTE, CANCER FACTS 1.2, THE NATIONAL CANCER INSTITUTE CANCER CENTERS PROGRAM (2004).

580   Id.

581   Id.

582   Id.; http://cancercenters.cancer.gov/grants_funding/comprehensiveness.html.

583   PTM HEALTHCARE MARKETING, INC., STRATEGIC MARKETING PLANS (2005).

584   CITY OF HOPE, CAUSE-RELATED MARKETING (2005).

585   PTM HEALTHCARE MARKETING, INC., STRATEGIC MARKETING PLANS (2005).

586   Gary Stoner, Ph.D., *Black raspberries fight cancer—full-length doctor's interview*, CANCER CHANNEL, Nov. 21, 2005.

587   NATIONAL CANCER INSTITUTE, STRATEGIC INVESTMENTS IN CANCER PREVENTION, EARLY DETECTION, AND PREDICTION (2006).

588   Id.

589   The vaccine Gardisil, which targets the HPV virus and helps prevent certain types of cervical cancer has been on the market since 2006. Research on vaccines for other cancers including breast cancers dependent upon the antigen a-lactalbumin continues.

590   NATIONAL CANCER INSTITUTE, STRATEGIC INVESTMENTS IN CANCER PREVENTION, EARLY DETECTION, AND PREDICTION (2006).

591   Dianne Partie Lange, *Vitamin E study reveals clue about prostate cancer*, LOS ANGELES TIMES, June 17, 2002; NATIONAL CANCER INSTITUTE, STRATEGIC INVESTMENTS IN ADVANCED TECHNOLOGIES (2006).

592   MICROSOFT CORPORATION, DIARRHEA BUG MAY PREVENT CANCER (2003).

593   http://news.bbc.co.uk/2/hi/science/nature/6261427.stm.

594   Linda Marsa, *Lotion may prevent cancer in sun-damaged skin*, LOS ANGELES TIMES, March 3, 2003; Linda Marsa, *Picking a poison for cancer*, LOS ANGELES TIMES, Nov. 25, 2002.

595   WHAT IS ONCOTYPE DX? (2004); Indeed, some drugs used to predict the recurrence of certain cancers have been found to actually help prevent some cancers. For example, Aromasin (or exemestane), an aromatase inhibitor which has been used to predict the recurrence of breast cancer, is now being used in high-risk post-menopausal women to help prevent the disease from developing in the first

place. Debra Sherman, *Aromasin cuts risk of breast cancer in some groups*, REUTERS, June 4, 2011.

596 DR. RALPH MERKLE, ZYVEX.COM, NANOTECHNOLOGY (2005); NANOTECHNOLOGY FOR CANCER PREVENTION, DIAGNOSIS AND TREATMENT, CANCERNANO 2009, SYMPOSIUM (2009).

597 NATIONAL CANCER INSTITUTE, STRATEGIC INVESTMENTS IN ADVANCED TECHNOLOGIES (2006); NATIONAL CANCER INSTITUTE, PROTEOMICS AND CANCER, FACT SHEET (2009).

598 NATIONAL CANCER INSTITUTE, STRATEGIC INVESTMENTS IN ADVANCED TECHNOLOGIES (2006).

599 Julian Guthrie, *Cancer-sniffing dogs have shown promise at detecting the disease in its early stages*, SAN FRANCISCO CHRONICLE, June 1, 2003.

600 Frangioni JV: New technologies for human cancer imaging. *J Clin Oncol* 26(24):4022-4021, 2008.

601 NATIONAL CANCER INSTITUTE, STRATEGIC INVESTMENTS IN ADVANCED TECHNOLOGIES (2006).

602 Id.; Rosie Mestel, *Mice are glowing green to help chemotherapy patients*, LOS ANGELES TIMES, Sept. 30, 2002, at S2.

603 AMERICAN CANCER SOCIETY, CANCER FACTS AND FIGURES 19 (2009).

604 Randy Dotinga, *Seaweed may help treat lymphoma*, HEALTH DAY, March 11, 2010; Hyperbaric Oxygen Therapy is known as HBOT. Roy Wood, *New strategy for attacking brain tumors*, THE CINNCINATI POST, June 18, 2004.

605 Linda Marsa, *Picking a poison for cancer*, LOS ANGELES TIMES, Nov. 25, 2002.

606 Rosie Mestel, *Pressing ahead to battle tumors*, LOS ANGELES TIMES, Dec. 23, 2002, at F1, F2; MAYOCLINIC.COM, THALIDOMIDE: RESEARCH ADVANCES IN CANCER AND OTHER CONDITIONS (2008).

607 Avastin also is known as Bevacizumab. In the United States its use has been confined to clinical trials after the Food and Drug Administration stated in 2010 that its benefits do not outweigh its significant risks in treating some advanced cancers. MED PAGE TODAY (2010-07-08), *FDA Panel Nixes Bevacizumab for Breast Cancer*. While aromatase inhibitors including Arimidex, Aromasin and Femara help prevent recurrences of estrogen-receptor positive breast cancer, they also carry risks that must be balanced with known benefits. Janet McConnaughey, *Cord blood could help battle leukemia in adults*, ROCKY MOUNTAIN NEWS, Nov. 25, 2004, at 49A; Peters C et al: Stem cell source and outcome after hematopoietic stem cell transplantation (HSCT) in children and adolescents with acute leukemia. *Pediatr Clin North Am* 57(1)27-46, 2010.

608 NATIONAL CANCER INSTITUTE, STRATEGIC INVESTMENTS IN ADVANCED TECHNOLOGIES (2006); Robert Langerth, *Conquering cancer*, FORBES, Nov. 11, 2002, at 119-128.

609 Id.

INDEX

About the Author

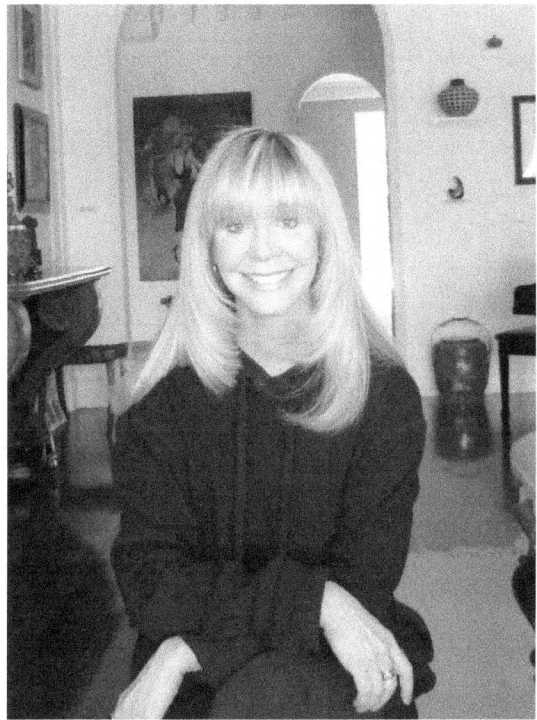

For more information, visit www.swilkinghoran.com

Ms. Horan received her Bachelor's Degree in Psychology from California State University, Northridge and her Juris Doctor Degree from Loyola Law School, Los Angeles. She has been an author, an attorney and an advocate for patient rights for the last twenty years. At present, she is living quietly and cancer free, with her attorney husband and Labrador Retriever in Los Angeles, California.

www.ingramcontent.com/pod-product-compliance
Lightning Source LLC
Chambersburg PA
CBHW051954280526
45793CB00005B/711